Step-Up

A High-Yield, Systems-Based Review
for the USMLE Step 1
Second Edition

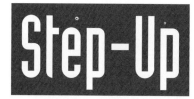

Step-Up

A High-Yield, Systems-Based Review for the USMLE Step 1, Second Edition

Samir Mehta, MD

Resident, Department of Orthopaedic Surgery
The Hospital of the University of Pennsylvania
University of Pennsylvania Health System
Philadelphia, PA

Edmund A. Milder, MD, LT MC USNR

Resident, Department of Pediatrics
Naval Medical Center
San Diego, CA

Adam J. Mirarchi, MD

Resident, Department of Orthopaedic Surgery
University Hospitals of Cleveland
Case Western Reserve University
Cleveland, OH

Eugene Milder, MD, LT MC USNR

Resident, Department of Ophthalmology
Naval Medical Center
San Diego, CA

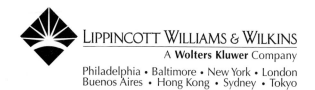

LIPPINCOTT WILLIAMS & WILKINS
A **Wolters Kluwer** Company

Philadelphia • Baltimore • New York • London
Buenos Aires • Hong Kong • Sydney • Tokyo

Editor: Neil Marquardt
Managing Editor: Emilie Linkins
Marketing Manager: Scott Lavine
Production Editor: Christina Remsberg
Compositor: Techbooks
Printer: Data Reproductions

Copyright © 2003 Lippincott Williams & Wilkins

351 West Camden Street
Baltimore, Maryland 21201-2436 USA

530 Walnut Street
Philadelphia, PA 19106

The publisher is not responsible (as a matter of product liability, negligence, or otherwise) for any injury resulting from any material contained herein. This publication contains information relating to general principles of medical care that should not be construed as specific instructions for individual patients. Manufacturers' product information and package inserts should be reviewed for current information, including contraindications, dosages, and precautions.

Printed in the United States of America

First Edition, 2000

Library of Congress Cataloging-in-Publication Data

CIP data has been requested and is available from the Library of Congress.

The publishers have made every effort to trace the copyright holders for borrowed material. If they have inadvertently overlooked any, they will be pleased to make the necessary arrangements at the first opportunity.

To purchase additional copies of this book, call our customer service department at **(800) 638-3030** or fax orders to **(301) 824-7390**. International customers should call **(301) 714-2324**.

Visit Lippincott Williams & Wilkins on the Internet: http://www.LWW.com.
Lippincott Williams & Wilkins customer service representatives are available from 8:30 am to 6:00 pm, EST.

04 05 06 07
2 3 4 5 6 7 8 9 10

Dedication

To my parents, Sudesh and Shobha, and to my sisters, Sonia and Sonul
—Samir Mehta

To my parents, James and Phyllis, and my siblings, Eugene, Shannon, and Robert
—Edmund A. Milder

To my parents, Anthony and Andrea, my brother, Alan, and my wife, Sharon
—Adam J. Mirarchi

To my parents, James and Phyllis, and my siblings, Edmund, Shannon, and Robert
—Eugene Milder

To our teachers
To our friends
And to the physicians of the future

The authors and publishers would like to thank the following people who reviewed the manuscript of the second edition:

Glen J. Barbee, MD
Family Practice
Huntington Beach, California

Emery H. Chang, MD
Resident, Internal Medicine and Pediatrics
Tulane University School of Medicine
New Orleans, Louisiana

Kyung Won Chung, PhD
David Ross Boyd Professor and Vice Chairman
Department of Cell Biology
University of Oklahoma College of Medicine
Oklahoma City, Oklahoma

Linda Costanzo, PhD
Professor of Physiology
Virginia Commonwealth University
Medical College of Virginia
Richmond, Virginia

Jennifer L. Cultrera
Class of 2003
University of Miami School of Medicine
Miami, Florida

Ivan Damjanov, MD, PhD
Professor of Pathology
University of Kansas School of Medicine
Kansas City, Kansas

Craig Flinders, DO
Resident, Family Practice
Wilson Memorial Regional Medical Center
Johnson City, New York

Anand Ramachandran M.D.
Clinical Assistant Professor of Ophthalmology
Ohio State University
Columbus, Ohio

William S. Strohl, PhD
Professor Emeritus
Department of Molecular Genetics and Microbiology
University of Medicine and Dentistry
Robert Wood Johnson Medical School
Piscataway, New Jersey

Table of Contents

Preface

Over the past several years, the NBME has transformed the USMLE Step 1 from a subject-based examination to one that approaches the body as a whole, yet subdivided into essential systemic components. While we were studying for our examinations, there were almost no systems-based review texts available. We realized there was a need for a comprehensive high-yield review text that takes a systems-based approach to the USMLE Step 1, and made this idea a reality after we experienced the Step 1 exam firsthand.

STEP-UP: A High-Yield, Systems-Based Review for the USMLE Step 1 was written with two major goals in mind: 1) to include only material pertinent for the Step 1 examination and 2) to present the material as efficiently as possible. Thus, while we tried to maintain a standard format, each chapter is an amalgamation of tables, figures, text, facts, and charts arranged in a manner we felt best conveyed the essential material. The transitions between sections are often rapid and the text is succinct to keep the student focused on only the relevant information. We realize that time is of the essence. This text also has a number of additional features. The "Quick Hits" in the margins (marked by the boxing glove) are key facts that are related to the text within the body of the book and provide information that is particularly relevant to the USMLE Step 1. These "Quick Hits" can give further information on a subject, help explain a difficult topic, or provide data that bridges more than one organ system. Furthermore, STEP-UP provides comprehensive "Bug" and "Drug"

tables in the appendix. These tables are invaluable resources for Step 1 preparation and also during the pre-clinical years.

The second edition of *STEP-UP: A High-Yield, Systems-Based Review for the USMLE Step 1*, while retaining the essential features of the first edition, has been changed in some important ways. First, the popularity of the case studies section "At the Bedside" led to our development of *STEP-UP to the Bedside: A Case-Based Review for the USMLE Step 1*. As such, the "At the Bedside" section from STEP-UP was expanded and transitioned to an entirely new book of case study review. Furthermore, we expanded coverage of the therapeutics portion of each system by integrating pharmacology directly into each system at the appropriate areas within the text. However, we retained the "Drug Index" at the end of the text for reference. Finally, figures, tables, and text have been revised to reflect the most current thinking in medicine. Many of these changes were implemented as a result of feedback from readers like yourself. We hope to continue this relationship with readers who use this text and future Step-Up texts.

Please feel free to forward comments to us at step_up@lww.com. We wish you the best of success!

Samir Mehta
Edmund A. Milder
Adam J. Mirarchi
Eugene Milder

Acknowledgments

We extend our thanks to the reviewers and contributors, listed below, who helped piece together the first edition. We extend a hand of gratitude to Scott Lavine, Emilie Linkins, and Neil Marquardt for their tireless effort and their vision to move ahead with the second edition of Step-Up.

The authors and publisher would also like to thank the following for their contributions to the first edition:

Reviewers
Sharon Ransom
Wendy A. Weeks
David B. Sykes

Contributors
Greg Anderson
Zara Cooper
Keith McNellis

Readers who provided suggestions and contributions: Cary Hsu, Manely G. Breving, Christine Tsang, Jeff Warber, Marina Pratt, Derek R. Johnson, Ted Lee, Garth Herbert, Ankoor Shah, Rana Malek, and Ngina Jemmott

Special thanks to Georgina Gercia for her numerous review suggestions and contributions to the second edition.

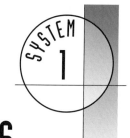
Basic Concepts

DNA, RNA, AND PROTEIN

I. Chemical components of DNA and RNA

A. Deoxyribonucleic acid (DNA) and ribonucleic acid (RNA) are made up of **nucleotides,** which contain:

    1. A **nitrogenous base**—either a purine or pyrimidine (Figure 1-1)

FIGURE
1-1   **Bases**

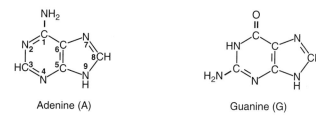

Purines

Adenine (A)   Guanine (G)

Pyrimidines

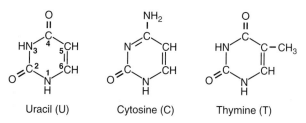

Uracil (U)   Cytosine (C)   Thymine (T)

C=carbon; H=hydrogen; N=nitrogen; O=oxygen

      a. **Purines** are formed from:
        (1) Aspartate
        (2) CO_2
        (3) Glutamate
        (4) Glycine
        (5) N10-Formyl-tetrahydrofolate
      b. **Pyrimidines** are formed from:
        (1) Aspartate
        (2) CO_2
        (3) Glutamate

2. A **pentose sugar**—either a **ribose** for RNA or a **2-deoxyribose** for DNA
3. One, two, or three phosphate groups: forming a -monophosphate, -diphosphate, or -triphosphate, respectively (Figure 1-2).

FIGURE 1-2 **Nucleotide structure**

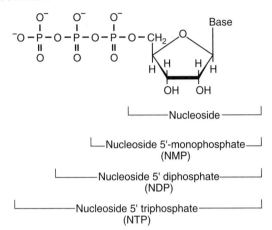

C=carbon; *H*=hydrogen; *O*=oxygen; *P*=phosphate

B. Nucleoside triphosphates (NTP) are linked together by a 3′–5′ phosphodiester bond to form single-stranded RNA or DNA.
C. **Adenine** (A) binds to **thymine** (T), while **guanine** (G) binds to **cytosine** (C) in DNA. **Uracil** (U) replaces thymine (T) in RNA.

II. DNA Replication

A. Is **semiconservative**—when two DNA molecules are created from the original helix, one strand of parental DNA is incorporated with each new daughter strand.
B. Takes place in the **S phase** of the cell cycle (Figure 1-3).

FIGURE 1-3 **The cell cycle**

M: mitosis: prophase–metaphase–anaphase–telophase

G₁: growth

S: synthesis of DNA

G₂: growth

G₀: quiescent G_1 phase

G_1 and G_0 are of variable duration. Mitosis is usually the shortest phase. Most cells are in G_0. Rapidly dividing cells have a shorter G_1.

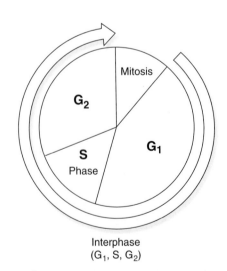

(Adapted from Bhushan V, Le T, Amin C: *First Aid for the USMLE Step 1*. Stamford, Connecticut, Appleton & Lange, 1999. p. 165.)

C. DNA strand separation requires several proteins:
1. **DnaA**—20 to 50 of these proteins aggregate at the origin of replication and begin to separate the DNA strands.

2. **Single-strand binding (SSB) proteins** bind cooperatively to further separate the two strands of DNA.

3. **DNA helicase** unwinds the DNA.

D. Supercoiling is prevented by **DNA topoisomerase** type I and II.

E. Replication process in prokaryotic cells (Figure 1-4)

FIGURE
1-4   **DNA synthesis**

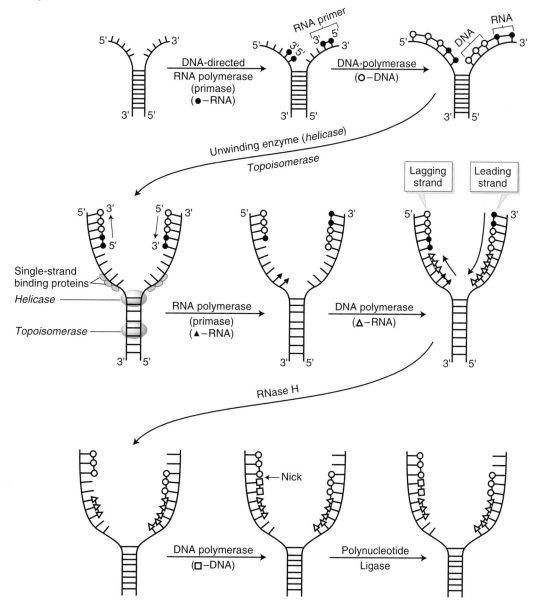

(Adapted from Marks DB: *BRS Biochemistry, 3rd edition.* Baltimore, Williams & Wilkins, 1999. Used by permission of Lippincott Williams & Wilkins.)

1. An RNA primer is placed on the separated DNA strands by RNA polymerase (also called **primase**) before replication can begin.

2. On the leading strand only one RNA primer is needed; on the lagging strand a new primer is required as the replication fork opens.

  a. Leading strand

    (1) The leading strand produces a continuously elongating strand of new DNA.

    (2) The leading strand of DNA is copied continuously from 5′ to 3′ in the direction of the replication fork.

DNA synthesis can be prevented by nucleoside analogs such as cytosine arabinoside, zidovudine, and acyclovir. These types of drugs are useful in antiviral and anticancer therapy.

In eukaryotic cells, replication is accomplished by POL enzymes similar to those in prokaryotic cells. POL α performs primase activity like prokaryotic primase, POL δ synthesizes the leading DNA strand, POL ε synthesizes the lagging strand, and POL β repairs and excises primers similarly to DNA polymerase I.

Xeroderma pigmentosum is a genetic disease in which cells cannot repair damaged DNA. People suffering from this disease cannot repair skin damage caused by sunlight and are predisposed to skin cancer.

  b. Lagging strand
     (1) The lagging strand of DNA is copied piecewise in the direction opposite of the replication fork.
     (2) The lagging strand produces small pieces of new DNA with RNA interspersed, called Okazaki fragments.
  3. The DNA chain is elongated by DNA polymerase III, which adds nucleotides with energy provided by breaking of the triphosphate bond.
  4. When DNA strand synthesis is complete, it is proofread.
     a. The proofreading function of DNA polymerase III (3'–5' exonuclease) allows it to correct mismatched base pairs.
     b. The improperly placed base is hydrolytically removed and replaced with the appropriate one.
  5. RNA primers are removed from the Okazaki fragments and leading strand.
     a. DNA polymerase I or III has **3'–5' exonuclease** activity that allows it to remove the RNA primer.
     b. Once the primer is removed, the space is filled with DNA.
  6. The break in the strand backbone is sealed by **DNA ligase.**
F. Repair
  1. Damage caused by ultraviolet light
     a. Ultraviolet light exposure results in **pyrimidine dimers** (especially thymine-thymine dimers).
     b. Dimers inhibit the replication process.
     c. Specialized **endonucleases** recognize a dimer and cleave it at its 5' end.
     d. An **exonuclease** then excises the dimer and leaves a gap in the DNA strand.
     e. The gap is filled with the appropriate nucleotides by DNA polymerase I.
     f. The strand is resealed by DNA ligase.
  2. Base alterations
     a. Bases may be changed spontaneously or slowly over time because of **alkylating agents** (cyclophosphamide and nitrosoureas).
     b. Specialized **glycosylases** remove the improper base and leave an empty (apyrimidinic or apurinic) space.
     c. The empty space is filled by specific endonucleases or polymerases in the same manner that dimers are repaired.

III. DNA Packaging
  A. Owing to the incredible length of DNA, it must be properly coiled inside the cell.
  B. **Histones** are a group of proteins designed to coil DNA.
     1. The high content of arginine and lysine gives histones a positive charge, which attracts them to negatively charged DNA.
     2. Histones organize themselves into a group of eight to make a **nucleosome** core; each core contains two each of type H2A, H2B, H3, and H4 histones.
     3. DNA twists approximately twice around each core.
     4. Between cores a histone of type H1 is attached to the DNA.
     5. The arrangement of histones and DNA is called a nucleosome and produces a characteristic "beads on a string" appearance.
     6. The nucleosomes coil around themselves to produce a nucleofilament.
     7. Nucleofilaments are further packaged and coiled into more compact structures when DNA is not being replicated.

IV. RNA Synthesis
  A. Initiation of transcription is influenced by a variety of factors:
     1. **RNA polymerase** binds to the promoter region of the DNA.

2. The **TATAAT** nucleotide sequence is a section of the promoter located upstream from the start of transcription; it is contained in the Hogness box of eukaryotes and the Pribnow box of prokaryotes.

3. The **CAAT box,** found in eukaryotes, and the −35 sequence, found in prokaryotes, are located further upstream from the TATAAT sequence and have promoter function.

B. After recognition of the promoter region by RNA polymerase, elongation begins.

1. Elongation of RNA occurs in a manner similar to DNA replication, but does not require a primer for initiation.

2. RNA polymerase does not have a proofreading function so it cannot correct mismatched base pairs that may occur.

C. In eukaryotic cells RNA undergoes **posttranslational modification;** in prokaryotic cells transcription and translation occur simultaneously.

1. RNA synthesized by eukaryotic **RNA polymerase II** is called **heterogeneous nuclear RNA (hnRNA)** and is found in the nucleus of the cell.

2. This hnRNA is **capped at the 5′ end** by a 7-methyl-guanine molecule provided by *S*-adenosylmethionine (SAM).

3. **A poly-A nucleotide tail is added to the 3′ end.**

4. Introns are cleaved out.

5. The molecule is now mature messenger RNA (mRNA) and is transported to the cytoplasm.

In eukaryotes, different RNA is synthesized by several different RNA polymerases. RNA polymerase I synthesizes ribosomal RNA, RNA polymerase II synthesizes messenger RNA, and RNA polymerase III synthesizes transfer RNA.

Point mutations include **silent mutations** (the same amino acid), **missense mutations** (a new amino acid), and **nonsense mutations** (stop codon). Insertions are the addition of extra amino acids, and deletions are the loss of amino acids.

V. Protein Synthesis (Figure 1-5)

FIGURE 1-5 **Protein synthesis**

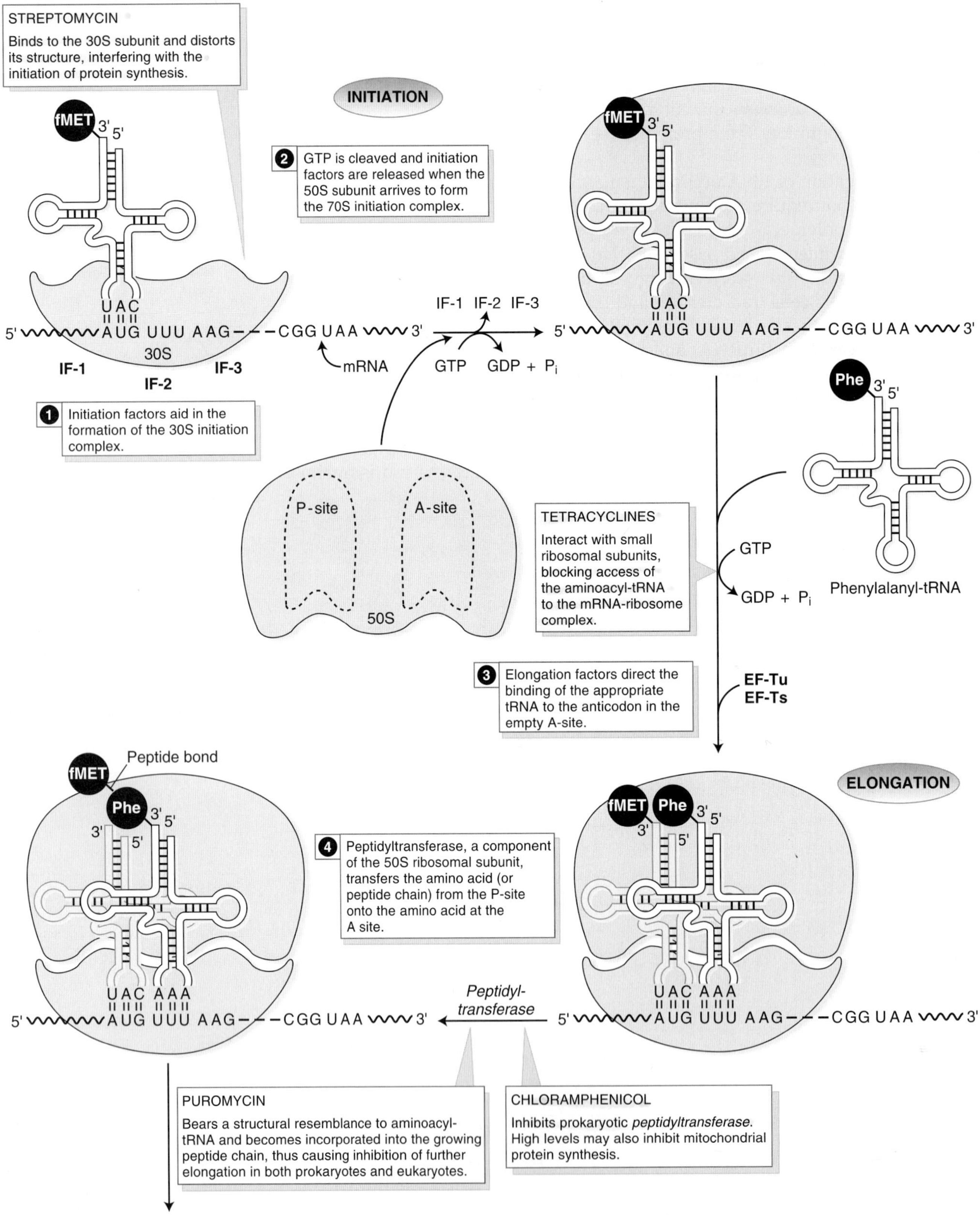

STREPTOMYCIN

Binds to the 30S subunit and distorts its structure, interfering with the initiation of protein synthesis.

INITIATION

2 GTP is cleaved and initiation factors are released when the 50S subunit arrives to form the 70S initiation complex.

fMET 3' 5'

U A C
| | | |
5' ~~~~~ A U G U U U A A G — — C G G U A A ~~~~ 3'
30S

IF-1   IF-3
IF-2

mRNA

IF-1 IF-2 IF-3

GTP   GDP + P_i

5' ~~~~~ A U G U U U A A G — — C G G U A A ~~~ 3'

fMET 3' 5'

U A C
| | | |

1 Initiation factors aid in the formation of the 30S initiation complex.

P-site   A-site

50S

TETRACYCLINES

Interact with small ribosomal subunits, blocking access of the aminoacyl-tRNA to the mRNA-ribosome complex.

GTP

GDP + P_i

Phe 3' 5'

Phenylalanyl-tRNA

3 Elongation factors direct the binding of the appropriate tRNA to the anticodon in the empty A-site.

EF-Tu
EF-Ts

ELONGATION

fMET

Peptide bond

Phe 3' 5'

3' | 5'

4 Peptidyltransferase, a component of the 50S ribosomal subunit, transfers the amino acid (or peptide chain) from the P-site onto the amino acid at the A site.

U A C   A A A
|| ||| |||||
5' ~~~ A U G U U U A A G — — C G G U A A ~~~ 3'

Peptidyl-transferase

fMET Phe 3' 5'
3' | 5'

U A C   A A A
|| ||| |||||
5' ~~~~ A U G U U U A A G — — C G G U A A ~~~ 3'

PUROMYCIN

Bears a structural resemblance to aminoacyl-tRNA and becomes incorporated into the growing peptide chain, thus causing inhibition of further elongation in both prokaryotes and eukaryotes.

CHLORAMPHENICOL

Inhibits prokaryotic *peptidyltransferase*. High levels may also inhibit mitochondrial protein synthesis.

Continued at top of next page

A=adenine; *Arg*=arginine; *C*=cytosine; *EF*=elongation factor; *fMET*=formyl methionine; *G*=guanine; *GDP*=guanine diphosphate; *GTP*=guanine triphosphate; *IF*=initiation factor; *P*=phosphate; *Phe*=phenylalanine; *RF*=release factor; *T*=thymine; *tRNA*=transfer ribonucleic acid; *U*=uracil
(Adapted from Champe PC and Harvey RA: *Lippincott's Illustrated Reviews: Biochemistry, 2nd edition*. Philadelphia, Lippincott-Raven Publishers, 1994. pp. 396–7. Used by permission of Lippincott Williams & Wilkins.)

FIGURE 1-5 Protein synthesis *(Continued)*

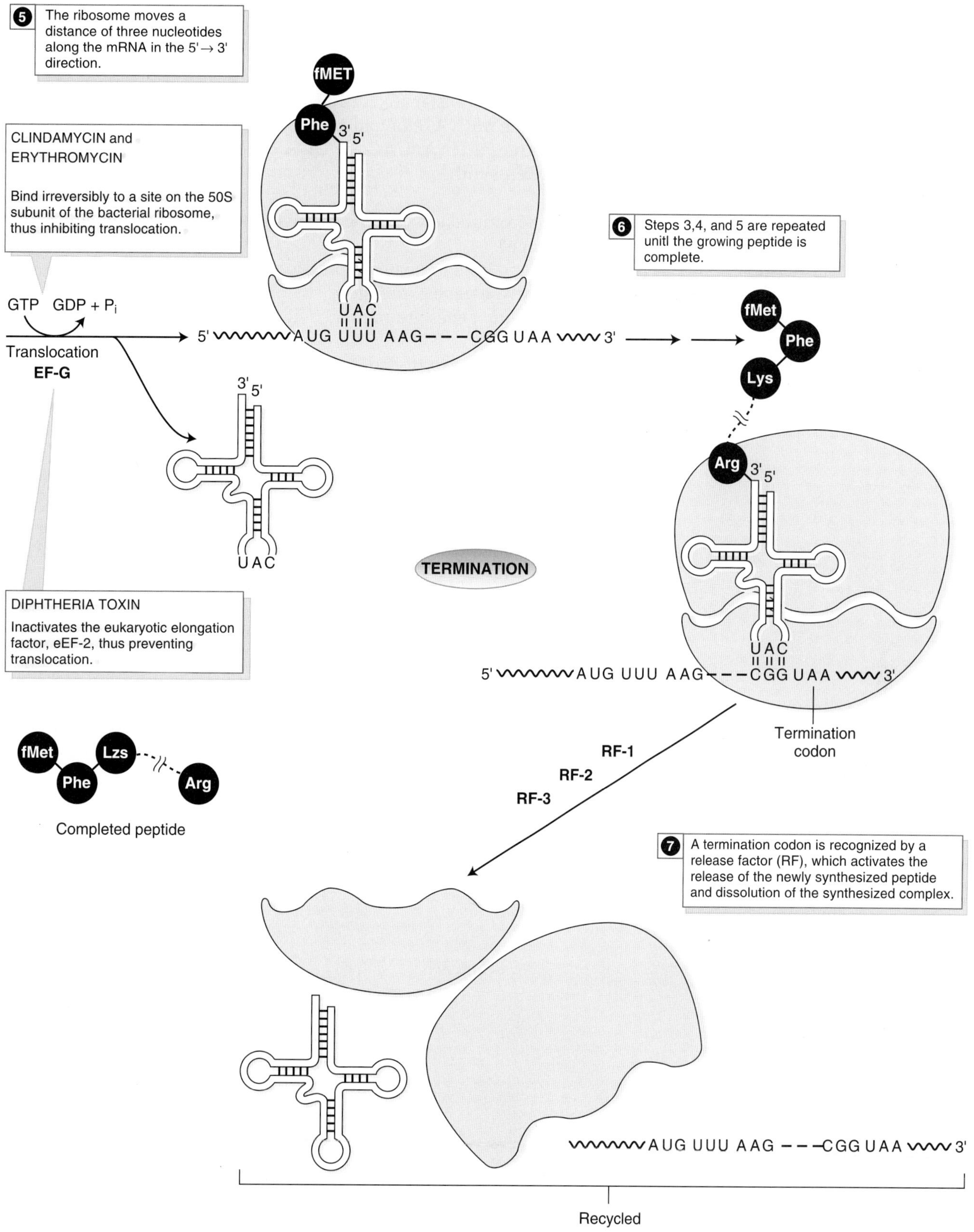

5 The ribosome moves a distance of three nucleotides along the mRNA in the 5' → 3' direction.

CLINDAMYCIN and ERYTHROMYCIN

Bind irreversibly to a site on the 50S subunit of the bacterial ribosome, thus inhibiting translocation.

GTP   GDP + P$_i$

Translocation
EF-G

DIPHTHERIA TOXIN

Inactivates the eukaryotic elongation factor, eEF-2, thus preventing translocation.

fMET

Phe   3' 5'

5' ~~~AUG UUU AAG — — — CGG UAA ~~~3'

U A C

6 Steps 3,4, and 5 are repeated unitl the growing peptide is complete.

fMet
Phe
Lys

Arg   3' 5'

TERMINATION

U A C

5' ~~~~~~AUG UUU AAG — — — CGG UAA ~~~3'

Termination codon

3' 5'

U A C

fMet   Lzs
Phe   Arg

Completed peptide

RF-1
RF-2
RF-3

7 A termination codon is recognized by a release factor (RF), which activates the release of the newly synthesized peptide and dissolution of the synthesized complex.

~~~~~~AUG UUU AAG — — CGG UAA ~~~3'

Recycled

A. Initiation is started with the binding of the ribosomal subunits to the mRNA.

B. The start codon **AUG** is the first codon to be recognized and translated; initiation factor 2 (**IF-2** in prokaryotes, **eIF-2** in eukaryotes) and guanosine 5'-triphosphate (GTP) are required.

C. A methionine is added as the first amino acid.

D. Elongation requires a transfer RNA (tRNA) with the appropriate **anticodon** to the codon on the mRNA, elongation factors, and GTP.

E. Termination requires a **UAA, UAG, or UGA** codon.

F. Regulation of RNA synthesis
   1. Eukaryotes
      a. Control is accomplished by gene **methylation, amplification,** and **rearrangement.**
      b. Histones play a role in gene suppression.
      c. Inducers activate gene expression.
      d. Some eukaryotic genes are regulated at transcription.
   2. Prokaryotes
      a. Protein synthesis is controlled at the level of transcription using operons.
      b. An **operon** is a set of adjacent genes that are activated or deactivated.
      c. Each operon has a **promoter** region upstream from the genes, an **operator** that activates or deactivates the genes, and a **repressor** protein that can bind to the operator and deactivate transcription (Figure 1-6).

FIGURE 1-6 Operons

Inducible operon (Lac operon)

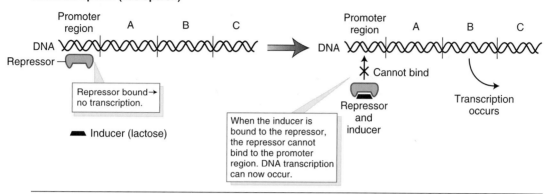

Promoter region

DNA

Repressor

Repressor bound → no transcription.

▬ Inducer (lactose)

Promoter region

✗ Cannot bind

Repressor and inducer

Transcription occurs

When the inducer is bound to the repressor, the repressor cannot bind to the promoter region. DNA transcription can now occur.

Repressible operon (tryptophan operon)

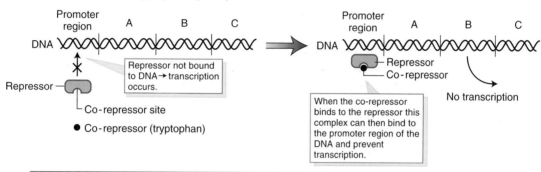

Promoter region

DNA

Repressor

Repressor not bound to DNA → transcription occurs.

Co-repressor site

● Co-repressor (tryptophan)

Promoter region

Repressor
Co-repressor

No transcription

When the co-repressor binds to the repressor this complex can then bind to the promoter region of the DNA and prevent transcription.

Positive control operon (arabinose operon)

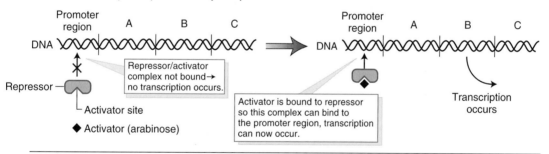

Promoter region

DNA

Repressor

Repressor/activator complex not bound → no transcription occurs.

Activator site

◆ Activator (arabinose)

Promoter region

Transcription occurs

Activator is bound to repressor so this complex can bind to the promoter region, transcription can now occur.

Catabolite repressor operon (Lac operon when glucose is present)

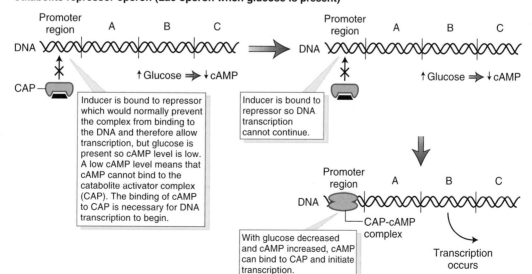

Promoter region

DNA

CAP

↑ Glucose ⟹ ↓ cAMP

Inducer is bound to repressor which would normally prevent the complex from binding to the DNA and therefore allow transcription, but glucose is present so cAMP level is low. A low cAMP level means that cAMP cannot bind to the catabolite activator complex (CAP). The binding of cAMP to CAP is necessary for DNA transcription to begin.

Promoter region

DNA

↑ Glucose ⟹ ↓ cAMP

Inducer is bound to repressor so DNA transcription cannot continue.

Promoter region

DNA

CAP-cAMP complex

Transcription occurs

With glucose decreased and cAMP increased, cAMP can bind to CAP and initiate transcription.

cAMP=cyclic adenosine monophosphate

VI. Posttranslational Folding of Proteins

A. Newly synthesized proteins have a linear structure **(primary structure)**.

B. On the basis of interactions between amino-acids, these linear structures can assume **secondary structures** such as an **α-helix** or **β-pleated sheet.**

C. The tertiary structure incorporates the secondary structures into a complete three-dimensional configuration. This is the final conformation of many proteins.

D. A quaternary structure is formed when several tertiary structures are arranged together. This occurs in hemoglobin, for example, in which two α and two β globular proteins form the complete hemoglobin molecule.

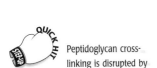

Disulfide bonds play a major role in maintaining the tertiary structure of proteins.

BACTERIAL MORPHOLOGY AND GENETICS

I. Cell Wall—the outermost component of all bacteria

A. Cell wall components

1. Peptidoglycan provides rigid support and protects against osmotic pressure changes, thick and multilayered in Gram-positive organisms, thin and single layer in Gram-negative organisms.

2. Gram-positive outer membrane is made up of teichoic acid.

3. Gram-negative outer membrane is made up of lipid-A (toxic component of endotoxin) and polysaccharide (major surface antigen).

4. Cytoplasmic membrane is a lipoprotein bilayer without sterols, the site of oxidative and transport enzymes.

Peptidoglycan cross-linking is disrupted by penicillin and cephalosporins.

B. Gram's stain

1. Separates most bacteria into two groups
   a. Gram-positive organisms stain blue.
   b. Gram-negative organisms stain red.

2. Procedure
   a. Crystal violet dye applied to the specimen stains all bacterial cells blue.
   b. Iodine, when added to the specimen, acts as a mordant and forms crystal violet-iodine complexes. Cells continue to appear blue.
   c. An organic solvent, such as ethanol, added to the specimen extracts the crystal violet-iodine complexes from Gram-negative organisms. Gram-negative organisms now appear colorless, whereas Gram-positive organisms remain blue.
   d. Safranin (red dye) is applied, staining the Gram-negative organisms red, while the Gram-positive organisms maintain their blue color.

II. Bacterial Genome

A. Bacteria have a **haploid** genome as compared with the **diploid** human genome.

B. A typical bacterial cell has a **circular** DNA molecule with a molecular weight of approximately 2×10^9 with about 5×10^6 base pairs, which code for approximately 2,000 proteins.

III. Mutation

A. Several types of mutations occur that can alter the bacterial genome.

B. Mutation is an important factor in bacterial survival as it allows the bacteria to change and adapt to their environment.

C. Mutations may be caused by a mistake committed by DNA polymerase, a chemical mutagen, ultraviolet light, a virus, or other cause.

D. Types of mutations

1. **Base substitution**
   a. One base replaces another
   b. Occurs at DNA replication

    c. Can generate a missense mutation, which causes the wrong amino acid to be placed in the protein, or it can generate a nonsense mutation, which is read as a stop codon.

    d. Base substitution also occurs in eukaryotic cells, but can be repaired by the processes described above.

  2. **Frameshift mutation**

    a. One or more bases are added or removed (not a multiple of 3).

    b. The reading frame is shifted on the mRNA molecule, causing massive errors in translation.

    c. Often causes protein to end prematurely as a result of creation of a stop codon

    d. Also occurs in eukaryotic cells

  3. **Transposons** (Figure 1-7)

FIGURE
1-7 **Transposons**

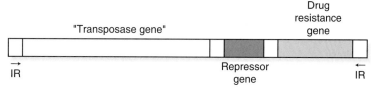

IR=inverted repeats

    a. Called "jumping genes" because they transfer pieces of DNA from one bacterium to another

    b. Transposons can integrate small pieces of DNA into the bacterial genome, plasmids, or bacteriophages.

    c. Integration of transposon DNA into the host genome can occur within a preexisting gene and render the host gene useless.

    d. Each transposon has four domains:

      (1) **Inverted repeats**—appear at the ends and mediate integration of the transposon into a DNA molecule

      (2) **Transposase**—the enzyme that controls integration and removal of the transposon

      (3) **Repressor gene**—controls synthesis of transposase and whichever gene is in the fourth domain

      (4) **Drug resistance gene**—often appears in the fourth gene domain

    e. Transposons replicate with the host DNA and are not capable of independent replication.

    f. When transposons integrate and remove themselves from a DNA molecule, they can cause profound mutations.

IV. Genetic Transfer

  A. Transfer within a cell

    1. Transposons can transfer information between different areas of the same DNA molecule.

    2. **Programmed rearrangements**

      a. These are performed by certain organisms including *Neisseria, Borrelia,* and *Trypanosomes.*

      b. Programmed rearrangements cause a silent gene to be expressed. Programmed rearrangements also allow the organism to evade the immune system.

● Transfer Between Cells (Table 1-1)

TABLE 1-1	Genetic Transfer Between Prokaryotic Cells	
Mode	**Mechanism**	**Notes**
Transduction	Transfer of DNA from one cell to another using a viral vector	**Generalized transduction** can transfer any gene and contains no viral DNA; **specialized transduction** can transfer only certain genes and contains viral DNA
Conjugation	Transfer of DNA from one bacterium to another via contact and exchange	Can transfer chromosomes or plasmids; uses a sex pilus

Conjugation is performed by fertility plasmid (F plasmid). A bacterium containing the F plasmid (the male) has a sex pilus, which can attach to an F plasmid-deficient bacterium (the female). Once attached, the female is reeled in and DNA is transferred.

VIRAL GENETICS

● Comparison of Cells and Viruses (Table 1-2)

In contrast to infectious bacteria and fungi, viruses are not cells. They do not have a nucleus or organelles and are not capable of reproducing independently. Current antiviral agents such as acyclovir or foscarnet can only suppress viral replication. Viral elimination requires a functioning host immune response.

Prions lack most of the features associated with cells or viruses. Prions are thought to be abnormally folded proteins that are capable of catalyzing similar folding in the host's proteins. Accumulation of these abnormally folded proteins can cause spongiform diseases characterized by vacuolization of brain tissues, such as kuru or Creutzfeldt-Jakob disease.

TABLE 1-2	Comparison of Cells and Viruses		
	Eukaryotes	**Prokaryotes**	**Viruses**
Size (in μm)	7	2–6	0.01–0.2
Membrane-bound	Present	Absent	Absent **organelles**
Ribosomes	80S	70S	Absent
DNA	46 chromosomes	1 circular chromosome	DNA or RNA; circular, single-strand, or multiple segments
Replication	Mitosis or meiosis	Binary fission	Production and assembly

I. Viral Structure (Figure 1-8)

    A. Nucleic acid

        1. May be DNA or RNA, but never both

        2. May be single or double stranded

        3. May be linear, segmented, or circular

        4. Most are haploid, but retroviruses are diploid

Viral structure is highly variable among viruses but constant for each particular virus.

FIGURE 1-8 Structure of viruses. A) Icosohedral Capsid, B) Helical Capsid.

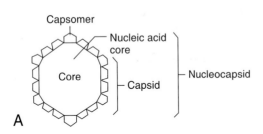

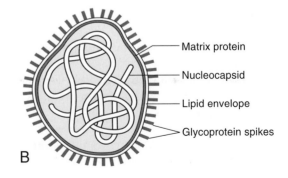

B. Capsid
  1. The protein coat around the nucleic acid core is composed of repeating units called **capsomeres.**
  2. The capsid assumes one of two shapes:
    a. **Helical**—hollow rod shape
    b. **Icosahedral**—multiple triangles arranged into a small sphere
  3. The capsid functions to protect the viral nucleic acid.
C. Envelope
  1. Surrounds the capsid of some viruses
  2. Causes the virus to be more susceptible to drying and lipid solvents
  3. Composed of virus-specific proteins and cell derived lipids
  4. Most **DNA viruses** derive their envelope from the host cell's **nuclear membrane,** whereas **most RNA viruses** derive their envelope from the host's **plasma membrane.**

II. Replication
  A. Attachment
    1. Viral surface proteins specifically attach to receptor proteins on the cell surface.
    2. The noncovalent interaction of proteins determines host range.
  B. Penetration
    1. The virus may be engulfed by the host via a pinocytotic vesicle (**viropexis**).
    2. Non-enveloped viruses may slip through the host membrane by direct **translocation.**
    3. The viral **envelope may fuse with the host cell membrane.**
  C. Uncoating
    1. DNA viruses partially uncoat in the cytoplasm and undergo final uncoating in the nucleus (to protect the DNA from endonucleases in the cytoplasm).
    2. RNA viruses uncoat in the cytoplasm.
  D. Expression and replication
    1. DNA viruses replicate in the nucleus (except poxvirus) using the host cell's RNA polymerase and other proteins.
    2. **Positive single-stranded RNA viruses** contain an mRNA genome, which **interacts directly with host ribosomes** for translation of a viral RNA polymerase, which completes replication.
    3. **Negative single-stranded and double-stranded RNA viruses** are packaged with a **viral RNA polymerase, which produces positive RNA** for transcription.
    4. Thousands of copies of viral proteins are produced.
    5. For the retrovirus life cycle, see discussion of human immunodeficiency virus (HIV) (System 8 "Reproductive System").
  E. Assembly
    1. DNA viruses are assembled in the nucleus (except for the pox viruses).
    2. RNA viruses are assembled in the cytoplasm (except for the influenza virus, which is assembled in the nucleus).
  F. Release
    1. Non-enveloped viruses usually cause **rupture the host cell membrane** which releases mature particles.
    2. Enveloped viruses are released via **budding,** in which each mature particle becomes surrounded by a portion of the host cell's membrane.

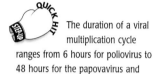
The duration of a viral multiplication cycle ranges from 6 hours for poliovirus to 48 hours for the papovavirus and adenovirus.

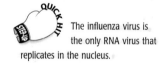
The influenza virus is the only RNA virus that replicates in the nucleus.

CONCEPTS IN PHARMACOLOGY

I. Absorption
A. There are many routes of administration (Figure 1-9).

FIGURE 1-9 **Routes of drug administration**

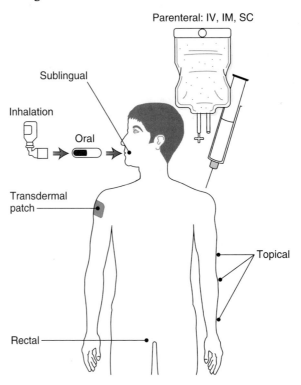

IM=intramuscular; IV=intravenous; SC=subcutaneous (Adapted from Mycek MJ, Harvey RA, and Champe PC: *Lippincott's Illustrated Reviews: Pharmacology, 2nd edition.* Philadelphia, Lippincott-Raven Publishers, 1996. p. 2. Used by permission of Lippincott Williams and Wilkins.)

If a drug is rapidly metabolized by the liver, the amount reaching the target tissues is significantly reduced. Such drugs include propranolol, lidocaine, verapamil, and meperidine.

Charged species do not cross the gastrointestinal membrane as readily as uncharged species. Therefore, the percent of drug in the uncharged state determines the rate of absorption.

$$pH = pK_a + log \frac{unprotonated}{protonated \ species}$$

When infusing a drug, it takes 4.3 half-lives to achieve 95% of the steady-state concentration.

Acidophilic drugs bind to albumin whereas basophilic drugs bind to globulins. The administration of a drug that binds to sites already occupied by a drug can displace the first drug. This leads to a surge in free drug, which in turn leads to increased activity and elimination.

B. **Oral** administration is the most common route.
C. Most drugs are absorbed in the **duodenum.**
   1. Drugs enter the portal circulation.
   2. They are subject to **first-pass metabolism** by the liver.
D. Other factors affect absorption:
   1. Intestinal pH
   2. Whether taken with food (slows transit allowing for further acid digestion)
   3. Whether the drug is a sustained-release preparation
   4. Whether gastrointestinal diseases or malabsorption syndromes are present

II. Distribution
A. Vd = TD/C
   where Vd = volume of distribution, TD = total drug in body,
   C = plasma concentration
B. Distribution occurs more rapidly with high blood flow, high vessel permeability, and a **hydrophobic drug.**
C. Binding to **plasma proteins** (albumin and globulins) accelerates absorption into plasma but slows diffusion into tissues.
D. Many disease states alter distribution.
   1. Edematous states (e.g., cirrhosis, heart failure, nephrotic syndrome) prolong distribution and delay clearance.

2. Obesity allows for greater accumulation of lipophilic agents within fat cells, increasing distribution and prolonging half-life.

3. Pregnancy increases intravascular volume, thus increasing Vd.

4. Hypoalbuminemia allows drugs that are protein-bound to have increased availability because of lack of albumin for binding.

III. Pharmacokinetics

A. The effect an agonist has on its receptors depends on concentration.

B. **Efficacy** is a measure of the maximum effect a drug can produce.

C. **Potency** is a measure of the amount of drug needed to produce a given effect (Figure 1-10).

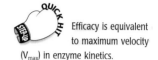

Efficacy is equivalent to maximum velocity (V_{max}) in enzyme kinetics.

FIGURE 1-10 **Dose-response curve**

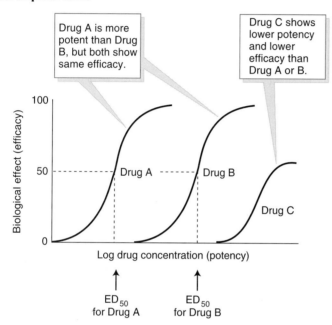

Drug A is more potent than Drug B, but both show same efficacy.

Drug C shows lower potency and lower efficacy than Drug A or B.

ED$_{50}$=dose effective in 50% of population

D. Effective Dose (ED) and Lethal Dose (LD)

1. ED is the dose of the drug that produces the desired effect.

2. ED_{50} is the dose of the drug that produces the desired effect in 50% of the population.

3. LD is the dose of the drug that produces death.

4. LD_{50} is the dose of the drug that produces death in 50% of the population.

5. Overlap of ED and LD determines therapeutic range (Figure 1-11).

FIGURE 1-11 **Therapeutic range**

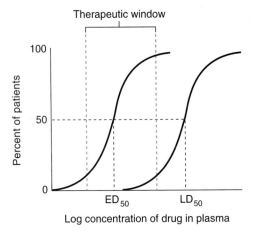

ED_{50}=dose effective in 50% of population; LD_{50}=dose that is lethal in 50% of population

E. Antagonists (Figure 1-12)

FIGURE 1-12 **Drug antagonism**

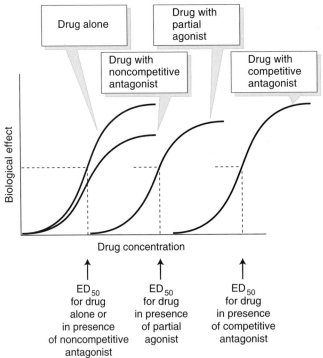

ED_{50}=dose effective in 50% of population

1. Competitive antagonist: competes for the same binding site as the agonist or drug
2. Noncompetitive antagonist
   a. Prevents binding of the agonist or drug to the receptor or prevents activation of the receptor by the agonist
   b. Decreases the efficacy of the agonist

3. Complete antagonist: prevents all pharmacologic action(s) of the agonist or drug
4. Partial agonist: binds to the same receptor site as the agonist or drug, but has a lower potency

F. A drug's **therapeutic index (TI)** is a measure of how safe it is to use: $TI = LD_{50}/ED_{50}$

G. Pharmacokinetics is affected by disease states:
1. Hyperthyroidism increases the heart's sensitivity to catecholamines.
2. Cirrhosis patients are more sensitive to sedative-hypnotics.
3. Patients with cirrhosis and congestive heart failure (CHF) will retain fluids if taking nonsteroidal anti-inflammatory drugs (NSAIDs) because of the role of prostaglandins in maintaining renal function.

IV. Metabolism

A. Drugs may be chemically altered to vary activity or aid excretion.
B. The enzymatic transformation of drugs usually follows one of two kinetics:
1. **First-order:** a constant **fraction** of drug is metabolized in a certain unit of time
2. **Zero-order:** a constant **amount** of drug is metabolized in a certain unit of time (e.g., ethanol)
C. The liver is the primary site of metabolism and uses two sets of reactions:
1. **Phase 1:** drugs are modified or portions are removed (cytochrome P-450 oxidation, enzymatic reduction, hydrolysis)
2. **Phase 2:** conjugation reactions add chemical groupings to the drug (e.g., glucuronidation, sulfate or glutathione conjugation, acetylation, methylation)
D. **Prodrugs** are drugs that are administered in an inactive form and are metabolically activated by the body.
E. Some drugs are metabolized to toxic products (e.g., acetaminophen).

QUICK HIT
Ethanol, barbiturates, and phenytoin induce cytochrome P-450 enzymes, whereas cimetidine and ketoconazole inhibit cytochrome P-450 enzymes, increasing and decreasing the metabolism of other drugs, respectively (e.g., warfarin). The macrolide antibiotics (e.g., erythromycin) inhibit cytochrome P-450 enzymes and increase the cardiac toxicity of cisapride.

V. Elimination

A. Most drugs are eliminated in the urine or bile.
B. Volatile drugs (e.g., ethanol) can be eliminated through the lungs.
C. **Renal excretion**
1. Substances with a molecular weight (MW) <5,000, free in the plasma, are filtered in the glomerulus.
2. Higher concentrations of a substance within the tubules may favor some reabsorption.
3. The proximal convoluted tubule (PCT) may actively secrete a drug.
4. Urine pH, the molecular size, lipid solubility, and negative logarithm of the acid ionization constant (pK_a) of the drug affect renal excretion.
D. **Biliary excretion**
1. Hepatocytes actively take up the drug from plasma, store it or metabolize it, and release it into the bile duct.
2. Some drugs are excreted in feces.
3. Some drugs are reabsorbed in the terminal ileum (**enterohepatic cycling**).

QUICK HIT
Filtration is dependent on the amount of free drug in the blood, whereas active secretion is dependent on the total plasma concentration (free and bound drug).

VI. Special Circumstances

A. Older patients
1. These patients often use multiple prescription and over-the-counter medications.
2. Decreased body size, body water, and serum albumin, along with increased body fat, alter drug distribution.
3. **Decreased phase 1 reactions,** liver mass, and liver blood flow all slow metabolism.
4. Decreased kidney mass, renal blood flow, glomerular filtration rate and tubular function hamper drug excretion.

B. Pediatric patients
  1. **Most drugs cross the placenta** to some extent, and their possible effects on the fetus are ranked as category A, B, C, D, and X (A = no risk, X = risk outweighs benefit).
  2. Absorption
     a. High gastric pH and delayed emptying affect enteral absorption.
     b. High surface area to volume ratio affects transdermal administration.
     c. Low muscle mass limits IM administration to the **vastus lateralis** in infancy.
  3. Albumin does not reach adult levels until 1 year of age.
  4. Both phases of metabolism are deficient to varying degrees until 1–2 years of age.
  5. Specific antibiotics avoided in childhood include **quinolones** (articular cartilage erosion and tendon damage) and **tetracycline** (depression of bone and teeth formation).

C. Pharmacogenetics
  1. Acetylation of isoniazid:
     a. **In patients who are slow acetylators,** there is increased incidence of neuropathy, bladder cancer, and familial Parkinson's disease.
     b. **Patients who are rapid acetylators** are the majority of the population.
     c. Also affects metabolism of hydralazine, dapsone, and phenytoin
  2. Succinylcholine sensitivity
     a. Atypical **pseudocholinesterase** does not hydrolyze succinylcholine as effectively
     b. Leads to prolonged paralysis (succinylcholine apnea)
     c. **Autosomal recessive**
  3. Ethanol metabolism
     a. **Aldehyde dehydrogenase** shows diminished activity in certain patients (50% of Chinese and Japanese)
     b. Acetaldehyde accumulation leads to facial flushing, headache, nausea, and vomiting.

D. Toxicology (Table 1-3)

TABLE 1-3 ● Toxicology

Poison	Therapy
Acetaminophen	*N*-Acetylcysteine
Aspirin	Alkalinization of urine
Benzodiazepine	Flumazenil
Carbon monoxide	100% oxygen
Cyanide	Sodium nitrite
Digitalis	Digitalis antibody or potassium (if serum potassium level is low)
Ethylene glycol, methanol, isopropyl alcohol	Ethanol
Heavy metals	Calcium EDTA (for lead); dimercaprol (for arsenic, mercury); penicillamine (for copper); deferoxamine (for iron)
Heparin	Protamine sulfate
Opioids	Naloxone
Propranolol	Glucagon
Tricyclic antidepressants	Gastric lavage, alkalinization of serum
Warfarin	Vitamin K

EDTA=ethylenediamine tetraacetic acid.

ANTI-INFECTIVE AGENTS

I. Antibiotics

A. β-Lactam agents
   1. Specific agents
      a. Penicillins (e.g., penicillin G, ampicillin, piperacillin)
      b. Cephalosporins (e.g., cefazolin, ceftriaxone)
      c. Carbapenems (e.g., meropenem)
      d. Monobactams (e.g., aztreonam)
   2. Mechanism of action: bactericidal
      a. **Inhibit cell wall synthesis**
      b. Act on penicillin-binding proteins (PBPs) in bacterial cell walls
      c. Require active cell division for bactericidal effect
   3. Spectrum of action: varies for each particular drug
      a. Gram-positive and Gram-negative bacteria
      b. Anaerobes and spirochetes
   4. Side effects/adverse reactions
      a. **Allergic reactions** (especially a rash with penicillins)
      b. Platelet aggregation dysfunction
      c. Thrombophlebitis (cephalosporins)
      d. Direct central nervous system (CNS) toxicity
      e. Superinfections including *Clostridium difficile* and yeasts such as *Candida* spp.
   5. Mechanisms of resistance
      a. Inactivation by **β-lactamase enzymes**
      b. Failure to reach PBP targets
      c. Poor binding to PBPs

B. Aminoglycosides (e.g., gentamicin, tobramycin, neomycin)
   1. Mechanism of action: bactericidal
      a. Bind to the **30S ribosomal subunits of bacteria**
      b. Subsequently interfere with protein synthesis
   2. Spectrum of action
      a. Broad-spectrum activity against Gram-negative bacilli
      b. Some activity against Gram-positive bacteria
      c. No anaerobic activity
   3. Side effects/adverse reactions
      a. **Ototoxicity**
      b. **Nephrotoxicity**
   4. Mechanisms of resistance
      a. Enzymatic modification of the aminoglycoside
      b. Altered ribosome binding sites
      c. Altered antibiotic uptake

C. Tetracyclines (e.g., tetracycline, demeclocycline, doxycycline)
   1. Mechanism of action: **bacteriostatic**
      a. Reversibly bind to the 30S ribosomal subunit
      b. Prevent the addition of new amino acids onto growing peptide chain
   2. Spectrum of action: broad-spectrum activity
      a. Gram-positive and Gram-negative bacteria, anaerobes, spirochetes, mycoplasma, rickettsiae, chlamydiae
      b. Some protozoa
   3. Side effects/adverse reactions
      a. Teeth discoloration
      b. **Depression of skeletal growth**
      c. Gastrointestinal distress
      d. **Hepatotoxicity**
      e. Photosensitivity

Gram-negative activity of cephalosporins: third-generation > second-generation > first-generation.

β-Lactam inhibitors, which have weak bactericidal activity but greatly inhibit β-lactamase, are used in combination with some penicillins to enhance their effectiveness (e.g., amoxicillin-clavulanate, ampicillin-sulbactam, piperacillin-tazobactam).

Tetracyclines are contraindicated in pregnancy and in children because of their effect on the teeth and bones.

4. Mechanisms of resistance
   a. Reduction of tetracycline influx
   b. Active tetracycline export from within the bacterial cell
D. Chloramphenicol
   1. Mechanism of action: usually bacteriostatic but bactericidal in some organisms
      a. Binds to the 50S ribosomal subunit
      b. Prevents the addition of new amino acids onto growing peptide chain
   2. Spectrum of action
      a. Gram-positive and Gram-negative bacteria
      b. Spirochetes, rickettsia, chlamydia, mycoplasma
   3. Side effects/adverse reactions: Chloramphenicol is rarely a first choice because of its adverse reactions.
      a. **Aplastic anemia**
      b. Reversible bone marrow depression
      c. **Gray baby syndrome:** abdominal distention, vomiting, flaccidity, cyanosis, circulatory collapse, death
   4. Mechanisms of resistance
      a. Impermeability of bacteria to drug
      b. Production of enzymes that inactivate the antibiotic
E. Macrolides (e.g., erythromycin, azithromycin, clarithromycin) and lincosamides (e.g., lincomycin and clindamycin)
   1. Mechanism of action: Bactericidal activity is relative to dose, and these agents are generally considered bacteriostatic.
      a. Bind to the bacterial 50S ribosomal subunit
      b. Consequently inhibit RNA-dependent protein synthesis
   2. Spectrum of action: broad-spectrum activity
      a. Gram-positive and Gram-negative bacteria. **Clindamycin is especially effective against anaerobes (chiefly *Bacteroides fragilis*).**
      b. Treponemes, mycoplasma, chlamydia, and rickettsia. Erythromycin is a good choice for cell wall–deficient organisms such as *Mycoplasma, Rickettsia, Chlamydia,* and *Legionella*
   3. Side effects/adverse reactions
      a. Gastrointestinal distress
      b. Allergic reactions
      c. Superinfections
         (1) *Candida* with erythromycin
         (2) *Clostridium difficile* **(pseudomembranous colitis) with clindamycin**
   4. Mechanisms of resistance
      a. Decreased permeability into bacterial cells
      b. Active efflux out of cells
      c. Alteration in a 50S ribosomal protein
      d. Enzymatic inactivation of antibiotic
F. Sulfonamides (e.g., sulfamethoxazole) and trimethoprim
   1. Mechanism of action: The **bacteriostatic** action is potentiated when sulfonamides and trimethoprim are used together.
      a. Competitively inhibits dihydrofolate reductase (trimethoprim)
      b. Competitively inhibits dihydropteroate synthetase (sulfonamides)
      c. **Blocks folic acid synthesis** in this way
   2. Spectrum of action: broad-spectrum activity
      a. Gram-positive and Gram-negative bacteria, *Chlamydia*
      b. *Actinomyces, Plasmodium, Toxoplasma*
   3. Side effects/adverse reactions
      a. Gastrointestinal distress
      b. Acute hemolytic anemia, aplastic anemia, agranulocytosis, and thrombocytopenia in individuals with glucose-6-phosphate dehydrogenase deficiency

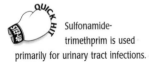
Although clindamycin is typically associated with pseudomembranous colitis (*C. difficile* infection), cephalosporins cause more cases of pseudomembranous colitis because of their greater use.

Sulfonamide-trimethoprim is used primarily for urinary tract infections.

c. Hypersensitivity reactions, including erythema multiforme (Stevens-Johnson syndrome)
4. Mechanisms of resistance
   a. Bacterial mutation, resulting in microbial overproduction of folic acid precursors
   b. Structural change in bacterial enzymes, with lowered affinity for sulfonamides and trimethoprim
   c. Decreased bacterial cell permeability

G. **Quinolones** (e.g., ciprofloxacin)
  1. Mechanism of action: bactericidal
   a. **Inhibit DNA gyrase** and DNA topoisomerase
   b. Block DNA synthesis in this way
  2. Spectrum of action: aerobic Gram-negative bacilli and Gram-negative cocci
  3. Side effects/adverse reactions
   a. Gastrointestinal distress
   b. Headache, dizziness
   c. Phototoxicity
   d. **Damages developing cartilage and tendons (contraindicated in children and pregnancy)**
  4. Mechanisms of resistance
   a. Mutation of bacterial enzymes
   b. Decreased permeability of bacterial wall to antibiotic

Quinolones are a good choice for urinary tract infections, the sexually transmitted diseases gonorrhea and chlamydia, and respiratory and gastrointestinal infections.

H. Other agents: vancomycin, teicoplanin, and the streptogramins quinupristin/dalfopristin)
  1. Mechanism of action
   a. Vancomycin and teicoplanin—**inhibit cell wall assembly**
   b. Quinupristin/dalfopristin—can be bactericidal or bacteriostatic depending on the organism; bind to the 50S bacterial ribosomal subunit
  2. Spectrum of action
   a. Vancomycin and teicoplanin: serious Gram-positive infections and some anaerobic infections
   b. Quinupristin/dalfopristin: serious infections caused by *Staphylococcus* or *Enterococcus*

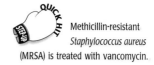

Methicillin-resistant *Staphylococcus aureus* (MRSA) is treated with vancomycin.

  3. Side effects/adverse reactions
   a. Vancomycin and teicoplanin:
    (1) **Red man syndrome** (flushing of the face, neck, and torso)
    (2) Fever, chills, and phlebitis at injection site
   b. Quinupristin/dalfopristin
    (1) Gastrointestinal distress
    (2) Pain at injection site
    (3) Arthralgia, muscle weakness
  4. Mechanisms of resistance
   a. Vancomycin and teicoplanin: gene-mediated alteration in cell wall peptidoglycans
   b. Quinupristin/dalfopristin
    (1) Drug-modifying enzymes
    (2) Efflux of antibiotic out of bacterial cell

II. Antimycobacterial and Antifungal Agents

A. Antimycobacterial agents: drugs active against *Mycobacterium tuberculosis*
  1. First-line agents: isoniazid, rifampin, pyrazinamide, ethambutol, streptomycin
  2. Bactericidal, except for ethambutol
  3. Initial therapy: three first-line agents for **6 to 9 months**

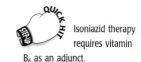

Isoniazid therapy requires vitamin B_6 as an adjunct.

B. Antifungal agents
  1. Amphotericin B
    a. Disrupts fungal membrane, leading to increased permeability
    b. Used for serious systemic fungal infections
    c. **Nephrotoxic**
  2. Triazoles (e.g., fluconazole)
    a. **Disrupt synthesis of ergosterol**, which is necessary for fungal membranes
    b. Fluconazole is used for candida infections and cryptococcal meningitis

III. Antiviral Agents
  A. Antiretrovirals (see System 8 for a more detailed discussion)
    1. Reverse transcriptase inhibitors (e.g., zidovudine [azidothymidine; AZT], didanosine [ddI], nevirapine)
      a. Act as either nucleoside/nucleotide analogs or inhibit the reverse transcriptase enzyme itself
      b. **Prevent creation of DNA copy of viral RNA**
    2. Protease inhibitors (e.g., saquinavir, indinavir)
      a. **Block the cleavage of viral polyproteins**
      b. Result in the production of immature, defective viral particles
  B. Acyclovir and ganciclovir
    1. Inhibit viral DNA polymerase, which blocks viral DNA synthesis
    2. **Suppress symptoms of herpes simplex virus infections** but are **not a cure**
  C. Amantadine and rimantadine
    1. Inhibit the replication of **influenza A**
    2. Can be used prophylactically and therapeutically
  D. Ribavirin
    1. Alters viral messenger RNA formation
    2. Used to treat **respiratory syncytial virus and pneumonia in children**
  E. Interferons (IFNs)
    1. Most cells produce IFN-α and IFN-β in response to viral infection.
    2. IFN-γ mediates the inflammatory response and has less antiviral action.
    3. IFNs are not directly antiviral but stimulate cellular mechanisms of viral resistance.
    4. IFNs also may cause some of the symptoms and tissue damage associated with viral infections.
    5. Used for Hepatitis B, C and some types of cancer.

QUICK HIT

Both acyclovir and ganciclovir are effective against herpes virus, but ganciclovir is also effective against cytomegalovirus.

ENZYME KINETICS

I. Enzymes
  A. An enzyme is a substance that **decreases the energy of activation for a reaction** (Figure 1-13).

FIGURE 1-13 Enzyme effect on a chemical reaction

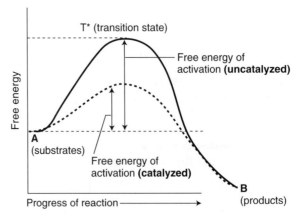

B. By lowering the energy of activation, enzymes increase the rate of reaction.
C. Enzymes **do not alter the equilibrium** of substrates and products, which is concentration-dependent.

II. Kinetics

A. **Velocity** (v) is the rate of reaction and is dependent on enzyme concentration, substrate concentration, temperature, and pH.
   1. Enzyme concentration: increased enzyme concentration leads to faster rate of reaction.
   2. Substrate concentration: increased concentration leads to increased rate of reaction, until a maximum is reached when all enzyme receptor sites are saturated.
   3. Temperature: increased temperature leads to increased rate of reaction up to a maximum, after which enzymes denature.
   4. pH: velocity of a reaction is maximum at its optimal pH. A pH that is either too high or too low leads to a slower reaction or may denature the enzyme.

B. Michaelis-Menten equation
   1. Enzymatically catalyzed reactions can be characterized by the Michaelis-Menten equation:

   $$v = V_m \times [S] / (K_m + [S])$$

   where v is the velocity of the reaction.
   V_m is the maximum velocity of the reaction.
   [S] is the substrate concentration.
   K_m is the Michaelis constant (the substrate concentration at which velocity is one-half of the maximum velocity of a given reaction; $v = 1/2\ V_m$).
   2. Effect of substrate concentration on reaction velocity (Figure 1-14)

FIGURE
1-14   **Effect of substrate concentration on reaction velocity**

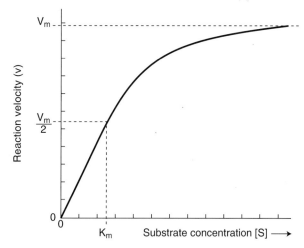

V_m = Maximum velocity
V   = Velocity
K_m = Michaelis constant, where $v = 1/2\ V_m$

C. Lineweaver-Burk plots (Figure 1-15)

FIGURE 1-15 Lineweaver-Burk plot

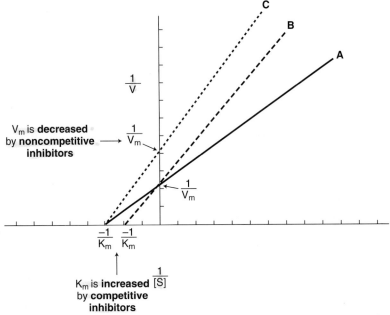

V_m is **decreased** by **noncompetitive inhibitors**

$\dfrac{1}{V_m}$

$\dfrac{1}{V}$

$\dfrac{-1}{K_m}$ $\dfrac{-1}{K_m}$

K_m is **increased** by **competitive inhibitors**

$\dfrac{1}{[S]}$

A = No inhibitor
B = Competitive inhibitor
C = Noncompetitive inhibitor

[S] = Substrate concentration
v   = Reaction velocity
V_m = Maximum velocity
K_m = Michaelis constant

$\dfrac{1}{V_m}$ is where the plot crosses the *y* axis

$\dfrac{-1}{K_m}$ is where the plot crosses the *x* axis

1. A Lineweaver-Burk plot is a linear representation of the Michaelis-Menten equation, which allows for easier interpretation of the maximum velocity of an equation
2. Lineweaver-Burk equation:

   $1/v = K_m / (V_m \times [S]) + 1/V_m$

   a. Competitive inhibitors increase the K_m
   b. Noncompetitive inhibitors decrease the V_m

BIOSTATISTICS AND EPIDEMIOLOGY

I. Sensitivity and Specificity (Table 1-4)

TABLE 1-4 **Sensitivity and Specificity**

	Disease States	
	Have disease	Do not have disease
Test Results		
+	True Positive (TP)	False Positive (FP)
−	False Negative (FN)	True Negative (TN)

Terminology	Equation	Definition
Sensitivity (positive in disease)	TP/(TP + FN)	Probability that a person having a disease will be correctly identified
Specificity (negative in healthy)	TN/(TN + FP)	Probability that a person who does not have a disease will be correctly identified
Positive-predictive value	TP/(TP + FP)	Probability that an individual who tests positive has disease
Negative-predictive value	TN/(TN + FN)	Probability that an individual who tests negative does not have the disease
Prevalence	TP + FN/(TP + FP + TN + FN)	Total number of cases in a population at a given time
Incidence	Generally calculated by: Prevalence × Length of disease process	Number of new cases of disease in the population over a given time

II. Cohort Studies

A. Observational and can be prospective or retrospective

B. After assessment of exposure to a risk factor, subjects are compared with each other for a period of time

C. Clinical treatment trial

1. Highest quality cohort study

2. Compares the therapeutic benefits of two or more treatments

D. **Relative risk**

1. Calculated only for cohort studies

2. Compares incidence rate in exposed group with incidence rate in unexposed individuals

III. Case-Control Studies

A. Retrospective and observational

B. Subjects with and without disorder are identified, and information on exposure to risk factors is assessed.

C. **Odds ratio**

1. Used to determine relative risk in case-control studies

2. Based on disease occurring with or without exposure

3. Odds ratio = TP × TN/FP × FN

where TP = true positives
TN = true negatives
FP = false positives
FN = false negatives

 High-sensitivity tests are better suited for screening purposes, whereas high-specificity tests are used as confirmatory tests.

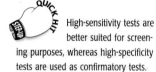 For chronic conditions (e.g., diabetes or cirrhosis), the prevalence is higher than the incidence because the long length of the disease process increases prevalence. For conditions that resolve quickly (i.e., strep throat) or are rapidly fatal (i.e., pancreatic cancer), the incidence and prevalence are approximately equal.

 The most rigorous form of a clinical trial is the **double-blind study** in which neither the subject nor the examiner knows which drug the subject is receiving. Single-blind, double-blind, crossover, and placebo studies are done to reduce bias.

IV. Testing and Statistical Methods
    A. Reliability versus validity
        1. **Reliability** refers to the reproducibility of test results either among examiners or among test-takers.
        2. **Validity** refers to the appropriateness of a test's measurements (i.e., the test measures what it is supposed to).
        3. **Sensitivity** and **specificity** constitute validity.
    B. Bell curve (Figure 1-16)

FIGURE 1-16 Bell curve

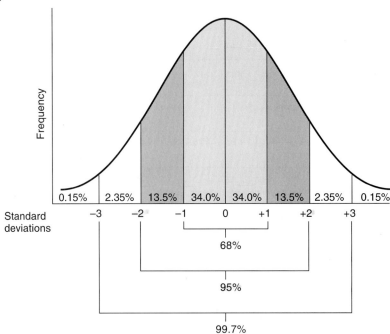

        1. In a **normal distribution,** the mean, median, and mode are **equal.**
          a. Mean: average
          b. Median: middle value in a sequentially ordered group of numbers
          c. Mode: number that appears most often in a group
        2. A bimodal distribution has two peaks.
        3. Skew refers to the way a peak may be offset.
          a. **Positive skew:** peak is to the left (most scores at low end; mean > median > mode)
          b. **Negative skew:** peak is to the right (most scores at high end; mean < median < mode)
    C. The **null hypothesis** (H_0)
        1. Postulates that there is no significant difference between groups
        2. **Probability (P) value:** the chance of a type I error occurring (rejecting the null hypothesis when the null hypothesis is actually true)
        3. If $P < .05$, then the null hypothesis can be rejected.
        4. Example
          a. A study is conducted on the influence of medical school on dating frequency.
          b. The null hypothesis would be that medical school students, when compared with 22- through 26-year-olds in the working population, have no difference in dating frequency.

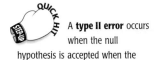

A **type II error** occurs when the null hypothesis is accepted when the null hypothesis is not true.

    c. If the *P* value of the study is less than 0.05 (meaning that there is a statistical difference), then the null hypothesis can be rejected.

    d. Furthermore, it can be stated that medical school decreases dating frequency.

V. General Statistics

A. Leading causes of mortality

    1. Ages 1–14 years: injuries

    2. Ages 15–24 years: accidents (majority are motor vehicle)

    3. Ages 25–64 years: cancer (lung > breast/prostate > colon)

    4. Ages 65+ years: heart disease

    5. **AIDS is the leading cause of death in males between 25 and 44 years of age.**

B. Aging

    1. The elderly comprise 12% of the U.S. population.

      a. They incur 30% of health-care costs.

      b. 5% are in nursing homes.

      c. **25% of suicides** are committed by the elderly population.

      d. 15% suffer from dementia.

    2. 75% of men and 50% of women 60–65 years of age have continued interest in sex.

    3. Life expectancy is 8 years longer for women.

C. Family

    1. 95% of people in the United States marry.

    2. Approximately 50% of marriages end in divorce.

    3. 50% of children live in an environment with two working parents.

    4. 20% of all families are single-parent households, but 50% of black families are single-parent households.

    5. Abuse

      a. 32% of children younger than 5 years of age are physically abused.

      b. 25% of children younger than 8 years of age are sexually abused.

    6. First sexual intercourse usually occurs around 16 years of age.

D. Disorders

    1. At least 25% of the people in the United States are obese.

    2. Insomnia occurs in 30% of people.

    3. Alcohol

      a. Highest use is by people 21–34 years of age.

      b. 13% of adults abuse alcohol.

    4. There is a 1.5% chance of becoming schizophrenic (equal occurrence rate in men and women and whites and blacks)

    5. 10% of men and 15%–20% of women have unipolar disorder (depression).

    6. 1% of all individuals have bipolar disorder.

Hard and fast statistical numbers are rarely sought after as answers on the USMLE Step 1 Examination. However, having a general idea of some select statistics may assist one in answering the vignette style questions.

Suicide is the second leading cause of death for people 15–24 years of age.

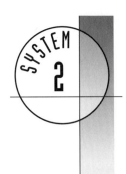
The Nervous System

DEVELOPMENT

I. Central Nervous System (CNS)

A. The CNS includes the **brain** and **spinal cord.**

B. It is **formed from the neural tube.**
1. The **basal plate** of the neural tube forms **motor neurons.**
2. The **alar plate** of the neural tube forms **sensory neurons.**
3. The basal and alar plates are **separated** by the **sulcus limitans.**

C. **Oligodendrocytes** are responsible for **myelination,** which begins 4 months after conception and is completed by the second year of life.

D. The distal end of the spinal cord, the conus medullaris, is at the level of the third lumbar vertebra **(L3)** at birth. As the body grows, the cord "ascends" to its final resting position at the first lumbar vertebra **(L1)** (Figure 2-1).

For developmental and anatomic reasons, symptoms of a disk herniation are referred to the myotome and dermatome **below** the lesion. For example, a herniation of the C4–C5 disk would cause impingement of the C5 nerve root.

FIGURE 2-1 **Adult derivatives of embryonic structures in the nervous system**

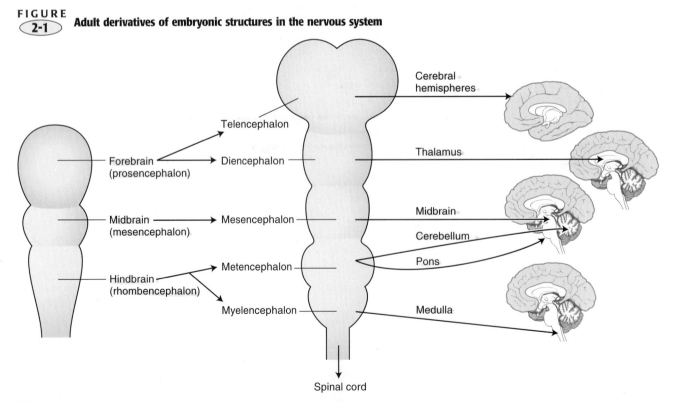

II. Peripheral Nervous System (PNS)

A. The PNS includes the **peripheral nerves** and the **autonomic** and **sensory ganglia.**

B. It is **derived from neural crest cells,** which give rise to:
   1. Schwann cells
   2. Pseudounipolar cells of the spinal and cranial nerve ganglia
   3. Multipolar cells of the autonomic ganglia
   4. Pia and arachnoid mater (not part of PNS)
   5. Melanocytes (not part of PNS)
   6. Epinephrine-producing chromaffin cells of the adrenal gland (not part of PNS)

C. **Schwann cells** are responsible for **myelination,** which begins 4 months after conception and is completed by the second year of life.

CONGENITAL MALFORMATIONS OF THE NERVOUS SYSTEM

Abnormal development of the embryonal components of the nervous system can result in some of the malformations described in Table 2-1.

TABLE 2-1 Congenital Malformations of the Nervous System	
Condition	**Clinical Features**
Fetal alcohol syndrome	• **Most common cause of mental retardation** • **Cardiac septal defects** • Facial malformations including widely spaced eyes and long philtrum • Growth retardation

Spina bifida	• Improper closure of posterior neuropore
	• Several forms
	  - **Spina bifida occulta** (mildest form)—failure of vertebrae to close around spinal cord (tufts of hair often evident)
	  - Spinal meningocele (spina bifida cystica)—meninges extend out of defective spinal canal
	  - Meningomyelocele—meninges and spinal cord extend out of spinal canal
	  - Rachischisis (most severe form)—neural tissue is visible externally

Hydrocephaly	• Accumulation of CSF in ventricles and subarachnoid space • Caused by congenital blockage of cerebral aqueducts • May be caused by **cytomegalovirus or toxoplasma infection** • Increased head circumference in neonates
Dandy-Walker malformation	• Dilation of 4th ventricle, leading to hypoplasia of cerebellum • Failure of foramina of Luschka and Magendie to open • May result from riboflavin inhibition, posterior fossa trauma, or viral infection
Anencephaly	• Failure of brain to develop • Caused by lack of closure of anterior neuropore • Associated with increased maternal α-fetoprotein (AFP) • Decreased head circumference in neonates
Arnold-Chiari malformation	• Herniation of the **cerebellar vermis** through the foramen magnum • Hydrocephaly • Myelomeningocele
CSF=cerebrospinal fluid.	

 The risk of spina bifida can be decreased by taking folate supplements during pregnancy.

Noncommunicating (obstructive) hydrocephalus is increased intracranial pressure caused by a block in CSF flow. In communicating (nonobstructive) hydrocephalus, there is normal flow of CSF, but abnormal absorption.

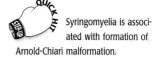 Syringomyelia is associated with formation of Arnold-Chiari malformation.

MAJOR RECEPTORS OF THE NERVOUS SYSTEM

I. Receptors of the Sympathetic and Parasympathetic Nervous Systems

A. The sympathetic and parasympathetic nervous systems exert their effects via various receptors scattered throughout the body (Table 2-2).

TABLE 2-2 Receptors of the Sympathetic and Parasympathetic Nervous Systems

Site of Action	Sympathetic Nervous System		Parasympathetic Nervous System	
	Receptor	*Effect on Site*	*Receptor*	*Effect on Site*
Smooth muscle; skin and viscera	α_1	Contract	Muscarinic	Relax
Smooth and skeletal muscle	α_1 β_2	Contract Relax	Muscarinic	Relax
Smooth muscle of the lung	β_2	Relax	Muscarinic	Contract
Smooth muscle of the gastrointestinal tract	β_2 α_1	Relax intestinal wall Contract sphincters	Muscarinic	Contract intestinal wall; relax sphincter
Heart; SA node	β_1	Increase heart rate	Muscarinic	Decrease heart rate
Heart; ventricles	β_1	Increase contractility and conduction velocity	Muscarinic	Small decrease in contractility
Eye; radial muscle	α_1	**Mydriasis** (dilation of pupil)	N/A	N/A
Eye; sphincter muscle	N/A	N/A	Muscarinic	**Miosis** (constriction of pupil)
Eye; ciliary muscle	β_2	**Relax**	Muscarinic	**Contract** (near vision)
Bladder	β_2 α_1	Relax wall Contract sphincter	Muscarinic	Contract wall: relax sphincter
Uterus	α_1 β_2	Contract Relax	Muscarinic	Contract
Penis	α_2	Ejaculate	Muscarinic	Erection
Sweat glands	Muscarinic	Secrete	N/A	N/A
Pancreas	α_2 β_2	**Decrease insulin secretion** **Increase insulin secretion**	N/A N/A	N/A N/A
Liver	α_1, β_2	Glycolysis, gluconeogenesis	N/A	N/A
Adipose tissue	β_1, β_3	Lipolysis	N/A	N/A

N/A=not applicable; *SA*=sinoatrial.

(text continues on page 37)

B. These effects are mediated by the substances in Figure 2-2.

FIGURE
2-2 Major receptors of the nervous system

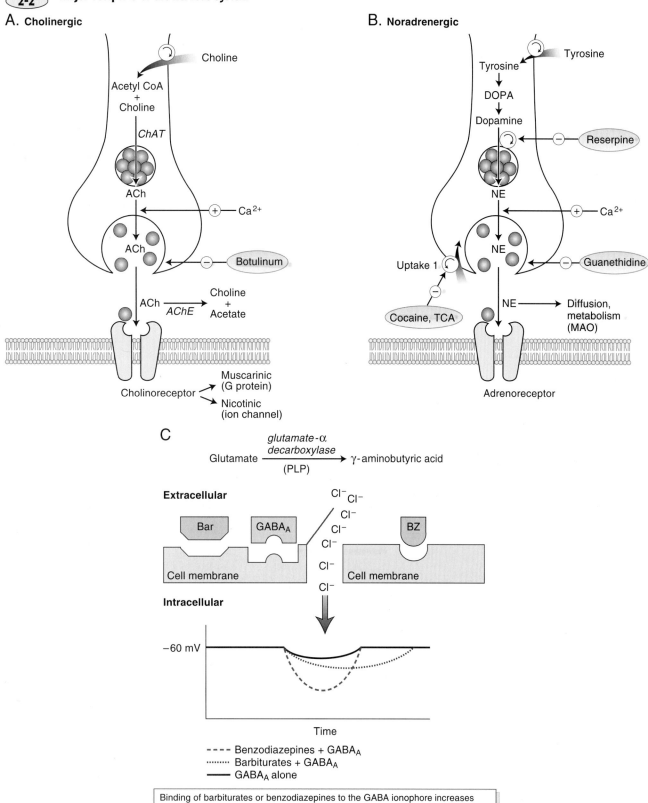

A. Cholinergic

Choline

Acetyl CoA
+
Choline

ChAT

ACh

$+$ Ca^{2+}

ACh

$-$ Botulinum

ACh → Choline + Acetate
AChE

Cholinoreceptor → Muscarinic (G protein)
→ Nicotinic (ion channel)

B. Noradrenergic

Tyrosine

Tyrosine
↓
DOPA
↓
Dopamine

$-$ Reserpine

NE

$+$ Ca^{2+}

NE

Uptake 1

$-$ Guanethidine

$-$ Cocaine, TCA

NE → Diffusion, metabolism (MAO)

Adrenoreceptor

C

Glutamate $\xrightarrow[\text{(PLP)}]{\textit{glutamate-}\alpha\ \textit{decarboxylase}}$ γ-aminobutyric acid

Extracellular

Cl$^-$ Cl$^-$
Cl$^-$
Cl$^-$
Cl$^-$
Cl$^-$
Cl$^-$

Bar   GABA$_A$ BZ

Cell membrane   Cell membrane

Intracellular

−60 mV

Time

- - - - Benzodiazepines + GABA$_A$
·········· Barbiturates + GABA$_A$
——— GABA$_A$ alone

Binding of barbiturates or benzodiazepines to the GABA ionophore increases chloride ion conductance. Barbiturates increase the duration of chloride channel opening while benzodiazepines increase the amplitude of depolarization.

ACh=acetylcholine; *AchE*=acetylcholinesterase; *BZ*=benzodiazepines; *Ca^{2+}*=calcium; *ChAT*=choline acetyl transferase *Cl$^-$*=chloride; *CoA*=coenzyme A; *DOPA*=dihydroxyphenylalanine; *GABA*=γ-aminobutyric acid; *MAO*=monoamine oxidase; *NE*=norepinephrine; *PLP*=phospholipid; *TCA*=tricyclic antidepressant

II. Neurotoxins and Their Effects (Figure 2-3)

FIGURE 2-3 Neurotoxins and their effects

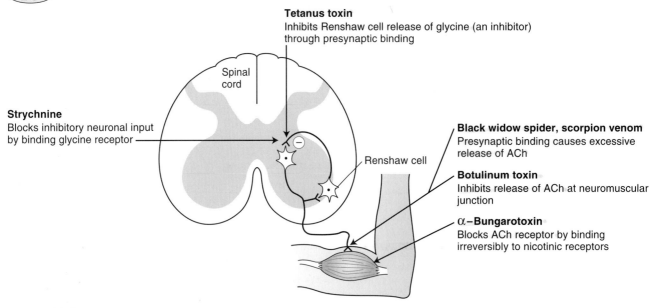

Tetanus toxin
Inhibits Renshaw cell release of glycine (an inhibitor) through presynaptic binding

Strychnine
Blocks inhibitory neuronal input by binding glycine receptor

Spinal cord

Renshaw cell

Black widow spider, scorpion venom
Presynaptic binding causes excessive release of ACh

Botulinum toxin
Inhibits release of ACh at neuromuscular junction

α–Bungarotoxin
Blocks ACh receptor by binding irreversibly to nicotinic receptors

ACh=acetylcholine

MENINGES, FLOW OF CEREBROSPINAL FLUID (CSF), AND PATHOLOGIC TRAUMA (Figure 2-4)

FIGURE 2-4 Meninges, flow of cerebrospinal fluid, and pathologic trauma

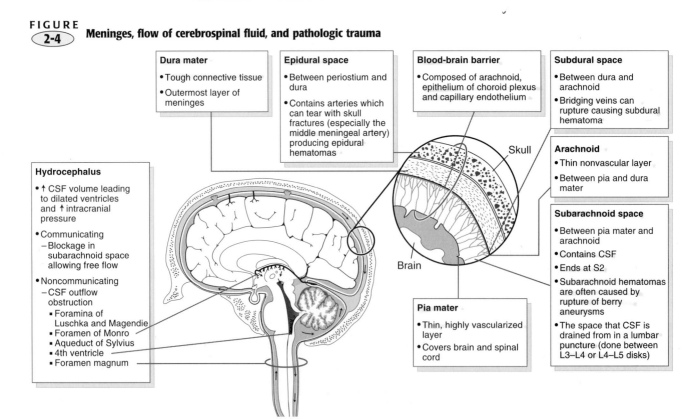

Dura mater
• Tough connective tissue
• Outermost layer of meninges

Epidural space
• Between periosteum and dura
• Contains arteries which can tear with skull fractures (especially the middle meningeal artery) producing epidural hematomas

Blood-brain barrier
• Composed of arachnoid, epithelium of choroid plexus and capillary endothelium

Subdural space
• Between dura and arachnoid
• Bridging veins can rupture causing subdural hematoma

Arachnoid
• Thin nonvascular layer
• Between pia and dura mater

Subarachnoid space
• Between pia mater and arachnoid
• Contains CSF
• Ends at S2
• Subarachnoid hematomas are often caused by rupture of berry aneurysms
• The space that CSF is drained from in a lumbar puncture (done between L3–L4 or L4–L5 disks)

Hydrocephalus
• ↑ CSF volume leading to dilated ventricles and ↑ intracranial pressure
• Communicating
 – Blockage in subarachnoid space allowing free flow
• Noncommunicating
 – CSF outflow obstruction
  ▪ Foramina of Luschka and Magendie
  ▪ Foramen of Monro
  ▪ Aqueduct of Sylvius
  ▪ 4th ventricle
  ▪ Foramen magnum

Skull

Brain

Pia mater
• Thin, highly vascularized layer
• Covers brain and spinal cord

CSF=cerebrospinal fluid; *L*=lumbar vertebra; *S*=sacral nerve

BLOOD SUPPLY TO THE BRAIN (Figure 2-5)

FIGURE
2-5   **Blood supply to the brain**

A. Arteries of the base of the brain and brain stem

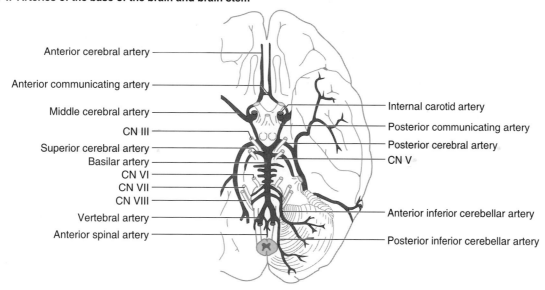

Anterior cerebral artery
Anterior communicating artery
Middle cerebral artery
CN III
Superior cerebral artery
Basilar artery
CN VI
CN VII
CN VIII
Vertebral artery
Anterior spinal artery

Internal carotid artery
Posterior communicating artery
Posterior cerebral artery
CN V
Anterior inferior cerebellar artery
Posterior inferior cerebellar artery

B. Arterial blood supply to the cortex

Lateral   Medial

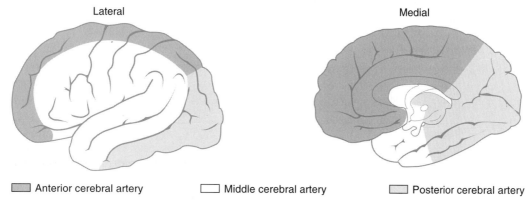

◼ Anterior cerebral artery   ☐ Middle cerebral artery   ◻ Posterior cerebral artery

CN=cranial nerve

FIGURE
2-5   **Blood supply to the brain** *(Continued)*

C. Venous drainage of the brain

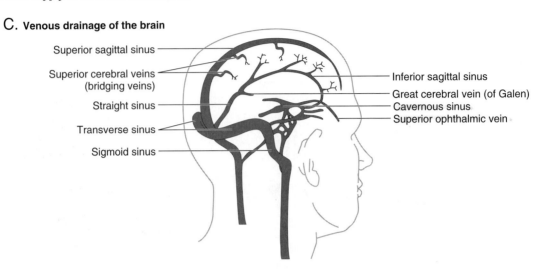

Superior sagittal sinus
Superior cerebral veins
(bridging veins)
Straight sinus
Transverse sinus
Sigmoid sinus

Inferior sagittal sinus
Great cerebral vein (of Galen)
Cavernous sinus
Superior ophthalmic vein

Cerebrovascular disease is the most common cause of CNS pathology and the third major cause of death in the United States (Table 2-3).

TABLE 2-3	Cerebrovascular Disease	
Disease	**Predisposing Factor**	**Common Sites**
Infarction (more frequent than hemorrhage)		
Thrombosis	Atherosclerosis	Arterial obstruction of internal and external carotid arteries in neck, vertebral and basilar arteries, vessels branching from circle of Willis to middle cerebral artery
Embolus	Cardiac mural thrombi Valvular vegetation Fat emboli	Middle cerebral artery: leads to contralateral paralysis, motor and sensory deficits, aphasias Smaller vessels: leads to **lacunar strokes**
Hemorrhage		
Intracerebral (bleeding into brain substance)	Hypertension, coagulation disorders, hemorrhage within tumor	Rupture of **Charcot-Bouchard** aneurysms (long-standing hypertension), basal ganglia, pons, frontal lobe, cerebellum
Subarachnoid (bleeding into subarachnoid space)	Associated with **berry aneurysm** in circle of Willis	Circle of Willis, bifurcation of middle cerebral artery

LESIONS OF THE CEREBRAL CORTEX (Figure 2-6)

FIGURE
2-6   Lesions of the cerebral cortex

A. Lateral view

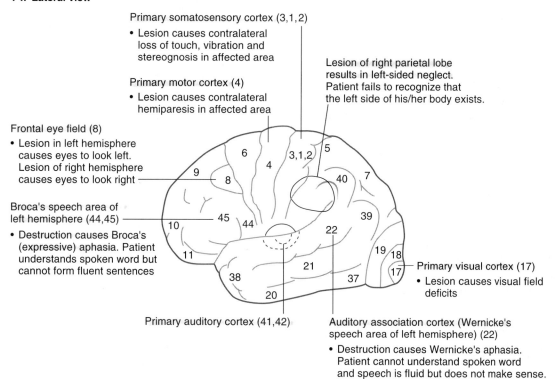

Primary somatosensory cortex (3,1,2)
- Lesion causes contralateral loss of touch, vibration and stereognosis in affected area

Primary motor cortex (4)
- Lesion causes contralateral hemiparesis in affected area

Lesion of right parietal lobe results in left-sided neglect. Patient fails to recognize that the left side of his/her body exists.

Frontal eye field (8)
- Lesion in left hemisphere causes eyes to look left. Lesion of right hemisphere causes eyes to look right

Broca's speech area of left hemisphere (44,45)
- Destruction causes Broca's (expressive) aphasia. Patient understands spoken word but cannot form fluent sentences

Primary visual cortex (17)
- Lesion causes visual field deficits

Primary auditory cortex (41,42)

Auditory association cortex (Wernicke's speech area of left hemisphere) (22)
- Destruction causes Wernicke's aphasia. Patient cannot understand spoken word and speech is fluid but does not make sense.

B. Medial view

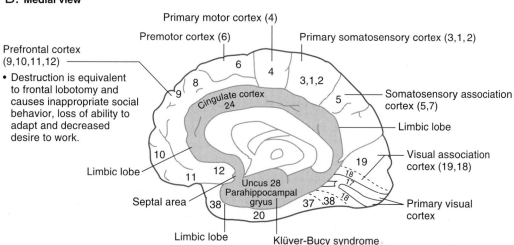

Primary motor cortex (4)

Premotor cortex (6)

Primary somatosensory cortex (3,1,2)

Prefrontal cortex (9,10,11,12)
- Destruction is equivalent to frontal lobotomy and causes inappropriate social behavior, loss of ability to adapt and decreased desire to work.

Cingulate cortex 24

Somatosensory association cortex (5,7)

Limbic lobe

Visual association cortex (19,18)

Limbic lobe

Uncus 28 Parahippocampal gryus

Primary visual cortex

Septal area

Limbic lobe

Klüver-Bucy syndrome

(Adapted from Fix JD: *High-Yield Neuroanatomy*. Baltimore, Williams & Wilkins, 1995. p. 102)

QUICK HIT Klüver-Bucy syndrome is a bilateral lesion of the amygdala nuclei. It results in hypersexuality, docility, and hyperorality.

IMPORTANT PATHWAYS OF THE SPINAL CORD (Figure 2-7)

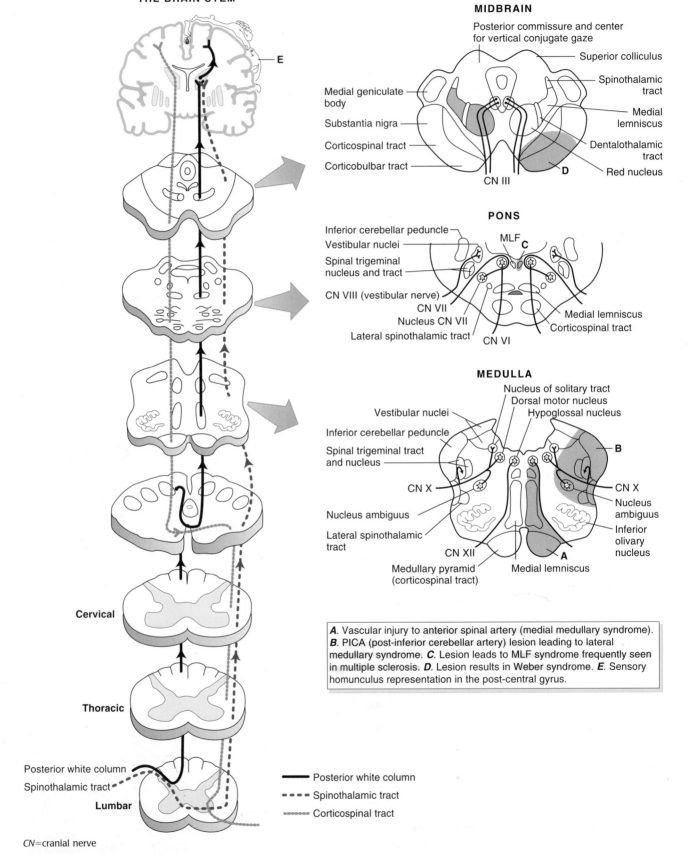

FIGURE 2-7 Important pathways of the spinal cord

THE BRAIN STEM

MIDBRAIN

Posterior commissure and center for vertical conjugate gaze
Superior colliculus
Spinothalamic tract
Medial geniculate body
Medial lemniscus
Substantia nigra
Corticospinal tract
Dentalothalamic tract
Corticobulbar tract
Red nucleus
CN III
D

PONS

Inferior cerebellar peduncle
Vestibular nuclei
MLF C
Spinal trigeminal nucleus and tract
CN VIII (vestibular nerve)
CN VII
Medial lemniscus
Nucleus CN VII
Corticospinal tract
Lateral spinothalamic tract
CN VI

MEDULLA

Nucleus of solitary tract
Dorsal motor nucleus
Hypoglossal nucleus
Vestibular nuclei
Inferior cerebellar peduncle
Spinal trigeminal tract and nucleus
B
CN X
CN X
Nucleus ambiguus
Nucleus ambiguus
Lateral spinothalamic tract
Inferior olivary nucleus
CN XII
A
Medullary pyramid (corticospinal tract)
Medial lemniscus

Cervical

Thoracic

A. Vascular injury to anterior spinal artery (medial medullary syndrome). *B*. PICA (post-inferior cerebellar artery) lesion leading to lateral medullary syndrome. *C*. Lesion leads to MLF syndrome frequently seen in multiple sclerosis. *D*. Lesion results in Weber syndrome. *E*. Sensory homunculus representation in the post-central gyrus.

Posterior white column
Spinothalamic tract
Lumbar

—— Posterior white column
- - - Spinothalamic tract
····· Corticospinal tract

CN=cranial nerve

I. Posterior White Column (Dorsal Column–Medial Lemniscus Pathway)

A. The posterior white column is the ascending pathway that conveys **discriminatory touch (two-point touch), vibration, proprioception,** and **stereognosis.**

B. The posterior white column receives information at all spinal cord levels from pseudounipolar cells of dorsal root ganglia. This information is conveyed from a variety of receptors:
  1. Meissner's corpuscles (rate of applied stimulus)
  2. **Pacinian corpuscles (vibration stimulus)**
  3. Joint receptors (joint position; proprioception)
  4. Muscle spindles (length of a muscle)
  5. **Golgi tendon organs (tension** on a muscle)

C. First-order neurons of the dorsal root ganglia enter at the dorsal horn and ascend in the **fasciculus gracilis (lower limb)** and **fasciculus cuneatus (upper limb)** and synapse in the nucleus gracilis and cuneatus, respectively.

D. Second-order neurons arise from these two nuclei, decussate at the level of the inferior medulla, and ascend as the **medial lemniscus.**

E. Medial lemniscus fibers synapse in the **ventral posterolateral (VPL) nucleus** of the thalamus, and third-order neurons project to the **cerebral cortex (areas 3, 1, 2).**

F. Lesions below the decussation produce ipsilateral loss of discriminatory touch, proprioception, and vibration, whereas lesions above the decussation produce contralateral loss of these sensations.

II. Spinothalamic Tract

A. The spinothalamic tract is the ascending pathway that conveys **pain** and **temperature** from the body.

B. It receives input from free nerve endings of fast (A-type) and slow (C-type) pain fibers.

C. First-order neurons originate in the dorsal root ganglion, enter the spinal cord, and synapse on second-order neurons in the dorsolateral tract of Lissauer (thoracic vertebra level 2 [T2] to lumbar vertebra level 3 [L3]).

D. Second-order neurons ascend while decussating through the **ventral white commissure** and continue to ascend in the lateral spinothalamic tract, terminating in the VPL nucleus of the thalamus.

E. Third-order neurons originate in the VPL and project to the **cerebral cortex (areas 3, 1, 2).**

F. Lesions of the spinothalamic tract produce contralateral loss of pain and temperature sensation beginning **one level below that of the lesion.**

III. Corticospinal Tract

A. The corticospinal tract is the descending pathway that originates in the **cerebral cortex (area 6; area 4; and areas 3, 1, 2).**

B. It mediates **voluntary movement** of striated muscle.

C. First-order neurons project to the posterior limb of the internal capsule, descend through the middle three fifths of the midbrain's **crus cerebri** and base of the pons, **decussate in the pyramids of the medulla,** and continue down the spinal cord as the corticospinal tract.

D. Corticospinal fibers synapse on second-order neurons of the ventral horn via interneurons.

E. Lesions above the pyramids (upper motor neurons [**UMN**]) produce **contralateral spastic paresis** and a positive Babinski's sign (upgoing toes).

F. Lesions below the pyramids (**UMN**) produce **ipsilateral spastic paresis** and a positive Babinski's sign.

G. Lesions of the second-order neurons (lower motor neuron [**LMN**]) produce **flaccid paralysis** and fasciculations.

Muscle spindles function as the afferent limb of the myotactic (stretch) reflex (e.g., tapping knee with reflex hammer). Ventral horn motor neurons function as the efferent limb.

Muscle spindles are arranged **in parallel** with the extrafusal muscle fibers; **Golgi tendon organs** are arranged in **series.**

IMPORTANT PATHWAYS OF THE BRAIN STEM AND CEREBRUM

I. **Trigeminothalamic Pathway**
   A. The trigeminothalamic pathway is the ascending pathway that conveys **pain** and **temperature from the face** (analogous to the spinothalamic tract).
   B. It receives input from free nerve endings of fast (A-type) and slow (C-type) pain fibers.
   C. First-order neurons originate in the trigeminal ganglion and synapse on second-order neurons in the spinal trigeminal nucleus (ventral trigeminothalamic tract) or principal sensory nucleus of the trigeminal nerve (dorsal trigeminothalamic tract).
   D. Second-order neurons of the ventral tract decussate while ascending; however, the dorsal tract neurons remain uncrossed, with termination in the VPM nucleus of the thalamus.
   E. Third-order neurons originate in the VPM and project to the **cerebral cortex (areas 3, 1, 2).**

II. **Corticobulbar Tract**
   A. The corticobulbar tract is the descending pathway that originates in the **cerebral cortex (area 6; area 4; and areas 3, 1, 2).**
   B. It mediates voluntary movement of the **muscles of facial expression** (analogous to the corticospinal tract).
   C. First-order neurons project to the genu of the **internal capsule,** descend through the middle three fifths of the midbrain's crus cerebri, and synapse in the nucleus of cranial nerve (CN) VII (facial nucleus).
   D. Second-order neurons innervate the muscles of facial expression (orbicularis oculi, orbicularis oris, buccinator, frontalis, platysma) via the facial nerve.
   E. The **upper face** (orbicularis oculi and frontalis muscles) receives **bilateral input** from the UMN and therefore is not affected by unilateral cortical lesions.
   F. The **lower face** (buccinator, orbicularis oris, platysma) receives only **contralateral input.**

Bell's palsy is an **LMN lesion** of the **facial nerve.** This lesion results in complete facial paralysis on the affected side and is characterized by loss of the nasolabial fold, drooling, and ptosis. It is often idiopathic and usually resolves spontaneously.

III. **Cerebellar Pathway**
   A. The cerebellar pathway controls posture and balance, maintains muscle tone, and coordinates motor activity.
   B. The **dentothalamic tract** is the major cerebellar tract.
      1. It originates in the dentate nucleus of the cerebellum.
      2. It projects to the ventrolateral nucleus of the thalamus (not the VPL) via the superior cerebellar peduncle.
      3. Thalamic fibers within the tract project to area 4 (primary motor cortex).
      4. Cerebral fibers within the tract project to corticospinal neurons.
      5. The pons receives cerebral fibers and sends fibers to the cerebellum where they terminate on mossy fibers.
   C. Damage to one side of the cerebellum results in ipsilateral findings. Patient will fall toward affected side **(positive Romberg sign).**

In Friedreich's ataxia (autosomal recessive), the most common congenital ataxia, the brain shows diffuse neuronal loss involving the posterior white columns, the dentate nuclei, and the spinocerebellar tract. These patients commonly have diabetes and heart disease.

IV. **Vestibulocochlear Pathways**
   A. **Auditory pathway**
      1. The auditory pathway originates from hair cells in the organ of Corti in the cochlea.
      2. Signals are sent down bipolar cell axons and are then relayed to the cochlear nuclei of the pons via the spiral ganglion.
      3. Signals are sent to higher CNS areas and relayed to the cerebral hemisphere via the **medial geniculate body of the thalamus.**
      4. Fibers terminate in the transverse temporal gyri **(areas 41 and 42).**

5. Because of the bilateral projection of information in the auditory pathway, one-sided lesions of this pathway at any point beyond the cochlear nuclei do not produce hearing loss.

6. Lesions of the cochlear nerve itself will produce ipsilateral hearing loss.

B. **Vestibular pathway**

1. Hair cells of the three **semicircular canals** encode **angular acceleration** and **deceleration.**

2. Hair cells of the **utricle** encode **linear acceleration.**

3. Information is passed via the vestibular nerve to the vestibular nuclei of the low pons.

4. Fibers then project to

   a. the spinal cord

   b. the cerebellum

   c. the thalamus

   d. CN III, IV, and VI via the medial longitudinal fasciculus (MLF).

5. **Nystagmus** is mediated by the vestibular and oculomotor nuclei, the MLF, and the muscles of ocular movement controlled by cranial nerves III, IV, and VI (Table 2-4).

 Tonotopic localization of sound in the cochlea is caused in part by the increasing thickness of the basilar membrane as it ascends toward the helicotrema. The **base** of the cochlea (closest to the oval window) is sensitive to **high frequency sounds.** The **apex** of the cochlea is sensitive to **low frequency sounds.**

 Linear acceleration sensed by the utricle and saccule can cause nausea and vomiting. Dimenhydrinate and scopolamine can prevent motion sickness. These drugs work best if used before the onset of symptoms.

TABLE 2-4   **Direction of Movement in Types of Nystagmus**

Form of Nystagmus	Direction of Movement During Fast Phase	Direction of Movement During Slow Phase
Rotary nystagmus (i.e., while spinning in a circle)	Same as direction of rotation	Opposite direction of rotation
Postrotary nystagmus (i.e., after spinning in a circle)	Opposite direction of rotation	Same as direction of rotation
Caloric nystagmus		
• Warm water placed in one ear	Toward the ear with warm water placed in it	Away from the ear with warm water placed in it
• Cold water placed in one ear	Away from the ear with cold water placed in it	Toward the ear with cold water placed in it

V. Visual Pathways (Figure 2-8)

FIGURE
2-8 Visual pathways. (A) Legend for lesions: 1) total blindness, 2) bitemporal hemianopsia—common lesion caused by superiorly growing pituitary tumor, 3) right hemianopsia, 4) right upper quadrantanopia, 5) right lower quadrantanopia, 6) right hemianopsia with macular sparing. (B) Light shined in one eye causes constriction of both pupils. (C) Abduction of one eye results in adduction of the other eye in individuals with an intact medial longitudinal fasciculus, and normal lateral conjugate gaze.

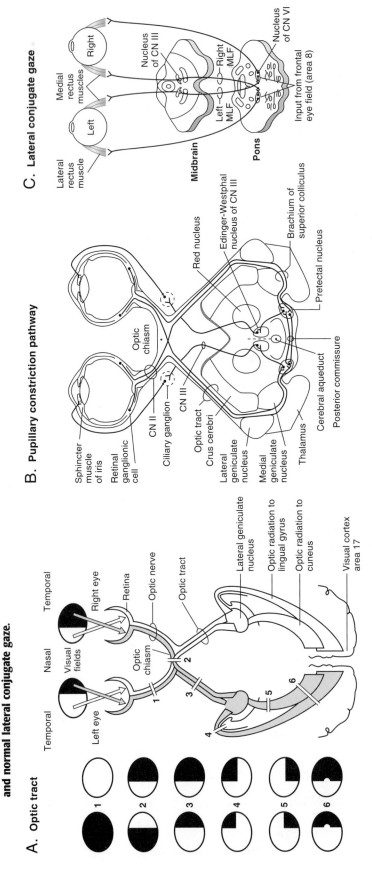

A. Optic tract

B. Pupillary constriction pathway

C. Lateral conjugate gaze

CN=cranial nerve; MLF=medial longitudinal fasciculus (Adapted from Fix JD: *High-Yield Neuroanatomy*. Baltimore, Williams & Wilkins, 1995. p. 74–75)

A. Muscles of the Eye (Figure 2-9)

FIGURE 2-9 Muscles of the eye

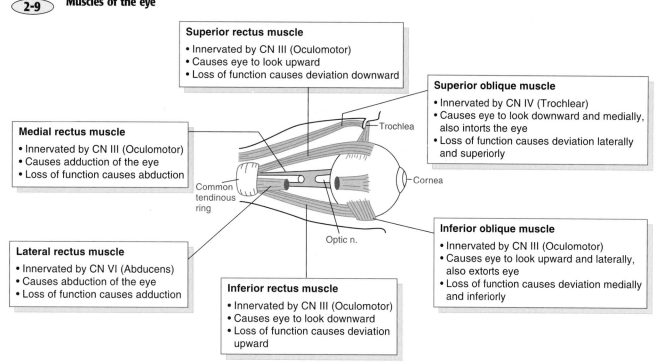

Superior rectus muscle
• Innervated by CN III (Oculomotor)
• Causes eye to look upward
• Loss of function causes deviation downward

Superior oblique muscle
• Innervated by CN IV (Trochlear)
• Causes eye to look downward and medially, also intorts the eye
• Loss of function causes deviation laterally and superiorly

Medial rectus muscle
• Innervated by CN III (Oculomotor)
• Causes adduction of the eye
• Loss of function causes abduction

— Trochlea

Common tendinous ring

— Cornea

Lateral rectus muscle
• Innervated by CN VI (Abducens)
• Causes abduction of the eye
• Loss of function causes adduction

Optic n.

Inferior oblique muscle
• Innervated by CN III (Oculomotor)
• Causes eye to look upward and laterally, also extorts eye
• Loss of function causes deviation medially and inferiorly

Inferior rectus muscle
• Innervated by CN III (Oculomotor)
• Causes eye to look downward
• Loss of function causes deviation upward

CN=cranial nerve (Adapted from Chung, Kyung Won: *BRS Gross Anatomy, 2nd edition.* Baltimore, Williams & Wilkins, 1991, page 302.)

B. **Horner's syndrome**
  1. This syndrome is caused by a lesion of the sympathetic trunk in the neck.
  2. Clinical features of the syndrome include ipsilateral **ptosis, anhydrosis, flushing of skin,** and **miosis.**
C. **Argyll Robertson pupil**
  1. This sign is seen in syphilis, systemic lupus erythematosus (SLE), and diabetes mellitus.
  2. It presents as a pupil that **accommodates** to near objects but **does not react to light.**
D. **Marcus Gunn pupil**
  1. This sign is caused by a relative deficit in the afferent portion of the light reflex pathway.
  2. Shining a light in the affected pupil causes minimal bilateral constriction, but shining light in the unaffected pupil causes normal constriction of both pupils.
E. **MLF syndrome**
  1. A bilateral lesion of the medial longitudinal fasciculus causes this syndrome.
  2. **Clinical features**
     a. When looking left, there is absence of right eye adduction and left eye nystagmus.
     b. When looking right, there is absence of left eye adduction and right eye nystagmus.
     c. Convergence is unaffected.
  3. MLF syndrome is often seen in **multiple sclerosis.**

Horner's syndrome is often caused by **Pancoast's tumor,** a lung neoplasm that invades the cervical sympathetic chain.

The Marcus Gunn pupil can be diagnosed using the **swinging flashlight test.** Shining a flashlight in the normal pupil causes constriction of both pupils. Swinging the flashlight quickly to the affected eye causes paradoxical dilation of the pupils.

F. **Uncal herniation**
1. The uncus of the temporal lobe is forced through the opening of the tentorium.
2. Clinical features (see Figure 2-8).
   a. Compression of CN III occurs, leading to
   b. Dilated ("blown") pupil
   c. Ophthalmoplegia (paralysis of one or more of the ocular muscles)
   d. Compression of the corticospinal tract occurs leading to ipsilateral hemiparesis.
   e. Compression of the posterior cerebral artery occurs, leading to contralateral homonymous hemianopsia.

VI. Taste
A. The **solitary** nucleus of the medulla receives taste sensation via the solitary tract from three sources:
1. The anterior two thirds of the tongue via the **chorda tympani** nerve of the facial nerve (CN VII)
2. The posterior third of the tongue via the **glossopharyngeal** nerve (CN IX)
3. The epiglottic region of the pharynx via the **vagus** nerve (CN X)
B. Neurons carrying taste sensations ascend in the ventral tegmental tract to the VPM nucleus of the thalamus.
C. The VPM nucleus of the thalamus sends fibers to the parietal lobe.

VII. Limbic System
A. Mediates behavior and emotion, specifically:
1. Feeding
2. Feeling (emotional)
3. Fighting
4. Fleeing
5. Sexual activity
B. Primarily controlled by the hypothalamus and autonomic nervous system
C. Other important areas include:
1. Anterior nucleus of thalamus
2. Cingulate gyrus
3. Mamillary bodies
4. Septal area
5. Hippocampus
6. Amygdala

Lesions of the mamillary bodies are produced from thiamine deficiency, commonly seen in chronic alcoholism. Damage results in **Korsakoff's syndrome**, characterized by confusion, severe memory impairment, and confabulation, which is **irreversible.**

The Nervous System

CLASSIC LESIONS OF THE SPINAL CORD (Figure 2-10)

FIGURE
2-10 Classic lesions of the spinal cord

Tabes dorsalis

- Seen in tertiary syphilis
- Bilateral loss of touch, vibration and tactile sense from lower limbs due to lesion of fasciculus gracilis

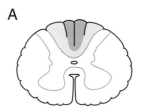

A

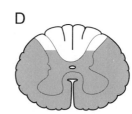

B

Amyotrophic lateral sclerosis

- Combined UMN and LMN lesion of corticospinal tract
- Spastic paresis (UMN sign)
- Flaccid paralysis with fasciculations (LMN)

Brown-Séquard syndrome

- Ipsilateral loss of touch and vibration and tactile sense below lesion due to posterior white column lesion
- Contralateral loss of pain and touch due to loss of spinothalamic tract
- Ipsilateral spastic paresis below lesion due to lesion of corticospinal tract
- Ipsilateral flaccid paralysis at level of lesion due to loss of LMN
- If lesion occurs above T1, Horner's syndrome on side of lesion will result

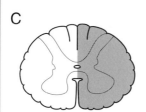

C

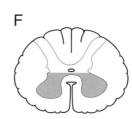

D

Spinal artery infarct

- Bilateral loss of pain and temperature one level below lesion due to loss of spinothalamic tract
- Bilateral spastic paresis below lesion due to lesion of corticospinal tract
- Bilateral flaccid paralysis at level of lesion due to loss of LMN
- Loss of bladder control due to lesion of corticospinal tract innervation of S2–S4 parasympathetics
- Bilateral Horner's syndrome if above T2

Subacute combined degeneration
(Vitamin B12 deficiency)

- Bilateral loss of touch, vibration and tactile sense due to posterior white column lesion
- Bilateral spastic paresis below lesion due to lesion of corticospinal tracts

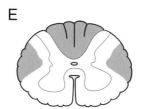

E

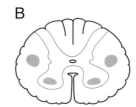

F

Syringomyelia

- Bilateral loss of pain and temperature one level below due to lesion of ventral white commissure (spinothalamic tract)
- Bilateral flaccid paralysis of level of lesion due to loss of LMN

LMN=lower motor neuron; *UMN*=upper motor neuron

FIGURE 2-11 Hypothalamus

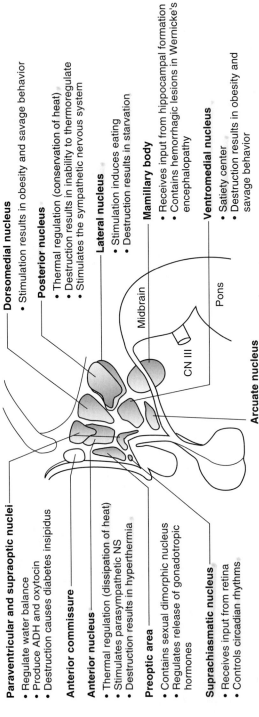

Paraventricular and supraoptic nuclei
- Regulate water balance
- Produce ADH and oxytocin
- Destruction causes diabetes insipidus

Anterior commissure

Anterior nucleus
- Thermal regulation (dissipation of heat)
- Stimulates parasympathetic NS
- Destruction results in hyperthermia

Preoptic area
- Contains sexual dimorphic nucleus
- Regulates release of gonadotropic hormones

Suprachiasmatic nucleus
- Receives input from retina
- Controls circadian rhythms

Dorsomedial nucleus
- Stimulation results in obesity and savage behavior

Posterior nucleus
- Thermal regulation (conservation of heat)
- Destruction results in inability to thermoregulate
- Stimulates the sympathetic nervous system

Lateral nucleus
- Stimulation induces eating
- Destruction results in starvation

Mamillary body
- Receives input from hippocampal formation
- Contains hemorrhagic lesions in Wernicke's encephalopathy

Ventromedial nucleus
- Satiety center
- Destruction results in obesity and savage behavior

Arcuate nucleus
- Produces hypothalamic releasing factors
- Contains DOPA-nergic neurons that inhibit prolactin release

Midbrain

Pons

CN III

ADH=antidiuretic hormone; *CN*=cranial nerve; *DOPA*=dihydroxyphenylalanine; *NS*=nervous system (Redrawn from Fix JD: *High-Yield Neuroanatomy*. Baltimore, Williams & Wilkins, 1995. p. 84)

THALAMUS (Figure 2-12)

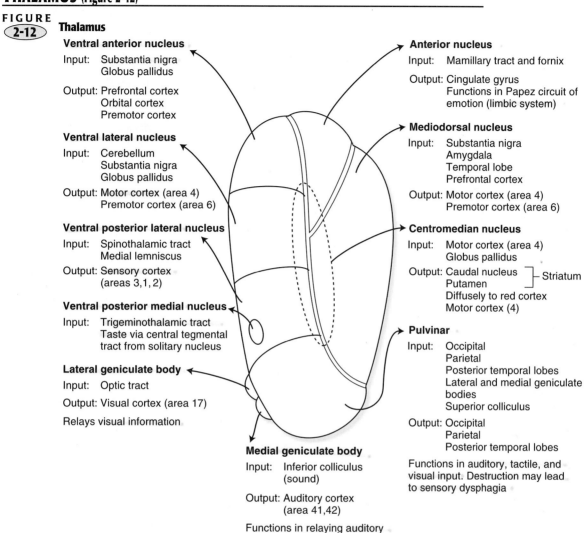

FIGURE 2-12 Thalamus

Ventral anterior nucleus

Input: Substantia nigra
Globus pallidus

Output: Prefrontal cortex
Orbital cortex
Premotor cortex

Ventral lateral nucleus

Input: Cerebellum
Substantia nigra
Globus pallidus

Output: Motor cortex (area 4)
Premotor cortex (area 6)

Ventral posterior lateral nucleus

Input: Spinothalamic tract
Medial lemniscus

Output: Sensory cortex
(areas 3,1, 2)

Ventral posterior medial nucleus

Input: Trigeminothalamic tract
Taste via central tegmental
tract from solitary nucleus

Lateral geniculate body

Input: Optic tract

Output: Visual cortex (area 17)

Relays visual information

Medial geniculate body

Input: Inferior colliculus
(sound)

Output: Auditory cortex
(area 41,42)

Functions in relaying auditory
information

Anterior nucleus

Input: Mamillary tract and fornix

Output: Cingulate gyrus
Functions in Papez circuit of
emotion (limbic system)

Mediodorsal nucleus

Input: Substantia nigra
Amygdala
Temporal lobe
Prefrontal cortex

Output: Motor cortex (area 4)
Premotor cortex (area 6)

Centromedian nucleus

Input: Motor cortex (area 4)
Globus pallidus

Output: Caudal nucleus ⎤
Putamen ⎦ Striatum
Diffusely to red cortex
Motor cortex (4)

Pulvinar

Input: Occipital
Parietal
Posterior temporal lobes
Lateral and medial geniculate
bodies
Superior colliculus

Output: Occipital
Parietal
Posterior temporal lobes

Functions in auditory, tactile, and
visual input. Destruction may lead
to sensory dysphagia

CRANIAL NERVES

The 12 cranial nerves arise from various nuclei within the brain stem and cortex and serve multiple functions in the body. Their extracranial course is important for locating lesions, which can be tested by asking the patient to perform simple tasks. Table 2-5 outlines important information about cranial nerves I though XII.

TABLE 2-5 Cranial Nerves

Nerve	Site of Exit From Skull	Function	Fiber Types	Common Lesions	Test
I-Olfactory	Cribriform plate	Smell	SVA	Cribriform plate fracture; Kallmann's syndrome	Smell
II-Optic	Optic canal	Sight	SSA	See Figure 2-8	Snellen chart; peripheral vision

(continued)

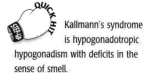

QUICK HIT

Kallmann's syndrome is hypogonadotropic hypogonadism with deficits in the sense of smell.

THE NERVOUS SYSTEM

The olfactory neurons are the only neurons in the adult that actively divide.

Injury to CN III (oculomotor) results in **ptosis** because of loss of the levator palpebrae superioris muscle, **exotropia** because of the unopposed pull of the lateral rectus, **dilation** of the pupil because of unopposed pull of the dilator pupillae muscle, and **impairment of near vision** as a result of loss of accommodation of the ciliary muscle.

Weber's syndrome is caused by a medial midbrain injury and results in ipsilateral CN III paralysis with contralateral spastic hemiparesis.

The trochlear nerve is particularly susceptible to head trauma owing to its course around the midbrain.

Tic douloureux (trigeminal neuralgia) is marked by severe stabbing bursts of pain in the distribution of CN V.

TABLE 2-5 Cranial Nerves (Continued)

Nerve	Site of Exit From Skull	Function	Fiber Types	Common Lesions	Test
III-Oculomotor	Superior orbital fissure	**Parasympathetic** to **ciliary and sphincter muscles;** medial rectus, superior rectus, inferior rectus, inferior oblique	GVE, GSE	Transtentorial (uncal) herniation; **diabetes;** Weber's syndrome	"H" in space; pupillary light reflexes; convergence
IV-Trochlear	Superior orbital fissure	Superior oblique muscle	GSE	Head trauma	"H" in space
V-Trigeminal			SVE, GSA	Tic douloureux (trigeminal neuralgia)	Facial sensation; open jaw **(deviates toward lesion)**
V1-Ophthalmic	-Superior orbital fissure	-Sensory from medial nose, forehead			
V2-Maxillary	-Foramen rotundum	-Sensory from lateral nose, upper lip, superior buccal area			
V3-Mandibular	-Foramen ovale	**-Muscles of mastication,** tensor tympani, tensor veli palantini; sensory from lower lip, lateral face to lower border of mandible			
VI-Abducens	Superior orbital fissure	Lateral rectus muscle	GSE	**Medial inferior pontine syndrome**	"H" in space
VII-Facial	Internal acoustic meatus	Parasympathetic to lacrimal, submandibular, and sublingual glands; **muscles of facial expression and stapedius, stylohyoid muscle, posterior belly of digastric muscle;** sensory from anterior 2/3 of tongue (including taste **via chorda tympani)**	GVE, SVE, GSA, SVA	**Bell's palsy**	Wrinkle forehead; show teeth; puff out cheeks; close eyes tightly

(continued)

TABLE 2-5 **Cranial Nerves** *(Continued)*

Nerve	Site of Exit From Skull	Function	Fiber Types	Common Lesions	Test
VIII-Vestibulocochlear	Internal acoustic meatus	Equilibrium; hearing	SSA	**Acoustic schwannoma**	Hearing; nystagmus (slow phase toward lesion)
IX-Glossopharyngeal	Jugular foramen	Parasympathetic to parotid gland; stylopharyngeus muscle; sensory from pharynx, middle ear, auditory tube, carotid body and sinus, external ear, posterior third of tongue (including taste)	GVE, SVE, GSA, GVA, SVA	Posterior inferior cerebellar artery (**PICA**) infarct	Gag reflex (no response ipsilateral to lesion)
X-Vagus	Jugular foramen	Parasympathetic to body viscera; laryngeal and pharyngeal muscles; sensory from trachea, esophagus, viscera, external ear, epiglottis (including taste)	GVE, SVE, GSA, GVA, SVA	Thyroidectomy, **PICA** infarct	Gag reflex (**uvula deviates away from lesion**)
XI-Accessory	Jugular foramen	Sternocleido-mastoid and trapezius muscles	SVE	**PICA** infarct	Turning head (weakness turning away from lesion); raising shoulder against resistance (ipsilateral)
XII-Hypoglossal	Hypoglossal canal	Intrinsic tongue muscles	GSE	Anterior spinal artery infarct	Tongue protrusion (**deviates toward lesion**)

GSA=general somatic afferent; *GSE*=general somatic efferent; *GVA*=general visceral afferent; *GVE*=general visceral efferent; *SSA*=special somatic afferent; *SVA*=special visceral afferent; *SVE*=special visceral efferent.

QUICK HIT

Medial inferior pontine syndrome results in ipsilateral lateral rectus paralysis with contralateral spastic hemiparesis and loss of sensation of pain and temperature.

THE NERVOUS SYSTEM

CONTENTS OF THE CAVERNOUS SINUS (Figure 2-13)

FIGURE 2-13 Contents of the cavernous sinus

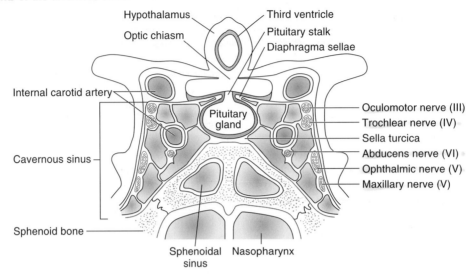

(Adapted from Bushan V, Le T, Amin C: *First Aid for the USMLE Step 1.* Stamford, Connecticut, Appleton & Lange, 1999. p. 110)

SLEEP (Figure 2-14)

FIGURE 2-14 The sleep cycle

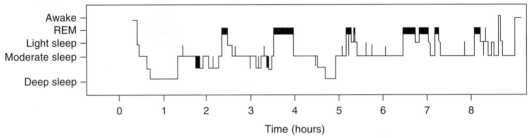

Stages of REM sleep in the young adult. As sleep progresses, slow wave sleep decreases and REM sleep episodes increase in duration and frequency. In the elderly, there is decreased slow wave sleep, increased awakenings, early sleep onset, and early morning awakenings. Solid bars indicate REM sleep.

REM=rapid eye movement

The time spent in stage 4 sleep decreases with aging and with the use of some drugs (i.e., benzodiazepines).

Slow wave sleep, which is the deepest, most relaxed sleep, is the sleep stage in which night terrors, bed-wetting, and sleepwalking occur.

I. Sleep-Wake Cycles

A. Based on circadian rhythms controlled by the suprachiasmatic nucleus of the hypothalamus

B. **Serotonin** released from the raphe nuclei of the brain stem is important in initiating sleep, whereas the **reticular activating system** maintains alertness.

C. **Stage 1** of sleep (when an individual is alert and relaxed) shows **alpha waves** on electroencephalograph (EEG).

D. **Stages 3 and 4** of sleep are called delta sleep and show **slow waves** on EEG.

E. Dreaming occurs during rapid eye movement (REM) sleep, which normally occurs at 90-minute intervals. During this period of "paradoxical sleep" the EEG registers beta waves, which mirror those seen in the alert individual in the waking state.

II. Common Sleep Disorders

A. Insomnia affects 30% of the population. It is associated with anxiety and leads to daytime sleepiness.

B. Narcolepsy is seen in 0.04% of the population and is characterized by sudden onset of sleep with rapid onset of REM sleep. It may be associated with hallucinations and cataplexy (sudden loss of muscle tone).

C. Central sleep apnea, affecting less than 0.5% of the population, involves an absence of respiratory effort (for a discussion of obstructive sleep apnea, see System 4, "The Respiratory System".)

SEIZURE TYPES

Seizures are paroxysmal events caused by abnormal and excessive discharges from CNS neurons triggered by a variety of causes (Table 2-6).

TABLE 2-6 Seizure Types

Type	Patient	Presentation	Pathology	Treatment
Simple partial seizures	All ages	Malfunction of one muscle or muscle group No loss of consciousness Sensory distortions	Single focus in brain No spread, localized muscular manifestations With chronicity, may progress to generalized muscular manifestations	Phenytoin; carbamazepine
Jacksonian seizures	All ages (subtype of simple partial)	Expanding area of motor malfunction	Original focus spreads to adjacent areas of cortex	Carbamazepine
Complex partial seizures	First seizure during first two decades of life may be caused by fever in children 6 months to 5 years of age (febrile seizure)	Incontinence Jaw movements (or other automatisms) Loss of consciousness Elaborate sensory distortions	Single focus	Phenytoin; carbamazepine
Absence (petit mal) seizures	Begin at 2–3 years of age Often end with puberty	1–5 second loss of consciousness Several episodes per day Blank stare with rapid blinking	Original focus rapidly **spreads across both hemispheres**	Ethosuximide, valproic acid
Tonic-clonic (grand mal) seizures	Most common type Encountered in different clinical settings, often in patients with metabolic disorders	Sudden loss of consciousness Loss of postural control and continence Tonic phase (static extension) Clonic phase (jerking movements) Recovery period with exhaustion and disorientation	Original focus rapidly spreads across both hemisphere	Phenytoin; carbamazepine

QUICK HIT Status epilepticus (characterized by continuous or rapidly recurring seizures with no return of consciousness) can be caused by any type of seizure and is potentially fatal. Treatment is intravenous diazepam.

The antiepileptic agents, which include several different medications, affect **ion channels** (Table 2-7). The side effects of these agents are often significant. Because it is frequently necessary to take these agents for long periods, it is important to understand these side effects.

Barbiturates and benzodiazepines are **sedative-hypnotics** that are often used to treat seizure activity. The more common examples are flurazepam, phenobarbital, temazepam, triazolam, and zolpidem.

CNS stimulants, which are at the other end of the spectrum from the sedative-hypnotics, usually cause sympathetic stimulation, resulting in increased alertness. They can also lower the seizure threshold. Common drugs of this type are amphetamine, caffeine, cocaine, dextroamphetamine, ephedrine, and methylphenidate.

TABLE 2-7 Antiepileptic Agents

Drug	Mechanism of Action	Type(s) of Seizure(s) Controlled	Side Effects
Carbamazepine	Blocks voltage-gated **sodium channels** by increasing the refractory period	Tonic-clonic (grand mal) Partial Jacksonian	Liver enzyme induction, ataxia, diplopia
Ethosuximide	Inhibits certain **sodium channels**, particularly in certain parts of thalamus that produce cyclic cortical discharges *[handwritten: T-type Ca²⁺ channels in thalamus]*	Absence	Headache, lethargy, diarrhea
Phenytoin	Blocks voltage-gated **sodium channels** by increasing refractory period	Tonic-clonic (grand mal) Partial	Liver enzyme induction, ataxia, diplopia, anemia, nystagmus, **hirsutism, gingival hyperplasia**
Valproic acid	May affect **potassium channels** to cause hyperpolarization of neuronal membranes	Absence Tonic-clonic (grand mal) Partial	Liver enzyme induction, diarrhea; rarely hepatotoxic
Barbiturates/ Benzodiazepines	Increase inhibitory effects of GABA by increasing duration (barbiturates) or frequency (benzodiazepines) of **chloride channel** opening	Alternative for several types of seizure disorder Status epilepticus	Liver enzyme induction, sedation, addiction

GABA=γ-aminobutyric acid.

DEGENERATIVE DISEASES

Degeneration in specific parts of the CNS can lead to focal or systemic loss of function. Many of the degenerative diseases affecting the CNS are irreversible, and are listed in Table 2-8.

TABLE 2-8 Degenerative Diseases

Disease	Etiology	Clinical Manifestation	Notes
Vitamin B₁₂ deficiency	Strict vegetarian diet; **pernicious anemia;** fundal gastritis type A; *Diphyllobothrium latum*	**Megaloblastic anemia; peripheral neuropathy; myelin degeneration of posterior white columns** and lateral corticospinal tracts	Megaloblastic anemia component of Vitamin B₁₂ deficiency can be treated with folate; however, this will not resolve the peripheral neuropathy component of the deficiency

(continued)

TABLE 2-8 Degenerative Diseases *(Continued)*

Disease	Etiology	Clinical Manifestation	Notes
Parkinson's disease	Unknown; similar symptoms may be caused by depression, hydrocephaly, MPTP intoxication	**Resting tremors; masked facies; muscular rigidity;** shuffling gait; **Lewy bodies; decrease in dopamine** caused by depletion of cells of substantia nigra and locus ceruleus	Usually appears after age 55; therapy with dopamine precursors or ACh inhibitors
Pick's disease	Autosomal dominant	Clinically resembles Alzheimer's; **Pick's bodies** seen; marked cerebral atrophy	Onset from 50 to 60 years of age; more frequent in women
Poliomyelitis	Poliovirus (RNA); fecal-oral; replicates in pharynx; spreads to CNS	Aseptic meningitis; **death of anterior horn cells** in spinal cord; paralysis	Killed (Salk) and live, attenuated (Sabin) vaccine available; Sabin vaccine given to children because of IgA response, longer action, and availability of oral form
Rabies	**Rhabdovirus** (RNA); spread via saliva	Laryngeal spasm resulting in fear of water; CNS excitability; **Negri body** inclusions; hippocampal degeneration	Treatment via passive and active immunization at distant sites
Spongiform encephalopathies (a) Animals: - Scrapie (sheep) - Borne Spargiphorm Encephalopathy (BSE; cows; aka mad cow disease) (b) Humans: - Cruetzfelat-Jacob Disease (CJD) - New variant CJD - Kuru	Prions: an abnormally folded variant of a normal cell protein; only infections agent with no nucleic acid	Vacuolization of brain tissue; dementia; ataxia; depositions of the abnormal protein; long incubation (years); rapid death after onset (months)	Diagnosed in autopsy; no treatment; new variant CJD acquired by eating BSE contaminated meat; Kuru spread by unit align of neurologic tissue; CJD has been spread by corneal transplant and on contaminated neurosurgical equipment
Tay-Sachs disease	Autosomal recessive; **deficiency of hexosaminidase A** with increase in GM_2 ganglioside	Mental retardation; **cherry-red spot on macula;** muscular weakness; seizures	Fatal; prenatal diagnosis possible; usually affects cells of CNS
Thiamine deficiency	Severe malnutrition (may be secondary to alcoholism)	**Degeneration of mamillary bodies** Wernicke's encephalopathy and Korsakoff's syndrome—psychosis manifested with confusion, ataxia, and confabulation Dry beriberi—polyneuropathy with peripheral sensorimotor loss Wet beriberi—dry beriberi with cardiovascular symptoms	**Wernicke's** encephalopathy **(reversible)** and **Korsakoff's** syndrome **(irreversible)** are both secondary to deficiency caused by alcoholism
Wilson's disease	Autosomal recessive; **decreased ceruloplasmin**	Copper accumulation; asterixis; dementia; liver cirrhosis; **Kayser-Fleischer ring** in cornea	Hepatolenticular **degeneration of the basal ganglia**

ACh=acetylcholione; *CSF*=cerebrospinal fluid; *CNS*=central nervous system; *GABA*=γ-aminobutyric acid; *MPTP*=1-methyl-4-phenyl-1,2,3,6-tetrahydropyridine.

QUICK HIT

Niemann-Pick disease, a deficiency of sphingomyelinase, also presents with **a cherry-red spot** on the macula.

Parkinson's disease, a movement disorder, results from deterioration of the **basal ganglia. Dopamine** production decreases; this increases the relative effects of **acetylcholine.** Treatment is purely symptomatic and is aimed at trying to restore the balance between the two hormones (Table 2-9).

TABLE 2-9	**Antiparkinsonian Agents**		
Drug	**Mechanism of Action**	**Side Effects**	**Notes**
Levodopa (L-dopa) (dopamine precursor)	More readily **crosses the blood-brain barrier** Converted to dopamine in the brain	Dyskinesias, postural hypotension, anorexia, depression, psychosis	Development of tolerance; wildly varying effectiveness **(on-off phenomenon)**, often necessitates drug holidays
Carbidopa	Inhibits conversion of L-dopa to dopamine by **DOPA decarboxylase**	Decreases systemic side effects of L-dopa such as anorexia and nausea	Given with L-dopa, **does not cross the blood-brain barrier;** inhibition of systemic conversion of L-dopa, which reduces L-dopa dosing approximately 75%
Amantadine	Unclear; may stimulate dopamine receptors, stimulate dopamine release, or inhibit its reuptake	Agitation, restlessness, psychosis, urinary retention	Rapid deterioration of effectiveness over a period of weeks
Selegiline	Selectively and irreversibly **inhibits MAO type B,** which metabolizes dopamine	Dyskinesias, hepatic conversion to amphetamine causes insomnia and anorexia	In high doses inhibition of MAO type A, which is prevalent in the gut; allowing absorption of ingested amines, which can cause **hypertensive crises**
Bromocriptine	Acts as a **dopamine receptor agonist**	Anorexia, nausea, vomiting, postural hypotension, psychosis	Given as an adjuvant with L-dopa, inhibits release of prolactin and growth hormone and is therefore used for **prolactinomas** and **acromegaly**
Benztropine	Blocks **muscarinic acetylcholine receptors**	**Atropine-like** side effects, inattention, psychosis	Used in combination with dopamine agonists and L-dopa

MAO=monoamine oxidase.

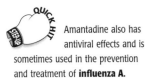

Amantadine also has antiviral effects and is sometimes used in the prevention and treatment of **influenza A.**

DEMYELINATING DISEASES

Loss of the neuronal sheath can lead to impaired nerve conduction, which in turn causes deficits and disease (Table 2-10).

TABLE 2-10	**Demyelinating Diseases of the Nervous System**		
Disease	**Etiology**	**Clinical Manifestation**	**Notes**
Amyotrophic lateral sclerosis (ALS, Lou Gehrig's disease)	No specific pattern of inheritance, though autosomal dominant in 5% of cases (similar symptoms with some heavy metal poisonings, infections, or tumors)	**Both upper and lower motor neuron signs;** loss of lateral corticospinal tracts and anterior motor neurons leading to muscle atrophy	Most common motor neuron disease; rapidly fatal course

(continued)

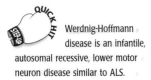

Werdnig-Hoffmann disease is an infantile, autosomal recessive, lower motor neuron disease similar to ALS.

TABLE 2-10 | **Demyelinating Diseases of the Nervous System (Continued)**

Disease	Etiology	Clinical Manifestation	Notes
Guillain-Barré syndrome	Postviral autoimmune reaction involving peripheral nerves	Muscle weakness and paralysis **ascending upward** from the lower extremities	Young adults; **albuminocytologic dissociation** pathognomonic (high albumin, low cell count)
Huntington's disease	Chromosome 4; **CAG triple base repeat** with anticipation	Degeneration of **caudate nucleus;** onset at 30–40 years of age; athetoid movements; muscular deterioration; dementia	Usually involves ACh and GABA neurons
Krabbe's disease	Autosomal recessive; decrease in β-galactocerebrosidase	Loss of myelin from globoid cells and peripheral nerves; mental retardation; blindness; paralysis; **globoid bodies** in white matter	Usually affects infants; **rapidly fatal**
Metachromatic leukodystrophy	Autosomal recessive defect of arylsulfatase A	Progressive paralysis and dementia; loss of myelin; accumulation of sulfatides; nerves stain **yellow-brown** in color; ataxia	Fatal in first decade
Multiple sclerosis	Unknown; more common in northern Europe; more common in women	Multiple focal areas of demyelination; variable course; **Charcot's triad:** intention tremor, scanning speech, nystagmus	Most common demyelinating disease; increased CSF immunoglobulin

ACh=acetylcholine; *CSF*=cerebrospinal fluid; *CNS*=central nervous system; *GABA*=γ-aminobutyric acid.

 The triad of jaundice, right upper quadrant (RUQ) pain, and fever is also known as Charcot's triad and is associated with cholangitis.

 Progressive multifocal leuko-encephalopathy (PML) is a demyelinating disease caused by JC virus infection of oligo-dendricytes. This is seen in patients with our immune deficiency.

 Subacute sclerosing panencephalitis (SSPE) is a demyelinating disease caused by measles virus that lacks in protein. Infection is chronic but progressive and ultimately fatal.

DISEASES CAUSING DEMENTIA

Dementia is a deterioration in cognitive ability in which mental faculties, such as attention span, judgment, memory, mood, and behavior, are affected. Dementia is a chronic condition (Table 2-11).

TABLE 2-11 | **Diseases Causing Dementia**

Disease	Etiology	Clinical Manifestation	Notes
Primary HIV dementia	Macrophages, infected with HIV, enter CNS	Onset before immunodeficiency; slow thinking; ataxia; *Toxoplasma gondii* on autopsy	**Most common CNS manifestation of HIV**
Alzheimer's dementia	Unknown; possibly **chromosome 21;** degeneration of nucleus basalis of Meynert; decreased choline acetyltransferase	Progressively worsening memory loss; **neurofibrillary tangles; senile plaques** (amyloid β/**A4** protein); Hirano bodies	**Most common cause of dementia;** age of onset is usually 65 years (younger in Down's syndrome patients)
Multi-infarct dementia	Cerebral atherosclerosis	Sudden onset; intermittent signs of dementia and motor deficits	**Second most common cause of dementia** (most common is Alzheimer's)

CNS=central nervous system.

 Dementia is a chronic loss of cognitive function without an altered level of consciousness. Delirium is an acute altered level of consciousness accompanied by disordered cognition.

 Toxoplasma gondii can infect the immunocompromised individual via three routes: undercooked meat, cat feces, or in utero. It is the most common CNS infection in AIDS patients.

ACUTE MENINGITIS

Meningitis is an infection of the meninges resulting in an inflammatory reaction characterized by severe headache, fever, photophobia, and positive **Kernig's** and **Brudzinski's signs.** Immunocompetent adults generally have *Streptococcus pneumoniae* or *Neisseria meningitidis* as the cause of their meningitis. Conditions predisposing an individual to acute bacterial meningitis as a result of pneumococcus include distant foci of infection (such as otitis, sinusitis, or pneumonia), sickle cell disease (owing to asplenism), alcoholism, or trauma with loss of meningeal integrity. Patients with a deficiency of complement components C5–C8 are at a greater risk of developing meningococcal meningitis. *Haemophilus influenzae* is a common cause of meningitis in children, although these numbers are decreasing because of widespread use of a capsular polyribitol phosphate vaccine conjugated to diphtheria toxoid (Table 2-12).

Prevnar is a new heptavalent pneumococcal conjugate vaccine that is being given to children. The goal is to prevent invasive pneumococcal infections. The seven serotypes used to make the immunization are thought to be responsible for the majority of severe, invasive pneumococcal infections. Common, less invasive infections such as otitis media likely will not be affected, because so many serotypes are not included in the vaccine.

TABLE 2-12	Common Causes of Meningitis in Various Age Groups
Age Group	**Causes**
Newborns	Group B streptococci *Escherichia coli* *Listeria*
Children	*Haemophilus influenzae B* *Streptococcus pneumoniae* *Neisseria meningitidis* Enteroviruses
Adolescents and Young Adults	Enteroviruses *Neisseria meningitidis* *Streptococcus pneumoniae* Herpes simplex virus
Elderly	*Streptococcus pneumoniae* Gram-negative rods *Listeria*

Immunocompromised adults are at risk for developing meningitis caused by *Listeria monocytogenes*. A lumbar puncture (LP) showing organisms with a thick capsule when stained with india ink suggests *Cryptococcus neoformans* is the causal organism and the infected individual is most likely immunocompromised as a result of HIV infection. LP is often performed to confirm a suspected diagnosis of meningitis. The LP usually shows increased neutrophils, increased protein, and decreased glucose if bacterial in origin. Also, organisms may be seen on gram stain. However, if the cerebrospinal fluid (CSF) contains increased lymphocytes and a normal glucose level, viral agents such as **enterovirus**, HIV, or herpes simplex virus should be considered (Table 2-13).

TABLE 2-13	Evaluation of Cerebrospinal Fluid To Determine Cause of Meningitis		
Laboratory Test	**Finding Indicating Bacterial Cause**	**Finding Indicating Viral Cause**	**Finding Indicating Fungal Cause**
CSF pressure	↑	N	↑
Lymphocytes	N	↑	↑
Neutrophils	↑	N	N
Glucose	↓	N	↓
Protein	↑	N	↑

↑=increased; ↓=decreased; *CSF*=cerebrospinal fluid; *N*=normal.

NERVOUS SYSTEM TUMORS

Nearly 50% of the tumors occurring within the nervous system are primary tumors. The other 50% are metastases to the brain from tumors elsewhere in the body. Table 2-14 lists nervous system tumors in order of clinical significance.

QUICK HIT — Tumors of the CNS are usually intracranial, with **adult tumors** commonly **supratentorial** and **childhood** tumors usually **infratentorial.**

QUICK HIT — Psammoma bodies are also seen in papillary adenocarcinoma of the thyroid, serous papillary cystadenocarcinoma of the ovary, and malignant mesothelioma.

TABLE 2-14 Nervous System Tumors

Tumor	Presentation	Significant Features
Glioblastoma multiforme (grade IV astrocytoma)	Cerebral hemisphere tumor; irregular mass with necrotic center surrounded by edema seen on CT; **pseudopalisading** arrangement of cells	**Most common primary intracranial neoplasm;** poor prognosis; neural tube origin
Meningioma	**Psammoma bodies;** slowly growing; originates in arachnoid cells; follows sinuses	Second most common primary CNS tumor; usually occurs in women; resectable; neural crest origin
Medulloblastoma	Ataxic gait; projectile vomiting; cerebellar mass; highly malignant; tightly packed cells in rosette pattern	**Most common intracranial tumor of childhood;** neural tube origin
Retinoblastoma (*Rb*)	Retinal tumor in children	**Two-hit theory** = *Rb* is a tumor suppressor gene (chromosome 13); tumor after deletion of both copies, neural tube origin
Craniopharyngioma	Papilledema; endocrine abnormalities; **bitemporal hemianopsia**	Enlarged sella turcica; **most common supratentorial brain tumor in children; ectodermal origin** (Rathke's pouch)
Schwannoma	Hearing loss; ataxic gait; positive Romberg's sign; increased intracranial pressure; hydrocephalus; benign	Usually occurs in the cerebellopontine angle and involves CN VIII; seen **bilaterally in NF-2;** third most common primary intracranial tumor; neural crest origin
Neuroblastoma	Occurs in cerebral hemispheres; related to neuroblastoma of adrenal gland	Increasing **N-myc amplification** directly proportional to worsening prognosis; seen in children; neural crest origin
Ependymoma	Hydrocephalus; blocked 4th ventricle; rosettes surround 4th ventricle	Seen in children; neural tube origin
Metastatic neoplasms	Headache; focal defects; formation of discrete nodules in brain	Nearly half of all intracranial neoplasm; usually bloodborne; commonly from lung, breast, GI, thyroid, kidney, GU, and melanoma

CNS=central nervous system; *CT*=computed tomography; *GI*=gastrointestinal; *GU*=genitourinary; *NF-2*=neurofibromatosis-type 2.

PSYCHIATRY AND BEHAVIORAL SCIENCE

I. Drugs of Abuse and Dependence (Table 2-15)

QUICK HIT

Substance abuse is defined as use of psychoactive substances for at least 1 month with interference in the user's life, but without meeting the criteria for dependence. Substance dependence involves craving, withdrawal, and tolerance.

QUICK HIT

Alcohol is the **most widely used drug** followed by nicotine. Caffeine is the most often used psychoactive substance followed by nicotine.

QUICK HIT

Dependence is mediated by dopamine, the neurotransmitter linked to the pleasure and reward center.

TABLE 2-15 Drugs of Abuse and Dependence

Drug	Mechanism	Intoxication Effect	Withdrawal Effects
Alcohol	Unknown; possible effect at GABA receptor directly on membranes	Sedation; hypnosis; slurred speech; ataxia; loss of motor coordination; Wernicke-Korsakoff syndrome	Malaise; tachycardia; tremors; seizures; **delirium tremens;** death
Amphetamine	Release of intracellular stores of catecholamines	Insomnia; irritability; tremor; hyperactive reflexes; arrhythmias; anorexia; psychosis	Lethargy; depression; hunger; craving for drug resulting in bizarre psychological behavior; anxiety
Barbiturates	**Potentiation of GABA** action on chloride by **increase of duration** of chloride channel opening	Mental sluggishness; anesthesia; hypnosis	Restlessness; anxiety; tremor; death
Caffeine	Translocation of Ca^{2+}; inhibition of phosphodiesterase (increase in cAMP, cGMP)	Insomnia; anxiety; agitation	Lethargy; irritability; headache
Cocaine	Blockade of norepinephrine, serotonin, and dopamine reuptake	Hallucinations; anxiety; arrhythmias; nasal problems; sudden death	Craving; depression; excessive sleeping; fatigue
LSD	5-HT agonist action in the midbrain	Pupillary dilation; increased blood pressure and body temperature; piloerection; hallucinations	Flashbacks
Marijuana	Unknown; THC is active compound; possible endogenous receptors in brain	Increased appetite; visual hallucinations; increased heart rate; decreased blood pressure Impairment of short-term memory and mental activity	
Nicotine	Low doses—ganglionic stimulation; high doses—ganglionic blockade	**Increased heart rate and blood pressure;** irritability; tremors; intestinal cramps	Irritability; anxiety; restlessness; headaches; insomnia; difficulty in concentrating
Opioids (heroin)	Inhibition of adenylate cyclase by opioid receptors within the CNS	Constipation; **pinpoint pupils;** potentially lethal via **respiratory depression;** sedation	Insomnia; diarrhea; sweating; fever; piloerection
Phencyclidine (PCP)	Inhibition of dopamine, serotonin, and norepinephrine reuptake	Hostile, bizarre behavior; hypersalivation; anesthesia	Sudden onset of violent behavior

cAMP=cyclic adenosine monophosphate; *cGMP*=cyclic guanosine monophosphate; *CNS*=central nervous system; *GABA*=γ-aminobutyric acid; *5-HT*=5-hydroxytryptamine (serotonin); *LSD*=lysergic acid diethylamide; *THC*=tetrahydrocanniabinol.

II. Defense Mechanisms (Table 2-16)

TABLE 2-16 **Defense Mechanisms**

Mechanism	Characteristics	Example
Acting out	Stress is dealt with through actions; immature	After the death of his brother, a priest breaks all the windows in his church
Denial	Not accepting the reality of a situation; immature	A single woman refuses to consider the possibility of pregnancy after having unprotected intercourse and missing two periods
Displacement	Feelings for causal source are transferred to another object; immature	A man kicks his dog after getting fired from his job
Dissociation	Loss of memory or change in personality as a result of stressor; immature	A woman who was sexually abused as a child develops another personality
Identification	Behavior patterned after another; immature	A teenager smokes pot because his favorite rock star does
Intellectualization	Reason is used to cope with anxiety; immature	A pediatrician starts reading textbooks and journal articles about his wife's cancer
Isolation of affect	Events are separated from emotion; immature	An airline passenger describes an emergency landing to his family without any emotion
Projection	One's own characteristics are applied to another; immature	A flirtatious man accuses his wife of cheating
Rationalization	Analytical reason is used to justify unacceptable feelings; immature	A man claims that his DUI arrest would never have happened if his softball team had won
Reaction formation	Feelings are denied and opposite actions are performed; immature	A woman who wants to cheat on her husband instead buys him a new car
Regression	Stress-induced behavior that involves returning to a childlike state; immature	Medical students have a food fight during their lunch break on the day of board examinations
Repression	Holding back an unacceptable feeling or idea from reaching consciousness; immature	A recent widower feels no sense of loss
Splitting	Feelings or stressors are placed in distinct, opposite compartments (i.e., either all good or all bad); immature	A woman in a doctor's office describes how much she hates the nurses, but loves the receptionist, hates her boss and coworkers, but loves the security guard
Altruism	One unselfishly assists others; mature	A woman donates her entire estate to her favorite charities upon her death
Humor	Humor is used to reduce stress; mature	While stuck in an elevator, a young man makes jokes to ease the tension
Sublimation	Unacceptable impulse is directed into a socially accepted action; mature	A boy getting into a lot of fights as a kid decides to become a professional boxer
Suppression	Conscious effort to suppress thoughts or feelings; mature	A recent widower actively refuses to think about his deceased wife while packing her things away

DUI=driving under the influence.

III. Personality Disorders (Table 2-17)

TABLE 2-17	Personality Disorders	
Disorder	**Characteristics**	**Example**
CLUSTER A Paranoid	Hostile; suspicious; mistrustful; usually male	A patient being prepared for surgery yells at the doctors on rounds because he feels they are gossiping about him
Schizoid	Voluntarily socially withdrawn without psychological problems; usually male	A 52-year-old computer programmer lives alone, is not married, has no friends, and is content
Schizotypal	Odd behavior, thoughts, and appearance without psychosis	A woman wears much layered clothing and inappropriately applied makeup, and only talks to people with brown-colored hair
CLUSTER B Histrionic	Dramatic; overemotional; sexually provocative; unable to maintain close friendships; usually female	A woman exaggerates her suffering over a mild cold, and behaves seductively toward physician
Narcissistic	Grandiosity, hypersensitivity to criticism, and lack of empathy	A resident refuses to put an IV line in an uninsured child because he feels it is beneath him and he only wishes to operate with the best surgeon in the hospital
Antisocial	Inability to conform to societal rules; criminal behavior; more often males	A multiple rapist has no concern for his victims or the law
Borderline	Unstable; impulsive; suicide attempts; usually female	After an argument with her boyfriend, a woman chases him out of her home with a frying pan and then calls him at home and tells him she loves him
CLUSTER C Avoidant	Shy; withdrawn; fear of rejection; usually female	A businesswoman defers speaking during presentations to her project partner and has few friends
Obsessive-compulsive	Rigid; perfectionist; stubborn; orderly. Found twice as often in males.	A businessman works long hours on a project, holding up both the project deadline and his personal life, in vain attempts to make it perfect.
Dependent	Defers decision-making; not comfortable with an authority position; insecure; usually female	A third-year resident often accepts on-call duty for other residents, never speaks up when talked down to by the junior residents, and has trouble writing orders
Passive-aggressive	Obstinate; inefficient; procrastinating; noncompliant	School student intentionally does poorly on homework because he does not like teacher

IV. Psychoses and Other Neuropsychiatric Disorders (Table 2-18)

TABLE 2-18 Psychoses and Other Neuropsychiatric Disorders

Disorder	Characteristics	Neurotransmitter(s) Involved	Treatment	Notes
Anorexia nervosa	Body weight <85% of predicted		Antidepressants; cyproheptadine; family therapy	Higher incidence in females and **upper middle socioeconomic classes;** amenorrhea; decreased libido
Attention-deficit hyper-activity disorder (ADHD)	Hyperactive; poor attention span; highly sensitive to stimuli		Amphetamines (methylphenidate)	More common in **male children**
Bipolar disorder	Rapid speech, decreased need for sleep, hyperenergetic state, impaired judgment followed by a state of depression	Decreased serotonin	**Lithium**	
Bulimia nervosa	Purging after binge eating; **normal weight;** abuse of laxatives		Behavioral therapy; psychotherapy fluoxetine; MAOI	Normal libido; no amenorrhea (unlike anorexics); erosion of tooth enamel
Delirium	Impaired cognitive processes; diurnal variation in mood (worse at night—**"sundowning"**); illusions and hallucinations	Autonomic dysfunction	Treat the underlying cause	**Most common** problem in hospitalized psychiatric patients
Dissociative disorders	Psychological factors resulting in memory loss and loss of function		Psychotherapy; hypnotherapy; medication for associated symptoms	Includes amnesia, fugue, identity disorder, depersonalization
Generalized anxiety disorder	Generalized, persistent anxiety; tension; insomnia; irritability	Decreased serotonin, norepinephrine, GABA	Buspirone; benzodiazepines; **SSRIs**	Anxiety for more than **6 months**
Major depressive disorder	**Early morning waking;** anhedonia; depressed mood; suicidal thoughts	Decreased norepinephrine and serotonin	SSRIs; TCAs or MAOIs; electroconvulsive therapy; hospitalization	Decreased REM latency and slow wave sleep; more common in women. See Table 2-19 for pharmacologic treatment options. *(continued)*

Dissociative disorders result in retrograde amnesia, whereas head trauma results in anterograde amnesia.

Münchausen syndrome is a factitious disorder in which the patient fakes illness in order to receive medical attention. An example would be a nurse purposely injecting himself or herself with insulin to receive medical attention. **Münchausen syndrome by proxy** is a syndrome whereby the attention-seeker feigns or creates illness in another, usually his or her child, to gain medical attention.

THE NERVOUS SYSTEM

THE NERVOUS SYSTEM

TABLE 2-18 **Psychoses and Other Neuropsychiatric Disorders (Continued)**

Disorder	Characteristics	Neurotransmitter(s) Involved	Treatment	Notes
Obesity	120% of total predicted body weight		Dieting and exercise; strict fad dieting ineffective; surgery not useful	Lower socioeconomic groups; genetics play a role; increased risk of disease
Obsessive-compulsive disorder	Recurrent thoughts and actions; patients are distressed by repetitive actions	Decreased serotonin	Behavioral therapy; clomipramine; trazodone; SSRIs	EEG changes
Panic disorder	Discrete, episodic periods of intense anxiety or discomfort; palpitations; chest pain; sweating; fear of dying	Decreased serotonin, norepinephrine, GABA	Imipramine; behavior therapy	Associated with mitral valve prolapse; young women predominantly affected; genetic component
Phobias	Irrational, situational fear	Decreased serotonin, norepinephrine, and GABA	Systemic desensitization; propranolol useful for physiologic manifestations	
Posttraumatic stress (PTSD)	Result of trauma; hypervigilance; nightmares; flashbacks	Decreased serotonin, norepinephrine, and GABA	Counseling; group therapy; benzodiazepines for symptoms	The first 3 months after the trauma disorder is acute PTSD; symptoms lasting longer than 3 months after the trauma is chronic PTSD
Schizophrenia	Autism; blunted affect; loose associations; ambivalence; auditory hallucinations; **negative symptoms** (i.e., flattened affect, lack of motivation, withdrawal); **positive symptoms** (i.e., hallucinations, hyperexcitability	Increased dopamine; increased norepinephrine in paranoid schizophrenia	Antipsychotics with a trial period of 3–5 weeks; clozapine has decreased extrapyramidal side effects (as opposed to haloperidol)	Occurs in young adults; enlarged lateral and 3rd ventricles; patients oriented ×3 (person, place, and time); types include disorganized, catatonic, and paranoid

(continued)

TABLE 2-18 **Psychoses and Other Neuropsychiatric Disorders (Continued)**

Disorder	Characteristics	Neurotransmitter(s) Involved	Treatment	Notes
Somatoform disorders	Symptoms of disease occur without related pathology		Psychotherapy and therapeutics may help; variable response	Patients truly believe in having illness whereas factitious disorders are the result of faking illness
Tourette's syndrome	Involuntary motor and vocal movements	Improper dopamine regulation	Haloperidol	Onset occurs in childhood

EEG=electroencephalograph; GABA=γ-aminobutyric acid; MAOI=monoamine oxidase inhibitor; SSRI=selective serotonin reuptake inhibitor; REM=rapid eye movement; TCA=tricyclic antidepressant.

V. Antidepressants (Table 2-19)

TABLE 2-19 **Antidepressants**

Class of Antidepressant (Specific Agent)	Mechanism of Action	Side Effects
Tricyclic antidepressants (TCAs) [e.g., amitriptyline, imipramine, nortriptyline]	Inhibit **reuptake** of NE and 5-HT at neuronal synapses	Sedation, tachycardia, antimuscarinic effects (e.g., dry mouth, fever)
Monoamine oxidase inhibitors (MAOI) [e.g., isocarboxazid, phenelzine, tranylcypromine]	Inhibit **degradation** of NE and 5-HT at neuronal synapses	**Hypertensive episodes** with ingestion of tyramine-containing foods, hyperthermia, convulsions
Selective serotonin reuptake inhibitors (SSRIs) [e.g., fluoxetine, paroxetine, sertraline]	Inhibit **reuptake** of 5-HT at neuronal synapses	Inhibits liver enzymes, nausea, agitation, sexual dysfunction, dystonic reactions

5-HT=serotonin; NE=norepinephrine.

 An **overdose** of a TCA, which causes delirium, coma, seizures, respiratory depression, and arrhythmias, is potentially fatal and difficult to treat. The large volume of distribution of a TCA makes dialysis relatively ineffective.

 Amitriptyline is somewhat more potent than imipramine and nortriptyline, which means that it often has more significant side effects.

 The use of the combination of SSRIs and MAOIs may produce a "**serotonin syndrome**." This constellation of hyperpyrexia, muscle spasm, and mental status changes may be fatal.

The **"amine theory"** attributes mood to levels of certain amines such as norepinephrine (NE) and serotonin (5-HT). It is theorized that low levels of these hormones leads to depression, and many of the antidepressants **boost amine levels.** Originally, the agents used as antidepressants boosted both NE and 5-HT levels. However, today drugs that selectively increase 5-HT levels are preferred because they have fewer side effects. The sites of action of the antidepressants are represented graphically (Figure 2-15).

FIGURE 2-15 Antidepressant sites of action

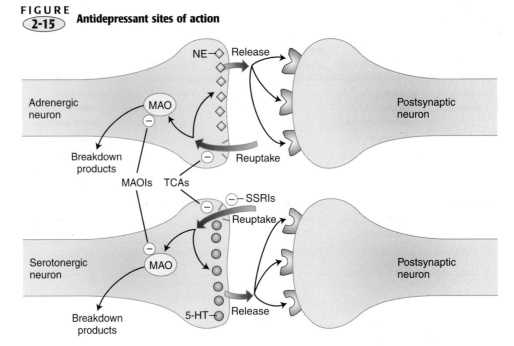

5-HT=5-hydroxytrptamine (serotonin); MAO=monoamine oxidase; MAOI=monoamine oxidase inhibitor; NE=norepinephrine; SSRIs=selective serotonin reuptake inhibitors; TCAs=tricyclic antidepressants

VI. Antipsychotics (Table 2-20)

Extrapyramidal effects, in their most severe form, may develop into **neuroleptic malignant syndrome,** a potentially fatal combination of severe rigidity, decreased perspiration, **hyperpyrexia,** and autonomic instability. Treatment involves immediate discontinuation of antipsychotic medications and administration of **dantrolene.**

TABLE 2-20 Antipsychotics

Class/Drug	Targeted Receptors (strongest to weakest)	Notes
Butyrophenone: Haloperidol	D_2, α_1	Used for **acute mania;** extrapyramidal side effects are more common
Lithium	Unclear	Used for **bipolar disorder;** inhibits regeneration of IP_3 and DAG; important for many second-messenger systems
Newer agents: Clozapine	D_4, α_1, 5-HT, muscarinic	Second-line agent used for refractory schizophrenia; small chance of agranulocytosis; weekly blood counts for patients on this agent
Risperidone	D_2, 5-HT, α_1, H_1	Second-line agent used for refractory schizophrenia
Thioxanthene: Thiothixene	D_2, α_1, H_1	No unique side effects or uses
Phenothiazines: Chlorpromazine	D_2, α_1, H_1	Atropine-like effects fairly common
Fluphenazine	D_2, α_1, H_1	**Extrapyramidal** side effects are more common
Thioridazine	Muscarinic, D_2, α_1	**Atropine-like effects** are very common; antimuscarinic effects exacerbate tardive dyskinesia, visual impairment has been reported

α_1=α_1-adrenergic; D_2=dopamine D_2; D_4=dopamine D_4; DAG=diacylglycerol; H_1=histamine H_1; 5-HT=serotonin; IP_3=inositol triphosphate.

Experts have theorized that an excess of **dopamine** in certain areas of the brain is in some way responsible for psychosis. The development of psychosis as a common side effect of treatment of Parkinson's disease with dopamine and dopamine agonists supports this belief. It is thought that most antipsychotics exert their effect by blocking **dopamine receptors.**

As a group, antipsychotics (excluding lithium) have several particular side effects in common. Antipsychotics may be **antiemetic,** they have a tendency to **lower the seizure threshold,** they cause **postural hypotension,** and they may cause **sedation.** In addition, they may also lead to **tardive dyskinesia,** a potentially irreversible syndrome of choreoathetoid movements. Tardive dyskinesia seems to be most common in older women who have received long-term treatment with high doses. However, it does occur in all kinds of patients, even after short-term, low-dose treatment. Finally, antipsychotics may cause **extrapyramidal effects,** which include parkinsonism and muscle rigidity.

VII. Nonpharmacologic Therapeutic Modalities (Table 2-21)

TABLE 2-21 Nonpharmacologic Therapeutic Modalities

Therapy	Characteristics	Notes
Biofeedback	Gaining control over physiology via continuous information; motivation and practice required	Used for hypertension, migraine headaches, and tension headaches
Classical conditioning	A **reflexive, natural behavior** is elicited in **response to a learned stimulus;** (e.g., ringing of a bell causing salivation)	**Aversive conditioning** pairs an unwanted response to a painful stimulus; stages include acquisition, extinction, and recovery
Cognitive therapy	**Negative thinking** is reorganized into self-affirming, positive thoughts	Short-term psychotherapy used to treat depression and anxiety
Electroconvulsive therapy (ECT)	Electric current introduced into brain to alter neurotransmitter function; improvement seen faster than with pharmacologic regimens	Used for **major depression;** safe; effective; retrograde amnesia is major side effect
Operant conditioning	Behavior that is not part of the natural repertoire is learned by altering the reward **(reinforcement)**	Reinforcement can be positive or negative; reward schedule includes continuous, fixed, or variable
Psychoanalysis	Intensive treatment based on recovering and integrating past experiences from the unconscious via free association; based on **Freud's theories**	**Id**—sexual drives and aggression; **ego**—controls instinct and interacts with the world; **superego**—morality and conscience
Systemic desensitization	Classical conditioning technique in which relaxation procedures are combined with increasing doses of anxiety-provoking stimuli	Used to **eliminate** phobias
Token economy	Positive reinforcement in which a reward is used to elicit a desired response	Seen often in mental hospitals or parents dealing with children

 QUICK HIT Behavior learned through a variable interval schedule of reinforcement is most difficult to extinguish. Behavior learned through a fixed schedule is easiest to extinguish.

ETHICS AND THE ROLE OF THE PHYSICIAN

The role of the nervous system in the manifestation of psychological problems is under debate. The occurrence of certain psychopathology has been linked to neurotransmitters and the lack of regulation in certain parts of the CNS.

Communication skills are essential to determine physical and psychological problems of patients. Establishing trust and confidence via facilitation, reflection, and an open-ended clinical interview allows the physician to gather physical, psychological, and social information. If an individual suffers from psychopathology, proper steps must be taken not to alienate, offend, or judge the patient. On the other hand, the individual's problems must be dealt with directly.

When presenting therapeutic options or advice, the physician should be forthright, direct, and honest. In making an assessment of any patient, the physician needs to be aware of the problems afflicting certain groups. For instance, it is important to remember that in elderly patients, sexual changes occur (i.e., men have slower erections and women have increased vaginal dryness and decreased vaginal length), sleep may decrease, suicide rate may increase, and depression becomes more prevalent.

Although the physician must be **nonmaleficent** (not intending to do harm) and **beneficent** (doing what's best for the patient), **patient autonomy** ultimately prevails in making the final decision about treatment. The physician must consider the patient's ability to make decisions based on communication skills, level of understanding about medicine, stability, consistency, and soundness of mind. Physicians have a **duty** to provide medical care to their patients, and if **breach** of this duty directly leads to **damage**, the physician has been **negligent** and therefore is **liable** for malpractice. The breach of duty owing to negligence and the damages caused by it represent a **tort.**

Before making a final decision regarding patient care, physicians should make an effort to obtain an **informed consent,** which indicates that the patient understands the risks and benefits of therapy. Disheartening as it may be, terminal disease may require the physician to explain to the patient and his family that further intervention is not appropriate inasmuch as maximal treatment has failed and it seems to be a reasonable conclusion that the goals of care will not be reached. **Advance directives** from the patient, either written or oral, may assist the physician in coming to a conclusion about when to terminate treatment measures.

Information about the patient must remain confidential unless the patient poses a risk to self or to others; information concerning the patient's own disease, diagnosis, or prognosis cannot be withheld from the patient, despite the wishes of the family.

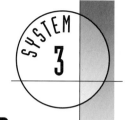

The Cardiovascular System

DEVELOPMENT

I. Heart

A. The cardiovascular system is derived from the mesoderm.

B. Paired **endocardial heart tubes** form in the cephalic region of the embryo.

C. Lateral and cephalocaudal folding causes the heart tubes to join together and lie in a ventral location, between the primitive mouth and the foregut.

D. The primitive heart dilates into five areas, shown in Figure 3-1. The five embryologic regions and their adult derivatives are as follows:

FIGURE 3-1 Embryological development of the heart

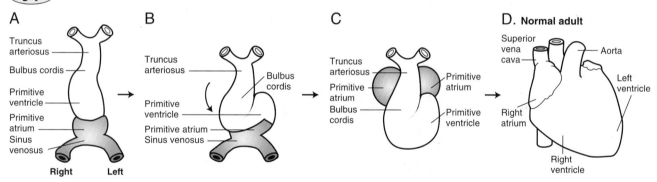

Folding of the developing heart (**A-C**) during weeks 5–8 into the normal adult heart (**D**).

(Adapted from Dudek RW, Fix JD: *BRS Embryology*, 2nd ed. Baltimore, Williams & Wilkins, 1998.)

1. **Truncus arteriosus** → proximal aorta and proximal pulmonary artery
2. **Bulbus cordis** → smooth parts of the right ventricle (conus arteriosus) and left ventricles
3. **Primitive ventricle** → right and left ventricles
4. **Primitive atrium** → right and left atria
5. **Sinus venosus** → smooth part of right atrium, the coronary sinus, and oblique vein

E. The lumen of the truncus arteriosus and bulbus cordis is divided into the aorta and pulmonary trunk by the **aorticopulmonary septum.**

F. The septum primum, septum secundum, and atriovenous (AV) cushion form the atrial septum.

G. The **foramen ovale** is a communication between the right and left atria that is formed by the walls of the septum primum and septum secundum.

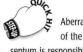
Aberrant development of the aorticopulmonary septum is responsible for tetralogy of Fallot.

The most common type of atrial septal defect is a patent foramen ovale.

1. It allows blood to flow from the venous side of the circulation to the arterial side without passing through the lungs as a result of higher pressure on the venous side during gestation.

2. **After birth,** the foramen ovale **closes** because of increased arterial pressure, which pushes the septum primum against the atrial septum.

H. The aorticopulmonary septum, the right and left bulbar ridges, and the AV cushion form the interventricular septum.

II. Arterial Vessels

A. **Aortic arches.** Initially, there are 6 paired aortic arches. Arches 3, 4, and 6 play a significant role in the adult.

1. Arch 3 helps to form the adult common carotid arteries bilaterally.

2. **Arch 4** helps to form the **aorta** on the left and the proximal subclavian artery on the right.

3. **Arch 6** helps to form the **ductus arteriosus** and part of the **pulmonary trunk.**

B. **Paired dorsal aortae** are paired vessels that run along the length of the embryo. They coalesce to form the descending aorta.

III. Venous Vessels

A. The paired vitelline, umbilical, and cardinal veins form the definitive adult structures.

B. The **vitelline veins** help form the ductus venosus and hepatic sinusoids, the inferior vena cava, the portal vein, and the superior and inferior mesenteric veins.

C. **Umbilical veins**

1. No adult vascular structures are formed by these veins.

2. The left umbilical vein connects to the ductus venosus and carries oxygenated blood from the placenta to the fetus.

3. Left umbilical vein gives rise to ligamentum teres hepatis.

4. Right umbilical vein regresses.

D. **Cardinal veins**

1. The anterior cardinal veins help form the internal jugular vein and the superior vena cava.

2. The posterior cardinal veins help form the inferior vena cava, common iliac veins, azygos vein, and renal veins.

The **umbilical circulation** is one of the only places in the body (along with the pulmonary circulation) where an **artery does not carry oxygenated blood.** The paired umbilical arteries carry deoxygenated blood to the placenta while the **umbilical vein** brings oxygenated blood back to the fetus.

IV. Fetal Circulation (Figure 3-2)

FIGURE
3-2   **Fetal circulation**

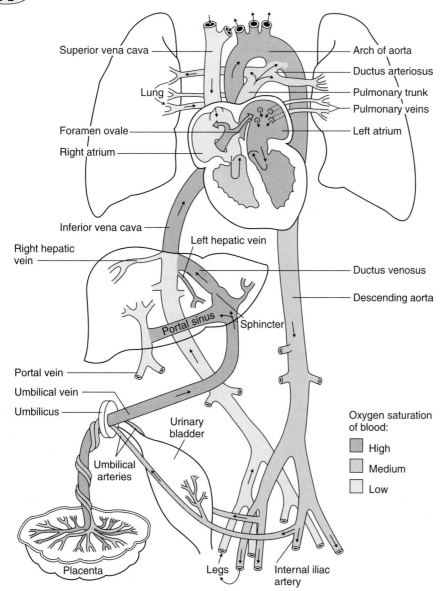

(Adapted from Lilly LS: *Pathophysiology of Heart Disease,* 2nd edition. Baltimore, Williams & Wilkins, 1997.)

V. Congenital Defects of the Heart and Great Vessels (Table 3-1)

Down's syndrome is associated with endocardial cushion defects, which may manifest as atrial septal defect (ASD) or ventral septal defect (VSD).

Paradoxical emboli are emboli that originate in the venous circulation and pass through a patent foramen ovale or ASD to produce symptoms on the arterial side.

In dextrocardia, the heart is located on the right side in the thorax. An isolated misplaced heart is often accompanied by multiple anomalies. If all of the body's organs are transposed (**situs inversus**—associated with **Kartagener's** syndrome; immotile cilia caused by a defect in the dynein arms resulting in lung disease and male sterility), the heart is often normal.

The ductus arteriosus closes in the first days of life. Exposure to oxygenated blood alters the production of prostaglandins (PGs). Indomethacin (PG synthesis inhibitor) induces closure of a patent ductus arteriosus (PDA), whereas alprostadil (PGE₁) therapy maintains patency.

Eisenmenger's syndrome is the change from a left-to-right shunt to a right-to-left shunt secondary to increasing pulmonary hypertension; it usually occurs as a result of a chronic, adaptive response to preexisting left-to-right shunts, such as a VSD.

TABLE 3-1 Congenital Defects of the Heart and Great Vessels			
Anomaly	**Pathology**	**Clinical Presentation**	**Notes**
Atrial septal defect (ASD)	**Secundum ASD** (defect of septum primum or septum secundum) Primum ASD (low) Sinus venosus ASD (high)	**Left to right shunt;** asymptomatic into 4th decade; murmur; right ventricular hypertrophy	Much higher incidence in females (3:1); 75–80% are secundum type
Coarctation of the aorta	Infantile (proximal to PDA); adult (constriction at closed ductus arteriosus, distal to origin of left subclavian artery)	Symptoms depend on extent of narrowing; infant presents with lower limb cyanosis and right heart failure at birth; adult asymptomatic with upper limb hypertension, rib notching on radiograph from collateral circulation through intercostal arteries, and **weak pulses in lower limbs**	Much higher incidence in males (3:1) and females with **Turner's syndrome**
Patent ductus arteriosus (PDA)	Failure of closure of the ductus arteriosus; may be caused by premature birth with **hypoxemia** or structural defects	Continuous **machinery murmur**	Second most common CHD
Tetralogy of Fallot	Defective development of the infundibular septum; results in **overriding aorta, ventricular septal defect, pulmonary stenosis, hypertrophy of the right ventricle**	Cyanosis (may not be present at birth); right-to-left shunt; **"boot-shaped heart"**	Survival to adulthood possible; patient assumes **squatting position** to relieve symptoms
Transposition of the great vessels	Aorta drains right ventricle; pulmonary artery from left ventricle; **separate pulmonary and systemic circuits**	Incompatible with life unless shunt present; cyanosis (present at birth)	Diabetic mother
Ventricular septal defect (VSD)	Membranous VSD Single muscular VSD	Left to right shunt; **loud holosystolic murmur means small defect;** large defects can present as heart failure at birth; small defects can close spontaneously	Much higher incidence in males; most common congenital heart defect (33%); 90% are membranous type

CHD=congenital heart defects; *PDA*=patent ductus arteriosus.

PHYSIOLOGY AND PATHOLOGY OF HEART FUNCTION

Properly timed and integrated myocyte contraction is essential to normal heart function. Cardiac myocytes (Figure 3-3) have **gap junctions** that allow for rapid relay of electrical signals between them. Electrical impulses are transmitted via the electrical conduction system composed of the sinoatrial (SA) node, AV node, and His-Purkinje cells (Figure 3-4). Normally, the SA node is the pacemaker of the heart. The node exhibits automaticity in which spontaneous **phase 4 depolarization** generates rhythmic action potentials (APs). These electrical signals propagate from the SA node through the atrial tissue and cause it to contract. Further propagation leads to excitation of the AV node, the ventricular bundles, and lastly the ventricular tissue. The nodal tissues are dependent on Ca^{2+} for their phase 0 depolarization whereas the cardiac muscular tissue uses Na^+ for phase 0 depolarization. The AV node transmits APs more slowly than the other cardiac tissues. This feature allows the atria to contract before the ventricles, with time for the ventricles to repolarize, fill with blood, and prepare to receive their next electrical signal. Furthermore, it also prevents excessively rapid beats from reaching and damaging the ventricular tissue. The conduction system of the heart can best be visualized on an electrocardiogram (ECG).

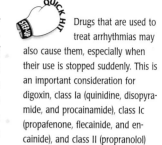

Drugs that are used to treat arrhythmias may also cause them, especially when their use is stopped suddenly. This is an important consideration for digoxin, class Ia (quinidine, disopyramide, and procainamide), class Ic (propafenone, flecainide, and encainide), and class II (propranolol) drugs.

FIGURE **Histology of cardiac myocyte. A longitudinal section of cardial muscle cells is shown.**

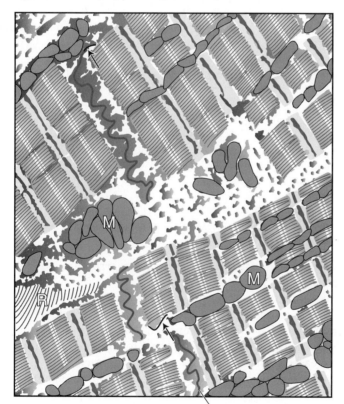

Intercalated disks

↑=location of gap junctions; *M*=mitochondria; *R*=reticular fibers.

FIGURE 3-4 Heart anatomy and signal conduction

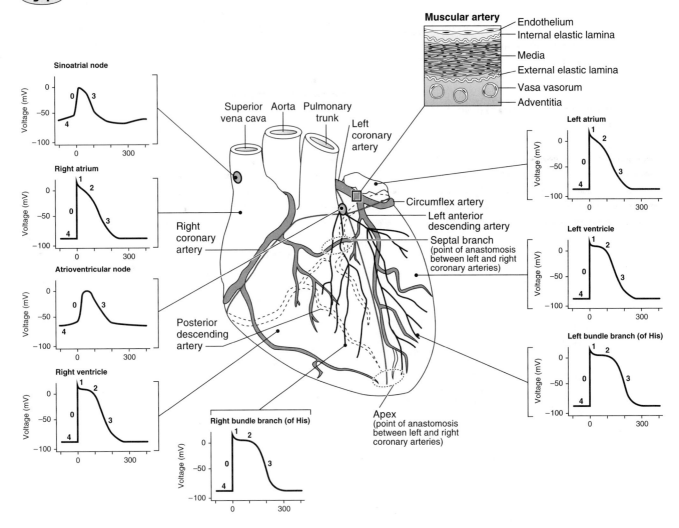

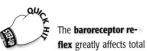

The **baroreceptor reflex** greatly affects total peripheral resistance. The carotid sinus baroreceptors, located at the bifurcation of the carotid arteries, sense arterial pressure. Afferent signals via cranial nerve (CN) IX induce efferent signals via CN X to influence heart rate. Increased arterial pressure causes an increase in vagal output and a reduction of heart rate and blood pressure. A decrease in arterial pressure causes a decrease in vagal output, resulting in an increase in heart rate and blood pressure.

ECG plots can determine disturbances, such as arrhythmias, along the cardiac conduction path (Figure 3-5) (Table 3-2)

Multiple mechanisms can affect the intrinsic mechanical properties of the heart. **Chronotropic** effects on the heart cause a change in heart rate by affecting the rate of depolarization of the SA node. **Inotropic** effects cause a change in contractility of the heart. Greater contractility allows the heart to squeeze harder and increase cardiac output. Increased intracellular Ca^{2+}, either drug-mediated (e.g., cardiac glycosides, diltiazem, verapamil, and nifedipine) or as a result of sympathetic β-receptor stimulation, allows for an increased inotropic effect. The preload and afterload also affect the function of the heart. Increased **preload** owing to increased filling of the ventricles lengthens the myocytes, which induces stronger contraction. **Afterload** of the left ventricle is equivalent to aortic pressure. It is influenced by the total peripheral resistance. A higher afterload means the left ventricle must work harder or cardiac output will fall. The cardiovascular system is constantly working to maintain homeostatic equilibrium.

Hormonal systems also respond to changes in homeostasis. A major influence on the cardiovascular system is exerted by the **renin-angiotensin-aldosterone (RAA) axis.** Whereas the baroreceptors attempt to maintain adequate pressures in the vascular system over a short-term period, the RAA system helps to regulate pressure

FIGURE 3-5 ECGs of important arrhythmias

Normal ECG

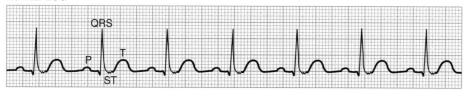

- P wave is atrial depolarization (atrial repolarization usually occurs during the QRS and remains unseen in ECG)
- PR interval (.12–.2 seconds) measures time between atrial and ventricular depolarization
- QRS interval (normally less than .1 second) reflects the duration of ventricular depolarization
- T wave is ventricular repolarization

Sustained ventricular tachycardia

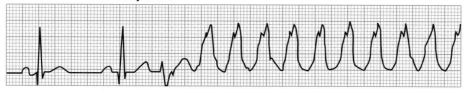

- Constant QRS morphology and fairly regular cycle length
- Initiating beat morphology may differ from ongoing VT
- AV dissociation a hallmark but not always present, nor easy to identify when present

Ventricular fibrillation

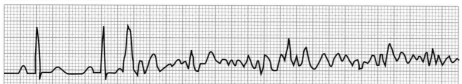

- Undulating baseline, no organized electrical activity
- Incompatible with life
- Atria may be dissociated, still in sinus rhythm

Atrial flutter

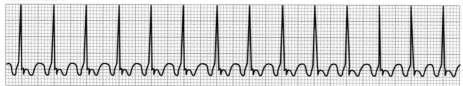

- A regular, saw-toothed pattern of atrial activity, usually very near 300/min
- Discrete, organized atrial activity on intracardiac electrograms
- Usually even-numbered AV conduction ratio (2:1, 4:1)

Atrial fibrillation

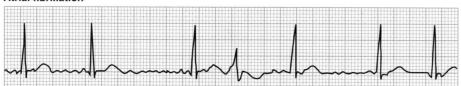

- Undulating, low amplitude atrial activity on ECG
- Intracardiac electrogram shows chaotic rapid spikes
- Variable conduction pattern as AV node is constantly bombarded with impulses; "long-short" sequences yield wide QRS complexes (aberrant, "Ashman" beats)

AV=atrioventricular; *ECG*=electrocardiogram; *VT*=ventricular tachycardia

(continued)

QUICK HIT

Torsades de pointes (twisting of the points): ventricular tachycardia often caused by antiarrhythmic drugs, especially quinidine. It is characterized by a long QT interval and a "short-long-short" sequence before the inception of tachycardia. The ECG shows a series of upward-pointing QRS complexes followed by a series of downward-pointing complexes.

FIGURE 3-5 ECGs of important arrhythmias *(Continued)*

Wolff-Parkinson-White syndrome

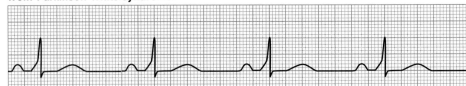

- Accessory atrioventricular conductions
- Anterograde or retrograde conduction
- Tachyarrhythmias
- Blurred QRS (referred to as δ-wave)

TABLE 3-2 Conduction Anomalies

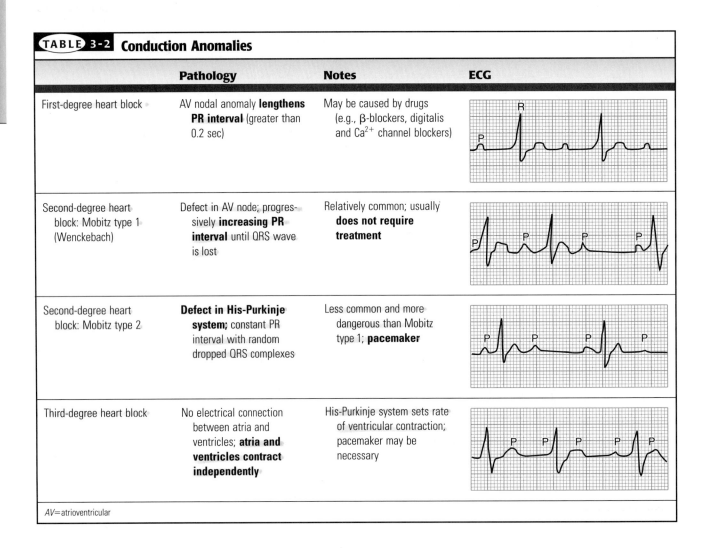

	Pathology	Notes	ECG
First-degree heart block	AV nodal anomaly **lengthens PR interval** (greater than 0.2 sec)	May be caused by drugs (e.g., β-blockers, digitalis and Ca²⁺ channel blockers)	
Second-degree heart block: Mobitz type 1 (Wenckebach)	Defect in AV node; progressively **increasing PR interval** until QRS wave is lost	Relatively common; usually **does not require treatment**	
Second-degree heart block: Mobitz type 2	**Defect in His-Purkinje system;** constant PR interval with random dropped QRS complexes	Less common and more dangerous than Mobitz type 1; **pacemaker**	
Third-degree heart block	No electrical connection between atria and ventricles; **atria and ventricles contract independently**	His-Purkinje system sets rate of ventricular contraction; pacemaker may be necessary	

AV=atrioventricular

over a longer period of time. The RAA axis responds to changes in arterial pressure by altering salt and water retention by the kidneys. Low blood pressure causes an increased release of renin, which converts angiotensinogen from the liver to angiotensin I. Angiotensin I travels to the lung where it is cleaved to angiotensin II (Ang II) by angiotensin-converting enzyme (ACE). Ang II stimulates constriction of arterioles and increases release of aldosterone (salt and water retention—see System 6 "Renal System"), both of which increase blood pressure. **Atrial natriuretic peptide** (ANP) also responds to blood pressure changes. An increase in blood pressure causes stretch of atrial myocytes, which then release ANP. ANP lowers blood pressure by relaxing smooth muscle, increasing salt and water excretion, and inhibiting renin release. **Antidiuretic hormone** (ADH), also known as arginine vasopressin (AVP), is involved in the response to changes in blood pressure. When released from the pituitary, it acts on the kidney to reduce urine output and retain water, while simultaneously constricting arterioles to increase total peripheral resistance (Figure 3-6).

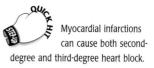

Myocardial infarctions can cause both second-degree and third-degree heart block.

FIGURE 3-6 Blood pressure control mechanisms

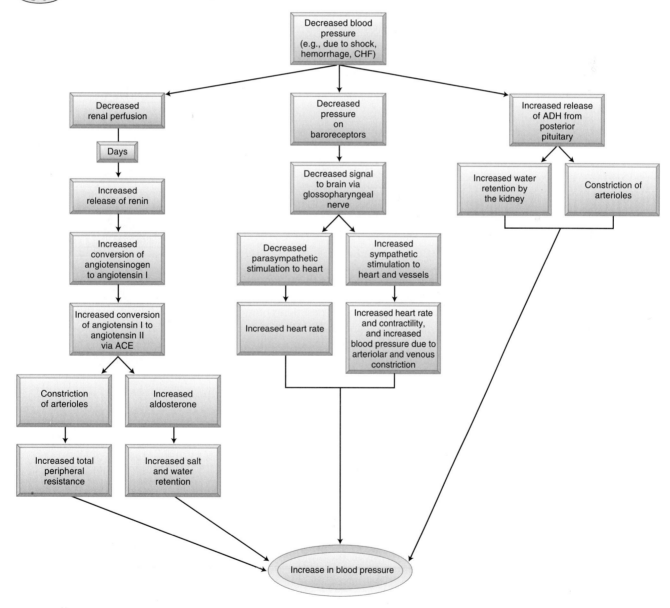

ACE=angiotensin-converting enzyme; *ADH*=antidiuretic hormone; *CHF*=congestive heart failure

Antiarrhythmics (Figure 3-7)

FIGURE 3-7 Antiarrhythmic drugs

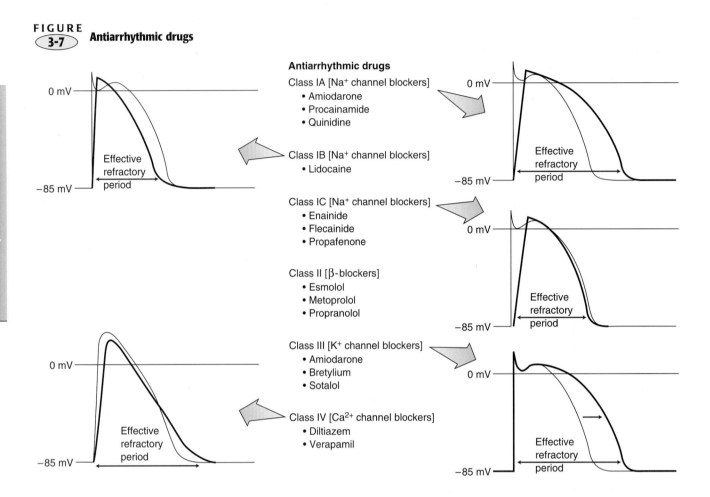

Antiarrhythmic drugs

Class IA [Na+ channel blockers]
• Amiodarone
• Procainamide
• Quinidine

Class IB [Na+ channel blockers]
• Lidocaine

Class IC [Na+ channel blockers]
• Enainide
• Flecainide
• Propafenone

Class II [β-blockers]
• Esmolol
• Metoprolol
• Propranolol

Class III [K+ channel blockers]
• Amiodarone
• Bretylium
• Sotalol

Class IV [Ca2+ channel blockers]
• Diltiazem
• Verapamil

The physiologic function of the heart can be represented in several ways (e.g., pressure-volume loops and the cardiac cycle) (Figure 3-8). The effects of cardiac output, total peripheral resistance, contractility, preload, and afterload are represented on the **Frank-Starling curve.** Cardiac output is measured using the Fick principle (Figure 3-9) and normal output is approximately 5 L/min.

FIGURE
3-8 **Physiologic cardiovascular relationships**

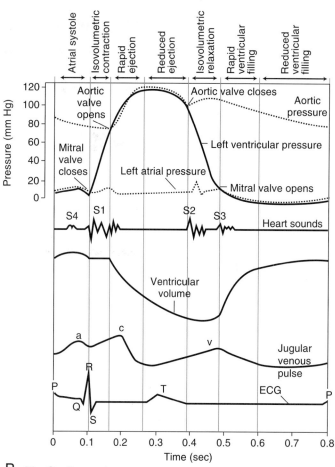

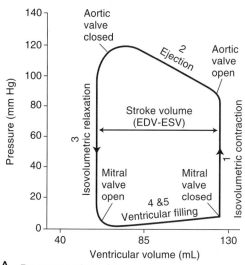

A. **Pressure-volume loop**

B. **The Cardiac cycle**

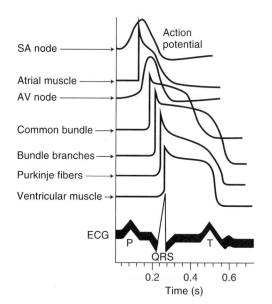

C. **Progression of the action potential through cardiac muscle cells**

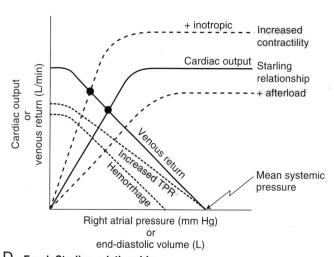

D. **Frank-Starling relationship**

AV=atrioventricular; *ECG*=electrocardiogram; *EDV*=end-diastolic volume; *ESV*=end-systolic volume; *SA*=sinoatrial; *TPR*=total peripheral resistance (Adapted from Bushan V, Le T, Amin C: *First Aid for the USMLE Step 1.* Stamford, Connecticut, Appleton & Lange, 1998. p. 284−285.)

FIGURE
3-9 **Important cardiovascular equations**

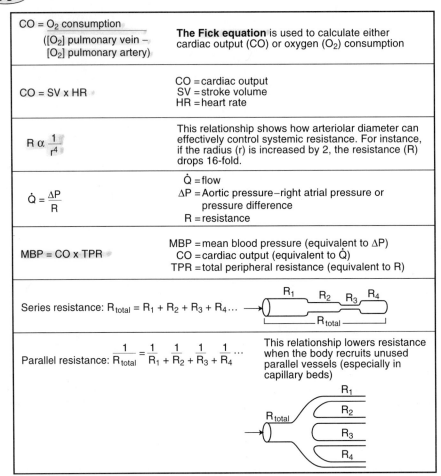

$CO = \dfrac{O_2 \text{ consumption}}{([O_2] \text{ pulmonary vein} - [O_2] \text{ pulmonary artery})}$	**The Fick equation** is used to calculate either cardiac output (CO) or oxygen (O_2) consumption
$CO = SV \times HR$	CO = cardiac output SV = stroke volume HR = heart rate
$R \propto \dfrac{1}{r^4}$	This relationship shows how arteriolar diameter can effectively control systemic resistance. For instance, if the radius (r) is increased by 2, the resistance (R) drops 16-fold.
$\dot{Q} = \dfrac{\Delta P}{R}$	$\dot{Q}$ = flow ΔP = Aortic pressure–right atrial pressure or pressure difference R = resistance
$MBP = CO \times TPR$	MBP = mean blood pressure (equivalent to ΔP) CO = cardiac output (equivalent to $\dot{Q}$) TPR = total peripheral resistance (equivalent to R)
Series resistance: $R_{total} = R_1 + R_2 + R_3 + R_4 \ldots$	
Parallel resistance: $\dfrac{1}{R_{total}} = \dfrac{1}{R_1} + \dfrac{1}{R_2} + \dfrac{1}{R_3} + \dfrac{1}{R_4} \ldots$	This relationship lowers resistance when the body recruits unused parallel vessels (especially in capillary beds)

ATHEROSCLEROSIS

I. Atherosclerosis is a disease of large and medium sized vessels characterized by the formation of atheromas (i.e., lesions that have a central lipid rich core surrounded by fibrous tissue) deposited in the intima of arteries.

II. It is the leading cause of mortality in the United States.

III. Risk Factors
   A. Major risk factors
   1. **Hyperlipidemia:** high blood cholesterol, high triglycerides, decreased high-density lipoproteins (HDL; <45) (see Table 3-3 later in the chapter)
   2. **Diabetes mellitus**
   3. **Cigarette smoking**
   4. **Hypertension**
   5. **Obesity**
   B. **Minor risk factors**
   1. Lack of physical activity
   2. Male sex
   3. Increased age
   4. Family history
   5. Oral contraceptives, decreased estrogens, or premature menopause
   6. Type A personality
   7. Elevated homocysteine level

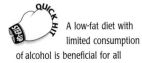

A low-fat diet with limited consumption of alcohol is beneficial for all patients with hyperlipidemia.

IV. Pathogenesis

A. Atheroma formation

1. Monocytes adhere to vessel walls, enter tissue, and become macrophages.
2. Macrophages are transformed into **foam cells** after engulfing oxidized low-density lipoprotein (LDL).
3. Foam cells accumulate in the intima.
4. Foam cells release factors causing the aggregation of platelets, the release of fibroblast growth factor, and the accumulation of smooth muscle.
5. After formation of plaque, calcification occurs.
6. The central core of the plaque consists mainly of cholesterol.

B. Complications

1. **Plaque rupture**
2. Development of fatty streaks
3. Ischemic heart disease or myocardial infarction
4. Stroke
5. Renal arterial ischemia
6. Death

Type IIb and type IV are the two most common dyslipidemias.

Vitamin E inhibits the oxidation of LDL and its subsequent absorption by macrophages. Compounds such as superoxide, nitric oxide, and hydrogen peroxide promote oxidation of LDL and blood vessel injury.

HDL works to remove cholesterol from tissues and plaques, therefore exerting a protective effect. HDL is increased by exercise.

FAMILIAL DYSLIPIDEMIAS (Table 3-3)

TABLE 3-3 **Familial Dyslipidemia**					
Familial Dyslipidemias	**Elevated**	**Blood Lipid Levels**	**Pathology (see System 5, Gastrointestinal System)**	**Clinical Picture**	**Treatment**
Hyperchylomicronemia I	Chylomicrons	↑↑TG	Lipoprotein lipase deficiency	Increased vascular and heart disease	Low-fat diet
Hypercholesterolemia IIa	LDL	↑Cholesterol	**Decreased LDL receptors**	Greatly increased vascular and heart disease; **xanthomas**	Cholestyramine/ colestipol, lovastatin (and niacin for homozygotes)
Combined hyperlipidemia IIb	LDL, VLDL	↑TG, ↑cholesterol	Hepatic overproduction of VLDL	Increased vascular and heart disease	Cholestyramine/ colestipol, lovastatin (and niacin for homozygotes)
Dysbetalipoproteinemia III	IDL, VLDL	↑TG, ↑cholesterol	Altered apolipoprotein E	Increased vascular and heart disease; xanthomas	Niacin and clofibrate or lovastatin
Hypertriglyceridemia IV	VLDL	↑↑TG, normal to ↑cholesterol	Hepatic overproduction (with possible decreased clearance) of VLDL	Increased vascular and heart disease; obese, **diabetic, pregnant,** and **alcoholic** patients	Weight loss; low-fat diet; niacin and clofibrate or lovastatin (if necessary)
Mixed hypertriglyceridemia V	VLDL, chylomicrons	↑↑TG, ↑cholesterol	Overproduction or decreased clearance of VLDL and chylomicrons	Obese and diabetic patients	Diet modification; niacin and clofibrate or lovastatin (if necessary)
LDL=low-density lipoproteins; *TG*=triglycerides; *VLDL*=very low density lipoproteins.					

THE CARDIOVASCULAR SYSTEM

Hypertrophy of the left ventricle is also caused by left-sided valvular disease, such as aortic stenosis and mitral regurgitation.

HYPERTENSION

I. Essential

A. **Most common** type (95% of cases)

B. Unknown etiology

C. Risk factors
   1. Family history
   2. Race (more common in blacks)
   3. Obesity
   4. Cigarette smoking
   5. Physical inactivity

D. **Characteristics**
   1. Blood pressure greater than 140/90 on **three separate occasions** or greater than 170/110 on one single visit

E. Chronic complications
   1. Hypertrophy of left ventricle
   2. Onion-skinning of vessel walls
   3. Retinal hemorrhages

F. **Essential hypertension predisposes to ischemic heart disease** (see next section).

II. Secondary hypertension refers to elevated systemic arterial pressure associated with a condition known to cause hypertension.

A. **Renal diseases.** These are the **most common cause** of secondary hypertension.
   1. Renal parenchymal disorders
   2. Unilateral renal artery stenosis
      a. **Atherosclerosis** (more common in black males and older individuals)
      b. **Fibromuscular dysplasia** (more common in white females and young people)
   3. The renin-angiotensin axis is activated.

B. **Endocrine causes**
   1. Primary aldosteronism
   2. Pheochromocytoma
   3. Hyperthyroidism
   4. Acromegaly
   5. Cushing syndrome

C. Coarctation of the aorta

Fibromuscular dysplasia of the renal artery causes a "beads on a string" sign on radiograph.

Treatment for emergent (malignant) hypertension (systolic blood pressure greater than 220 mm Hg or diastolic pressure greater than 120 mm Hg) includes IV sodium nitroprusside or IV β-blockers.

III. Malignant (emergent) hypertension

A. Accelerated course results in end-organ damage in days

B. End-organ damage occurs to the following organ systems:
   1. Cardiovascular—vascular damage, aortic dissection
   2. Pulmonary—pulmonary edema
   3. Renal— "flea-bitten kidneys," azotemia
   4. Ocular—fundal hemorrhages, papilledema
   5. Central nervous system (CNS)—encephalopathy, seizures, coma

C. Early death because of cerebrovascular accidents (CVA) is the result of this type of hypertension.

D. **Young black males** are the usual victims of this type of hypertension.

ANEURYSMS (Table 3-4)

TABLE 3-4 Aneurysms		
Type of Aneurysm	**Etiology**	**Characteristics**
Arteriovenous fistula	Abnormal communication between arteries and veins; usually secondary to **trauma**	Ischemic changes; aneurysm formation; **high output cardiac failure**
Atherosclerotic	**Atherosclerotic** disease; coronary artery disease	Usually in the **abdominal** aorta; located between renal arteries and iliac bifurcation
Berry	Congenital medial weakness at the bifurcations of the cerebral arteries	Saccular lesions in cerebral vessels (especially at the **circle of Willis**); hemorrhage into **subarachnoid** space
Dissecting	**Hypertension;** cystic medial necrosis; **Marfan's**	**Tearing pain;** longitudinal separation of tunica media of aortic wall
Syphilitic	Tertiary syphilis; obliteration of the vasa vasorum; necrosis of the media	Involves **ascending** aorta and aortic root; aortic valve insufficiency
Mycotic (infectious)	Inflammation secondary to bacterial infection; usually salmonella	Involves abdominal aorta

ANTIHYPERTENSIVE AGENTS

I. α-Blockers

A. α-Adrenergic receptors are the primary controllers of vascular tone used primarily to lower blood pressure.
   1. α_1-Selective agents commonly used in the treatment of hypertension include **prazosin, doxazosin,** and **terazosin**
   2. Little impact on the heart, but they have selective effects, which are evident in their side-effect profiles

B. Side effects
   1. Postural hypotension with reflex tachycardia (most common)
   2. Nasal congestion and headache
   3. Rebound hypertension if stopped abruptly

C. **Phenoxybenzamine** and **phentolamine** are nonselective α-blockers that can be used in the diagnosis and treatment of the symptoms of pheochromocytoma

II. β-Blockers

A. β-Blockers can be divided into three subgroups
   1. Nonselective β-blockers (β_1 and β_2): **propranolol,** timolol, and nadolol
   2. β_1-Selective agents: **metoprolol,** atenolol, acebutolol, and esmolol
   3. β_2-Selective agents will be discussed in Chapter 4, "The Respiratory System."

B. This important class of drugs has many clinical uses.
   1. Cardiac uses (most common)
      a. **Hypertension**
      b. **Stable angina**
      c. Prophylaxis after a myocardial infarction
   2. Less common uses
      a. Symptomatic treatment of hyperthyroidism
      b. Prophylaxis against migraine headaches
      c. Anxiety disorder

Berry aneurysms are commonly associated with adult polycystic kidney disease, an **autosomal dominant** disease; the gene is located on chromosome 16.

Syphilis is a sexually transmitted disease caused by *Treponema pallidum* (a spirochete) that is characterized initially (primary stage) by a painless, hard chancre. Untreated syphilis progresses to secondary and tertiary stages which are characterized by rashes, lymphadenopathy, **condylomata lata, Argyll Robertson pupils (pupils constrict with accommodation but not with light)**, and aortic root aneurysms.

Exercise tolerance testing ('stress testing') is a good way to diagnose subacute coronary occlusion. **Thallium 201** scans reveal perfusion defects. Technetium (^{99m}Tc) scans are useful for imaging MIs.

Cocaine use can also result in coronary vasospasm resulting in myocardial ischemia. In general, cocaine works by inhibiting the reuptake of endogenous catecholamines (dopamine, norepinephrine, epinephrine and serotonin). On the other hand, amphetamines stimulate the release of endogenous catecholamines.

THE CARDIOVASCULAR SYSTEM

C. Therapeutic effects of β-blockers on various organ systems (Table 3-5)

TABLE 3-5	Therapeutic Effects of β-Blockers*	
Organ System	**Effect**	**Clinical Implication**
Cardiac (**β₁**)	Negative inotropic and chronotropic effects; slowing of SA and AV nodes	Decreases cardiac output Bradycardia can limit dosing AV nodal slowing is useful in SVT
Pulmonary (**β₂**)	Constriction of airway smooth muscle	β-Blockers are contraindicated in patients with COPD
Endocrine	Decreased glycogenolysis Decreased glucagon release	β-Blockers must be used with caution in diabetic patients taking insulin who are at risk for hypoglycemia
Ocular	Decreased aqueous humor production by processes of ciliary body	β-Blockers, such as timolol, can be used topically for glaucoma

AV=atrioventricular; *COPD*=chronic obstructive pulmonary disease; *SA*=sinoatrial; *SVT*=supraventricular tachycardia.
*Those effects known to be predominantly caused by either β₁ or β₂ blockers are listed as such.

    D. Adverse effects
        1. Sexual dysfunction in males
        2. Arrhythmias if the drug is stopped abruptly
        3. Bronchoconstriction
        4. Blocking hypoglycemic response in a diabetic

III. Calcium-Channel Blockers
    A. Second-line antihypertensive agents
    B. Act by binding to the L-type calcium channel of vascular smooth muscle cells and myocytes
    C. Block the entry of calcium into these cells
    D. These agents affect both vascular tone and the heart itself. Effects on the heart include negative inotropy and slowing of the conduction system.
    E. Calcium-channel blockers are often divided into two groups.
        1. Dihydropyridines
          a. Examples: **nifedipine** and **amlodipine**
          b. Greater effect on vascular smooth muscle than on the heart
        2. Nondihydropyridines
          a. Examples: **diltiazem** and **verapamil**
          b. Increasingly greater effects on the myocardium
    F. Adverse effects include **hypotension,** headache, **constipation,** and exacerbation of gastroesophageal reflux.

IV. Other Antihypertensive Agents
    A. Clonidine
        1. Along with α-methyldopa, a centrally acting antihypertensive agent
        2. This agent acts as an **agonist at presynaptic α₂ receptors,** thereby decreasing central sympathetic tone.
        3. Adverse effects include sedation and **rebound hypertension** if the drug is stopped abruptly.
    B. Sodium nitroprusside
        1. Given intravenously, this agent is the drug of choice for **hypertensive emergencies.**
        2. Given orally, this drug is toxic because it results in cyanide production.
        3. Affects both arterial and venous smooth muscle
    C. Vasodilators (**hydralazine, minoxidil**)
        1. Dilate both arteries and veins (predominantly arteries), lowering blood pressure

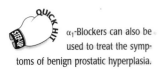

α₁-Blockers can also be used to treat the symptoms of benign prostatic hyperplasia.

a. **Reflex tachycardia** that results can actually precipitate attacks of angina.
b. These agents are not first-line agents for hypertension.
c. Often used along with β-blockers and diuretics.
2. Adverse reactions to hydralazine include headache, arrhythmias, and a **lupuslike reaction.**
3. Adverse effects of minoxidil include sodium retention and hypertrichosis.

ISCHEMIC HEART DISEASE

I. Defined as an inadequate supply of oxygen relative to demand.

II. Ischemic heart disease is most often caused by atherosclerosis.

III. Four types of ischemic heart disease
A. **Angina pectoris**
1. Paroxysmal attacks of retrosternal pain, heaviness, or squeezing chest pain occur and may radiate to the neck, jaw, left shoulder, or arm. Angina pectoris is often associated with diaphoresis and nausea.
2. Imbalance between cardiac perfusion and cardiac demand is characteristic. Ninety percent occlusion of coronary vessel produces symptoms.
3. **Three types** of angina pectoris
a. **Stable angina**
(1) **Most common** form
(2) Induced by exercise
(3) Relieved by rest
(4) Results from chronic stenosis of coronary arteries
b. **Prinzmetal's (variant) angina**
(1) **Episodic** pain occurs at rest.
(2) Attacks are **unrelated to activity, blood pressure,** or **heart rate,** but are related to coronary artery **vasospasm.**
(3) Significant artery stenosis is often present.
c. **Unstable angina**
(1) This type occurs at rest or with **increasing frequency, severity,** or **duration.**
(2) It is preceded by less and less activity.
(3) It produces pain of longer and longer duration.
(4) It is induced **by ruptured atherosclerotic plaque** with subsequent thrombosis and embolization.
(5) Activated platelets help cause thrombosis and vasospasm.
(6) Microinfarcts may be caused.
4. **Treatment of stable angina**
a. Nitrates
(1) These drugs are converted within the cell to **nitric oxide,** a smooth muscle relaxant.
(a) The relaxation of vascular smooth muscle causes widespread venous dilation.
(b) This lowers preload and therefore reduces the workload and oxygen demand of the heart.
(c) To a lesser extent, the relaxation of coronary arteries provides ischemic myocardium with increased oxygen.
(2) Sublingual **nitroglycerin** is the treatment of choice for acute episodes of angina.
(3) A long-acting nitrate such as **isosorbide dinitrate** can be used for angina prophylaxis.
(4) Unwanted side effects of nitrate therapy include **headache** and **tachyphylaxis,** postural hypotension, and facial flushing.
b. Calcium-channel blockers
c. β-Blockers ⟶ rapid tolerance

 β-Blockers mask many of the symptoms of hypoglycemia (tremors, sweating, palpitations) that are mediated by epinephrine. This, as well as the endocrine effects, puts individuals with insulin-dependent diabetes taking β-blockers at increased risk for profound hypoglycemia.

 Diltiazem can be used to control the ventricular response rate in atrial fibrillation because it slows AV nodal conduction.

B. **Myocardial infarction (MI)**
1. Lack of adequate perfusion to cardiac tissue leads to myocyte death in affected area.
2. MI is most often caused by **atherosclerosis** with plaque rupture and thrombus.
3. The sub-endocardium is most vulnerable to ischemia (because of decreased blood flow during systole) and therefore most likely to infarct.
4. In a transmural infarct (see below), the full thickness of the ventricular wall is affected within 3–5 hours.
5. **Two types** of myocardial infarction are possible.
   a. **Nontransmural** (non-Q-wave) **infarcts** (circumferential)
      (1) Diffuse coronary atherosclerosis is found.
      (2) This causes overall reduction of coronary flow.
      (3) Rupture or thrombosis eventually results, followed quickly by clot lysis.
      (4) Loss of perfusion to inner one third of muscular wall of ventricle occurs.
      (5) **ST-segment depression** is seen on ECG.
   b. **Transmural infarct**
      (1) Atherosclerotic plaques rupture.
      (2) Platelet-mediated thrombosis occludes vessel.
      (3) Occluded vessel stops flow of blood to entire muscular wall.
      (4) **ST-segment elevation** is seen on ECG.
6. Cardiac enzymes are released when myocytes are damaged (Figure 3-10).

The **left anterior descending** artery is the most common artery involved in acute MI. Infarcts of this artery affect the left ventricle near its apex, or the anterior portion of the interventricular septum.

ST elevation is pathognomonic for transmural (Q-wave) infarcts. However, ST depression is not pathognomonic for nontransmural (non–Q-wave) infarcts, as it can also be produced by digitalis drugs.

FIGURE 3-10 **Myocardial infarction enzyme release and timeline of histologic changes**

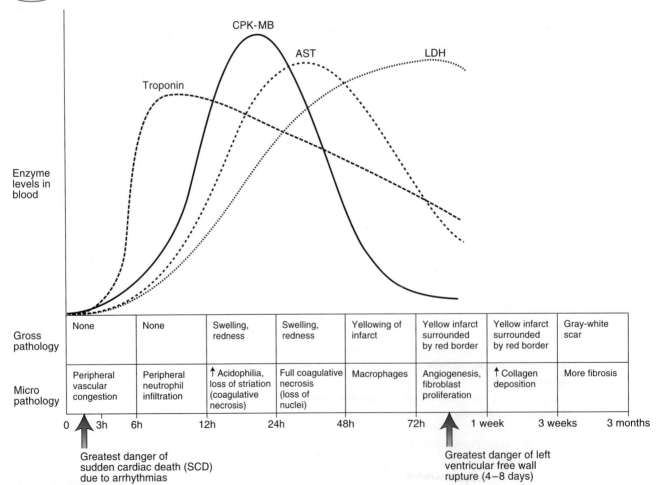

AST=aspartate aminotransferase; CPK-MB=creatine kinase-MB; LDH=lactate dehydrogenase

7. Complications
   a. Arrhythmia
   b. Heart block
   c. Myocardial rupture occurs most commonly during first week post-MI.
   d. Papillary muscle rupture
   e. Mural thrombus with possible embolization
   f. Aneurysm
   g. Death
8. Remodeling and scar formation occur over a period of 3–6 months after an infarct (see Fig 3–10).

C. **Chronic ischemic heart disease (CIHD)**
   1. **Congestive heart failure (CHF)** that results from ischemic cardiac damage leads to CIHD.
   2. Hypertrophy of the heart and cardiac decompensation occur as a result of infarction.
   3. CIHD is most often found in the elderly.

D. **Sudden cardiac death**
   1. This is unexpected death from cardiac failure occurring less than **2 hours post-MI.**
   2. This is caused less commonly by a congenital anomaly.
   3. Marked atherosclerosis is usually present.
   4. The mechanism of death is almost always because of **arrhythmia.**

 Reentry is the most common cause of arrhythmias. Reentry requires a circuit, refractory tissue (unidirectional block), slow conduction velocity, and an initiating event (usually a premature beat).

 Cor pulmonale is right-sided heart failure secondary to lung disorders that lead to pulmonary arterial hypertension.

CONGESTIVE HEART FAILURE (Table 3-6) (Figure 3-10) (Figure 3-11)

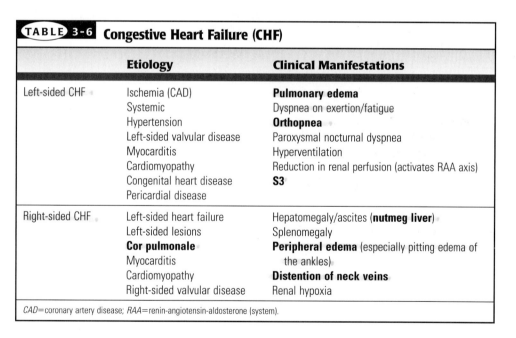

TABLE 3-6 Congestive Heart Failure (CHF)

	Etiology	Clinical Manifestations
Left-sided CHF	Ischemia (CAD) Systemic Hypertension Left-sided valvular disease Myocarditis Cardiomyopathy Congenital heart disease Pericardial disease	**Pulmonary edema** Dyspnea on exertion/fatigue **Orthopnea** Paroxysmal nocturnal dyspnea Hyperventilation Reduction in renal perfusion (activates RAA axis) **S3**
Right-sided CHF	Left-sided heart failure Left-sided lesions **Cor pulmonale** Myocarditis Cardiomyopathy Right-sided valvular disease	Hepatomegaly/ascites (**nutmeg liver**) Splenomegaly **Peripheral edema** (especially pitting edema of the ankles) **Distention of neck veins** Renal hypoxia

CAD=coronary artery disease; *RAA*=renin-angiotensin-aldosterone (system).

Congestive heart failure is a clinical diagnosis in which the heart is unable to pump an adequate amount of blood to meet the metabolic needs of the body. A number of factors play a role in congestive heart failure, including hormonal changes (RAA and sympathetic activation), peripheral vasoconstriction, and myocardial dysfunction. One of the final common pathways in CHF is hypoperfusion of the kidneys and activation of the RAA axis, which leads to sodium and water retention. Treatment is directed at blocking the RAA axis, or increasing cardiac performance and therefore renal perfusion. **Therapeutic agents** in CHF include ACE inhibitors, Ang II receptor blockers (ARBs), digitalis, diuretics, and dobutamine.

FIGURE
(3-11) **Congestive heart failure**

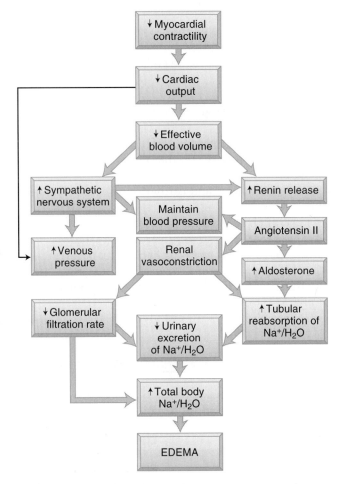

I. ACE Inhibitors

A. First-line treatment for CHF

B. ACE inhibitors are able to lower blood pressure (lower afterload), improve cardiac performance, and prevent the aldosterone-mediated salt and water retention typical of CHF.

C. Specific agents

1. **Enalapril** decreases mortality in CHF.

2. Other ACE inhibitors include **captopril** and **lisinopril.**

D. Adverse effects of ACE inhibitors

1. Reversible renal failure

2. **Angioedema,** hyperkalemia, **dry cough,** orthostatic hypotension

3. ACE inhibitors are fetotoxic and contraindicated in pregnancy.

II. ARBs

A. These agents block the RAA axis at the Ang II receptor, producing the same benefits as ACE inhibitors.

B. Examples of ARBs are **losartan** and **valsartan.**

C. These drugs have all the same effects as the ACE inhibitors except that they do not increase levels of bradykinin, as do the ACE inhibitors.

III. Digitalis

A. Treats CHF by increasing cardiac performance—digitalis treats CHF by increasing the intracellular concentration of calcium in cardiac myocytes, therefore increasing contractility

B. Blocks sodium-potassium pump
   1. This increases the intracellular sodium concentration.
   2. Activity of a sodium-calcium antiporter is decreased.
   3. Decreased activity of this antiporter raises intracellular calcium levels.
C. Digitalis improves the symptoms of CHF, but unlike ACE, it has not been shown to decrease mortality.
D. Digitalis also has a low therapeutic index, which means that the toxic dose is closer to the therapeutic dose.
E. Common adverse reactions
   1. **Nausea** and headache
   2. **Arrhythmias** (more serious)

IV. Diuretics, the other major treatment modality for CHF, are not discussed here (see System 6).

INTRINSIC DISEASES OF THE HEART

I. Myocarditis
A. This is defined as **inflammation of the cardiac muscle.**
B. **Etiology**
   1. **Viral etiology** is the most common cause (usually **coxsackie B** virus)
   2. HIV (via toxoplasmosis and metastasis of Kaposi's sarcoma) may cause myocarditis.
   3. Bacterial causes include *Staphylococcus aureus* or *Corynebacterium diphtheriae.*
   4. Chagas' disease
   5. Lyme disease
   6. Hypersensitivity reactions
C. **Physical examination**
   1. **Muffled S1**
   2. **Audible S3** heart sound
   3. Murmur of **mitral regurgitation**
   4. Cardiomegaly

II. Endocarditis
A. Inflammation of heart lining and connective tissue
B. **Causes**
   1. **Rheumatic heart disease**—endocarditis may be caused by rheumatic fever (see below)
   2. **Infective endocarditis**
      a. Etiology
         (1) Bacteria, usually Gram-positive cocci, or fungi (*Aspergillus* or *Candida*) are the most common causes.
         (2) Damage, surgical repair, prosthetic heart valves, or congenital abnormalities are predisposing conditions.
         (3) Vegetative growth (usually on atrial surface of valves) can throw **septic thrombi** to brain or peripheral circulation.
         (4) Endocarditis is complicated by ulcerations of valves or rupture of chordae tendineae.
      b. Characteristics
         (1) Clinical features
            (a) Petechiae
            (b) **Janeway lesions** (peripheral hemorrhages with slight nodular character)
            (c) **Osler's nodes** (small, tender nodules on fingers and toe pads)

 Trypanosoma cruzi causes Chagas' disease and is transmitted by the reduviid bug (kissing bug).

 Borrelia burgdorferi, a spirochete, causes Lyme disease and is transmitted by the *Ixodes* tick. Stage 1 is marked by erythema chronicum migrans. Stage 2 is marked by cardiac and neurologic involvement. Stage 3 involves arthritis.

 Doxorubicin, daunorubicin, and anthracyclines used to treat sarcomas, breast cancer, lung cancer, and acute lymphocytic leukemia, result in dose-dependent, irreversible cardiotoxicity.

 Culture-negative endocarditis can result from the **HACEK** group of organisms: *Haemophilus, Actinobacillus, Cardiobacterium, Eikenella, Kingella.*

(d) **Splinter hemorrhages** (subungual linear streaks)
(e) Roth's spots (retinal hemorrhages)
(f) Splenomegaly
(2) The mitral and aortic valves are frequently involved.
(3) The presence of **right-sided** valvular lesions, usually of the tricuspid, suggests **intravenous (IV) drug abuse.**

C. Types
1. **Acute endocarditis**
   a. Cause is most often *Staphylococcus aureus.*
   b. Onset is rapid.
   c. Clinical features include fever, anemia, embolic events, and heart murmur.
   d. Treatment is with IV antibiotics.
2. **Subacute endocarditis**
   a. Cause is most often the viridans Streptococci.
   b. Results from poor dentition or oral surgery in patients with preexisting heart disease.
   c. Onset is over a period of 6 months.
   d. Treatment is with IV antibiotics.
3. **Nonbacterial (marantic) endocarditis**
   a. This type is associated with metastatic cancer.
   b. Sterile fibrin deposits appear on valves.
   c. Sterile emboli cause cerebral infarct.
4. Libman-Sacks endocarditis
   a. This is a manifestation of systemic lupus erythematosus **(SLE).**
   b. It is caused by auto-antibody damage to valves.
   c. **Vegetations form on both sides** of the valve.
5. Carcinoid syndrome
   a. This syndrome is characterized by increased serotonin and other secretory products from a carcinoid tumor.
   b. Plaques build on **right-sided valves** of the heart.

III. Rheumatic Heart Disease
A. This is a systemic inflammatory disorder with cardiac manifestations.
B. Pathogenesis
   1. Rheumatic heart disease usually occurs 1–4 weeks after a bout of tonsillitis caused by group A β-hemolytic streptococci.
   2. **Antigenic mimicry** occurs between streptococcal antigens and human antigens in the heart.
   3. This results in immunologic origin for rheumatic heart disease.
C. **Epidemiology**
   1. Children 5–15 years of age have the highest incidence of rheumatic fever.
   2. Incidence is decreasing since the advent of penicillin.
D. Cardiac manifestations of rheumatic fever include the following conditions:
   1. Pancarditis—inflammation of all structures of the heart
   2. Pericarditis with effusions
   3. Myocarditis
      a. Leads to cardiac failure
      b. **Most common cause of early death** in rheumatic fever
   4. Endocarditis
      a. Usually afflicts the **mitral** and **aortic** valves (areas of high stress)
      b. Mitral—aortic—tricuspid—pulmonary shows the order in which the valves become involved.
      c. Early nonembolic vegetations occur.
      d. With fibrosis and calcification, valvular damage leads to chronic rheumatic heart disease.

Prosthetic valves predispose individuals to endocarditis caused by *Staphylococcus epidermidis.*

Primary tumors of the heart are very rare. Metastatic (secondary) tumors are more common. Atrial myxomas are the most frequently occurring primary tumors.

Antiphospholipid syndrome, common in SLE, results from antibodies to phospholipids primarily producing a hypercoagulable state leading to thrombotic disorders and multiple spontaneous abortions.

THE CARDIOVASCULAR SYSTEM

E. **Other manifestations** of rheumatic fever
1. **Migratory polyarthritis**
2. Sydenham's chorea
3. Subcutaneous nodules
4. Erythema marginatum
5. Recent infection by group A streptococci (indicated by elevated antistreptolysin O titers)
6. **Aschoff body**
   a. Lesion characterized by focal interstitial myocardial inflammation
   b. Fragmented collagen/fibrinoid material
   c. Anitschkow myocytes: large activated histiocytes
   d. Aschoff cells: granuloma with giant cells

IV. Cardiomyopathies (Table 3-7)

TABLE 3-7 Cardiomyopathies

	Pathology	Etiology	Clinical Manifestations	Notes
Dilated	Dilated ventricles; right and left heart failure; pulmonary edema	**Idiopathic;** alcoholics; thiamine deficiency; peripartum; **coxsackievirus B;** *Trypanosoma cruzi;* TCAs; lithium, doxorubicin	Premature ventricular contractions; **decreased ejection fraction;** JVP; cardiomegaly; hepatomegaly	**Most common** form
Restrictive	**Stiffened heart muscle;** may result in right and left heart failure; tricuspid regurgitation	Senile or primary amyloidosis; sarcoidosis; hemochromatosis	Peripheral **edema;** ascites; JVD	Differentiate from hypertrophic cardiomyopathy
Hypertrophic	Ventricular and ventricular septal hypertrophy; mitral regurgitation	Usually **Autosomal dominant;** young **athletes**	Dyspnea; syncope; **S4;** systolic murmur; cardiomegaly on chest radiograph	Relieved by **squatting;** exacerbated by physical exertion; sudden death

JVD=jugular venous distention; *JVP*=jugular venous pressure; *TCA*=tricyclic antidepressant.

 Idiopathic dilated cardiomyopathy is the most common form of cardiomyopathy. Treatment includes digitalis, ACE inhibitors, heart transplant, and sometimes chronic anticoagulation.

 Senile amyloidosis is derived from transthyretin. Primary amyloidosis is caused by the amyloid light chain (AL) protein from immunoglobulin light chains. This is seen in plasma cell disorders (see System 10, "Hematopoietic and Lymphoreticular System").

 Mitral valve prolapse (MVP) is the most frequently occurring valvular lesion, often found in young women or Marfan's patients, and related to tissue laxity. The murmur is exaggerated by the **Valsalva** maneuver, but reduced by **squatting.** These patients require endocarditis prophylaxis before surgical or dental procedures.

 A midsystolic click is often indicative of mitral prolapse.

V. Valvular Heart Diseases (Table 3-8)

TABLE 3-8 Valvular Heart Disease

Valvular Disease	Etiology	Physical Examination	Clinical Manifestations	Schematic Representation
Mitral stenosis	Usually **rheumatic heart disease**	Cyanosis; **opening snap;** diastolic rumbling murmur	Dyspnea; orthopnea; left atrial enlargement; mid-to-late diastolic murmur	
Mitral regurgitation	**Rheumatic heart disease** (50% of cases); mitral valve prolapse; hypertrophic cardiomyop-athy; papillary muscle dysfunction (secondary to myocardial infarction)	Splitting of S2; **S3;** systolic murmur	Arrhythmias; infective endocarditis; dilated left atrium; holosystolic murmur	
Aortic stenosis	Thickening and **calcification** of valve; bicuspid aortic valves	Delayed pulses; carotid thrill; **crescendo-decrescendo systolic ejection murmur**	Syncope; angina; death; do not administer β-blockers	
Aortic regurgitation	Rheumatic heart disease; syphilitic aortitis; nondissect-ing aortic aneurysm; Marfan's syndrome	Wide pulse pres-sure; water-hammer pulse; **S3; blowing, decrescendo diastolic murmur**	Left ventricular enlargement; dyspnea; early diastolic murmur	

VI. Murmurs (Table 3-9)

TABLE 3-9 Murmurs					
Systolic			**Diastolic**		
Ejection	*Holosystolic*	*Late-Systolic*	*Early*	*Mid-to-Late*	*Continuous*
• Aortic valve stenosis • Hypertrophic cardiomyopathy • Pulmonic valve stenosis	• Mitral regurgitation • Tricuspid regurgitation • Ventricular septal defect	• Mitral valve prolapse	• Aortic valve regurgitation • Pulmonic valve regurgitation	• Mitral stenosis	• Patent ductus arteriosus

VII. Peripheral Vascular Diseases (Table 3-10)

TABLE 3-10 Peripheral Vascular Diseases				
Disease	**Pathology**	**Vessels Affected**	**Clinical Manifestations**	**Notes**
Churg-Strauss	Eosinophils, vasculitis	Small and medium sized arteries	**Asthma; elevated plasma eosinophils;** heart disease	May be associated with p-ANCA
Henoch-Schönlein purpura	**IgA** immune complex–mediated acute vasculitis; renal deposits in mesangium	Arterioles; capillaries; venules	Hemorrhagic urticaria; palpable purpura; fever; RBC casts in urine; **atopic** patient	Often associated with an **upper respiratory infection; children**
Kaposi's sarcoma	Viral origin; common malignancy in AIDS patients	Cutaneous and visceral vasculature	Malignant vascular tumor, especially in **homosexual** men	Probably results from re-activation of latent HHV-8 infection
Kawasaki's disease	Acute necrotizing inflammation	Large, medium, and small vessels	Fever; conjunctival lesions; lymphadenitis; coronary artery aneurysms	Affects **young children**
Rendu-Osler-Weber syndrome	**Autosomal dominant;** hereditary hemorrhagic telangiectasia	Dilatation of venules and capillaries	Epistaxis; GI bleeding	Increased frequency in **Mormon** population
Polyarteritis nodosa (PAN)	Antineutrophil antibodies (**p-ANCA**) lead to necrotizing degeneration of media; aneurysms	Small and medium sized arteries	Fever; weight loss; abdominal pain (GI); hypertension (renal)	Associated with **hepatitis B infection**
Takayasu's arteritis (pulseless disease)	Inflammation leading to stenosis; **aortic arch** and the origins of great vessels	Medium and large arteries	**Loss of carotid, radial, and ulnar pulses;** fever; night sweats; deficits arthritis; visual	Pathology referred to as "aortic arch syndrome"; young **Asian females**

(continued)

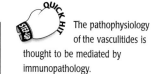

The pathophysiology of the vasculitides is thought to be mediated by immunopathology.

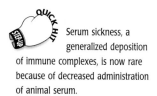

Serum sickness, a generalized deposition of immune complexes, is now rare because of decreased administration of animal serum.

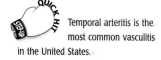

Temporal arteritis is the most common vasculitis in the United States.

TABLE 3-10 **Peripheral Vascular Diseases** *(Continued)*

Disease	Pathology	Vessels Affected	Clinical Manifestations	Notes
Temporal arteritis (giant cell arteritis)	Nodular inflammation of branches of carotid (especially **temporal**)	Medium and large arteries	**Headache;** absence of pulse in affected vessels; **visual deficits;** polymyalgia rheumatica	Significant elevation of **erythrocyte sedimentation rate; usually elderly population**
Thromboangiitis obliterans (Buerger's disease)	Acute, full-thickness inflammation of vessels; may extend to nerves; occlusive lesions in extremities	Small and medium arteries and veins	Cold, pale limb; pain; **Raynaud's phenomenon;** gangrene	Typical patient is a young **Jewish** man who **smokes heavily**
Von Hippel-Lindau disease	**Autosomal dominant;** localized to chromosome 3	Visceral vasculature	**Hemangioblastomas** of the cerebellum, brainstem, and retina; hepatic, renal, and pancreatic cysts	Increased incidence of **renal cell carcinoma**
Wegener's granulomatosis	Antineutrophil antibodies (**c-ANCA**) causes necrotizing, **granulomatous lesions** in **kidney, lung** and upper respiratory tract.	Small arteries; small veins	Cough; ulcers of sinuses and **nasal septum;** RBC casts in urine	More common in males

GI=gastrointestinal; *HHV-8*=human herpesvirus 8; *RBC*=red blood cells.

The needle for a pericardiocentesis passes through the skin, superficial fascia, pectoralis major muscle, external intercostal membrane, internal intercostal membrane, fibrous pericardium, and parietal layer of serous pericardium.

DISEASES OF THE PERICARDIUM

I. Cardiac Tamponade

A. This is an accumulation of fluid in the pericardial sac that causes cardiac filling defects because of compression of the heart.
   1. Blood is usually indicative of a traumatic perforation of the heart or aorta or rupture owing to an MI.
   2. Serous transudate may accumulate as a result of edema or CHF.
B. The most common causes are neoplasms, idiopathic pericarditis, and uremia.
C. Principal features of cardiac tamponade
   1. Intracardiac pressure is elevated.
   2. **Ventricular filling** is limited.
   3. Cardiac output is reduced.
   4. Decreased or absent heart sounds on auscultation
D. **Pulsus paradoxus** is a greater than normal (10 mm Hg) decline in systolic arterial pressure on inspiration.
E. **Treatment** involves pericardiocentesis (removal of fluid from the pericardial cavity).

II. Pericarditis

A. Pericarditis is defined as an inflammation of the pericardium (fiberoserosus membrane) covering the heart.
B. Causes
   1. Usually idiopathic
   2. **Coxsackievirus A or B**

3. Tuberculosis
4. Uremia
5. SLE
6. Scleroderma
7. Post-MI (Dressler's syndrome)
C. Physical examination
1. Jugular venous distention (JVD)
2. Increase of jugular venous pressure (JVP) with inspiration (**Kussmaul's sign**)
3. Pericardial **friction rub**
4. **Distant heart sounds**
D. Characteristics
1. Pain exacerbated by inspiration
2. Pain relieved by sitting
3. Cardiomegaly
4. Hypotension
5. **ST elevation** on ECG
E. Persistent, acute pericarditis leads to chronic, constrictive pericarditis.
1. Both acute and chronic pericarditis mimic right-sided heart failure.
2. Both acute and chronic pericarditis lead to obliteration of pericardial cavity.
3. Fibrous tissue proliferation and calcification result.

SHOCK

I. Shock is defined as a metabolic state in which oxygen delivery is not adequate to meet oxygen demand.

II. Signs and Symptoms
  A. Tachycardia
  B. Hypotension
  C. Oliguria
  D. Mental status changes
  E. Weak pulses
  F. Cool extremities

III. Types of Shock (Table 3-11)

 An MI also produces ST elevation. However, in an MI, ST elevation is followed by depression of the ST segment and QRS changes.

Autoregulation of blood flow in the heart is altered to meet the demands of tissue metabolism via nitric oxide and adenosine. Autoregulation also occurs in the kidney and brain.

 Septic shock is associated with vasodilation, hypotension, and warm extremities.

TABLE 3-11	Shock	
Type of Shock	**Mechanism**	**Clinical Causes**
Cardiogenic	Pump failure	Cardiac arrhythmias; heart failure; intracardiac obstruction; myocardial infarction
Hypovolemic	Volume loss	Blood, electrolyte, fluid, or plasma loss; burns; severe vomiting; or diarrhea
Obstructive	Extracardiac obstruction of blood flow	Aortic dissection; cardiac tamponade; pulmonary embolism
Septic	Increased venous capacitance	Gram-negative endotoxemia; direct toxic injury; DIC
Neurogenic	Massive peripheral vasodilation	Severe cerebral, brain stem, or spinal cord injury
Anaphylactic	Increased venous capacitance stimulated by histamine release	Type I hypersensitivity reaction to exogenous stimulus (e.g., food allergy, bee sting)
DIC=diffuse intravascular coagulation.		

IV. Clinical Manifestations of Shock
A. Acute tubular necrosis
B. Necrosis in the brain
C. Fatty change in the heart and liver
D. Patchy hemorrhages in the colon
E. Pulmonary edema

CARDIOVASCULAR MANIFESTATIONS OF SYSTEMIC DISEASES (Table 3-12)

Marasmus (calorie deficiency) and kwashiorkor (protein deficiency with or without calorie deficiency) are profound states of malnutrition.

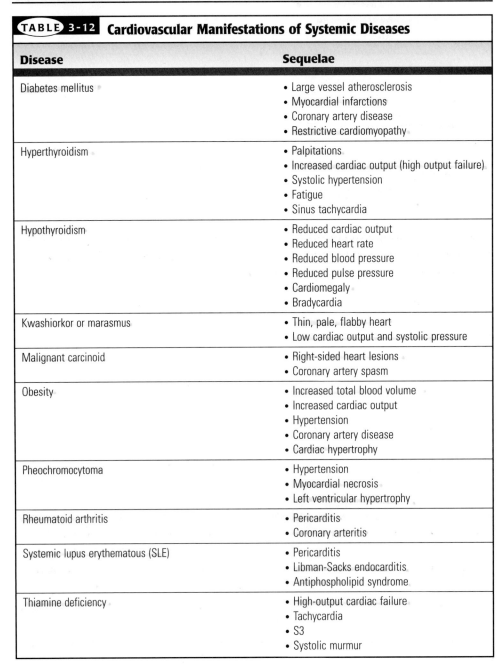

TABLE 3-12	Cardiovascular Manifestations of Systemic Diseases
Disease	**Sequelae**
Diabetes mellitus	• Large vessel atherosclerosis • Myocardial infarctions • Coronary artery disease • Restrictive cardiomyopathy
Hyperthyroidism	• Palpitations • Increased cardiac output (high output failure) • Systolic hypertension • Fatigue • Sinus tachycardia
Hypothyroidism	• Reduced cardiac output • Reduced heart rate • Reduced blood pressure • Reduced pulse pressure • Cardiomegaly • Bradycardia
Kwashiorkor or marasmus	• Thin, pale, flabby heart • Low cardiac output and systolic pressure
Malignant carcinoid	• Right-sided heart lesions • Coronary artery spasm
Obesity	• Increased total blood volume • Increased cardiac output • Hypertension • Coronary artery disease • Cardiac hypertrophy
Pheochromocytoma	• Hypertension • Myocardial necrosis • Left ventricular hypertrophy
Rheumatoid arthritis	• Pericarditis • Coronary arteritis
Systemic lupus erythematous (SLE)	• Pericarditis • Libman-Sacks endocarditis • Antiphospholipid syndrome
Thiamine deficiency	• High-output cardiac failure • Tachycardia • S3 • Systolic murmur

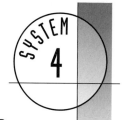

The Respiratory System

DEVELOPMENT

I. The lung bud forms from the foregut during week 4 of embryologic development.

II. The lining of the lower respiratory tract is derived from endoderm, whereas the connective tissue cartilage and muscle are derived from mesoderm.

III. Normal development causes the lung bud to completely separate from the esophagus at the level of the larynx.

IV. Incomplete separation causes a tracheoesophageal (TE) fistula (Figure 4-1).

FIGURE
4-1   Tracheoesophageal fistula

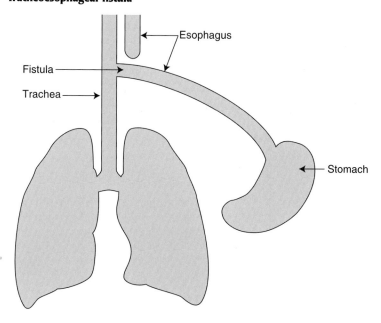

A. In the most common form of TE fistula, the esophagus ends in blind pouch and air enters the stomach.
B. Signs and symptoms of the most common form of TE fistula:
1. Copious secretions
2. Possible aspiration with respiratory distress
3. Inability to pass nasogastric tube

93

V. Stages of bronchial development

A. **Pseudoglandular period** (5–17 weeks)

1. During this period, the primary bronchi are formed, followed by secondary, tertiary, and segmental bronchi.
2. Bronchi appear as glandlike structures organized in tubules.
3. Respiration is not yet possible in this stage.

B. **Canalicular period** (15–25 weeks)

1. Respiratory bronchioles and terminal sacs begin to develop.
2. Vascular structures begin to form around sacs.
3. Respiration is possible only in the very latest weeks.

C. **Terminal sac period** (24 weeks to birth)

1. Vascular structures and terminal sacs continue to proliferate.
2. Cells differentiate into type I (blood–air barrier) and type II (surfactant-producing) pneumocytes.
3. Respiration is possible **after week 25.**
4. The amount of surfactant is the primary determinant of survival.

D. **Alveolar period** (29 weeks—8 years of age)

1. The majority of alveoli develop after birth.
2. As the child grows, the lung increases in size as a result of proliferation of respiratory bronchioles and terminal sacs.

VI. Diaphragm muscle

A. This is the primary muscle used for breathing.
B. The diaphragm muscle separates the pleural and peritoneal cavities.
C. It is formed from fusion of the following structures:

1. **Septum transversum**
2. Paired **pleuroperitoneal membranes**
3. **Dorsal mesentery** of the **esophagus**
4. **Body wall**

D. It is innervated by the phrenic nerve (C3, C4, and C5).
E. Improper formation of this muscle can lead to a **diaphragmatic hernia,** a condition with serious complications.

1. Abdominal contents are forced into the pleural cavity.
2. Lung hypoplasia results.
3. Hernias appear most often on the **left side** (posterolateral).
4. Diaphragmatic hernia is associated with polyhydramnios.
5. Diaphragmatic hernia presents at birth as a flattened abdomen, cyanosis, and inability to breathe.

The primary molecule of surfactant is dipalmitoyl-phosphatidylcholine (lecithin). A lecithin-to-sphingomyelin ratio of 2:1 is the normal ratio of surfactant molecules in a newborn. A ratio below 2:1 can result in neonatal respiratory distress, especially in cesarean section delivery.

The sternocleidomastoid and the internal and external intercostals are accessory muscles of respiration. They are used when there is an increased demand for oxygen (such as in exercise) or in disease states.

PHYSICS AND FUNCTION OF THE LUNG

I. Lung volumes

A. Capacities and volumes in the normal lung (Figure 4-2)

FIGURE 4-2 **Lung volumes**

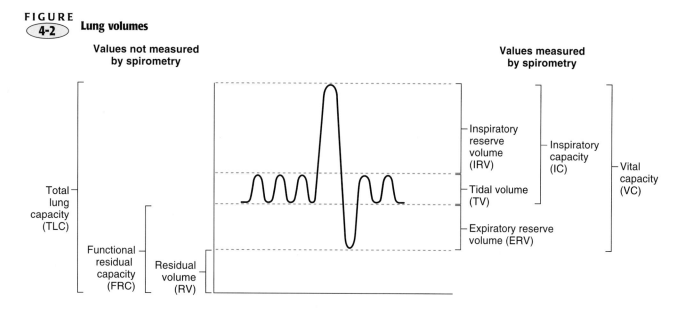

B. Volumes and pressure during the breathing cycle (Figure 4-3)

FIGURE 4-3 **Breathing cycle**

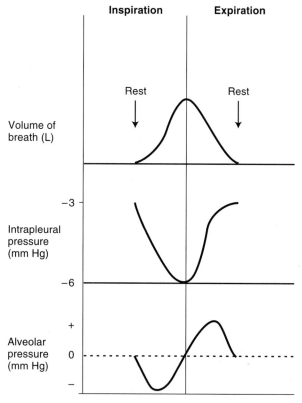

(Redrawn from Costanzo LS. BRS Physiology. Baltimore: Williams & Wilkins, 1995:113.)

C. Spirometry tracing—normal versus diseased (Figure 4-4)

FIGURE
4-4 **Spirometry tracings: normal versus diseased**

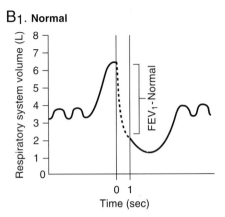

B₁. **Normal**

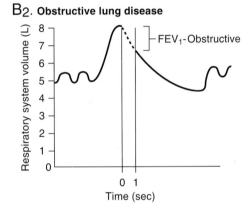

B₂. **Obstructive lung disease**

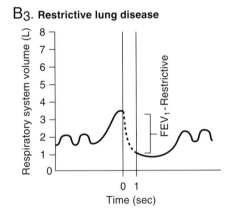

B₃. **Restrictive lung disease**

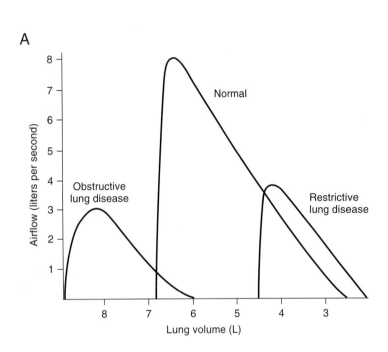

A

FEV_1=forced expiratory volume in 1 second

II. Compliance

A. Defined as $\Delta V/\Delta P$, where V is volume and P is pressure, compliance describes the ability of the chest wall and lung to expand when stretched.

1. At functional residual capacity (FRC), the lungs have a tendency to collapse.

2. This force is balanced by the chest wall, which has a tendency to expand.

3. Low compliance implies a stiff chest wall or lung (seen in **pulmonary fibrosis**).

4. High compliance implies a flaccid lung (seen in **emphysema;** see Figure 4-4).

B. **Surfactant** plays an important role in lung compliance.
1. Alveoli have a tendency to collapse.
2. An alveolus with a small radius has more collapsing pressure than an alveolus with a large radius, according to **Laplace's law:**

$$P \propto T/r$$

where P is pressure required to prevent alveolar collapse, T is surface tension, and r is alveolar radius.
3. Surfactant reduces the pressure and prevents collapse by reducing the intermolecular forces between liquid molecules lining the alveoli.
4. Surfactant increases compliance and allows the alveoli to expand.
5. **Neonatal respiratory distress** occurs in premature infants (<37 weeks) because **type II** (surfactant-producing) **pneumocytes** are not yet fully developed and fail to produce sufficient surfactant.
6. Atelectasis (collapsed alveoli) results from neonatal respiratory distress syndrome.

III. Airway resistance

A. Airway resistance (R) is inversely proportional to the fourth power of the radius (r) (formula: $R \propto 1/r^4$); thus, any mechanism that decreases the radius of the bronchi will greatly affect the airway resistance.
B. **The airway radius** is under the control of the parasympathetic and sympathetic nervous systems.
1. **Parasympathetic nervous system**
a. Causes **constriction** of the airways
b. Mediated by direct stimulation, airway irritation, and slow-reacting substance of anaphylaxis (SRS-A)
c. Stimulates mucus secretion
2. **Sympathetic nervous system**
a. Causes **dilation** of airways
b. Used as treatment for allergy and asthma (β_2-agonists)
c. Functions in fight-or-flight autonomic reflexes; dilates airways to help provide oxygen in times of stress

IV. Ventilation and perfusion

A. **Ventilation/perfusion ($\dot{V}/\dot{Q}$) ratio:** the ratio of the rate of alveolar ventilation to the rate of pulmonary blood flow.
B. Varies over the entire lung (higher in the apices, lower in the bases in an upright patient), but is 0.8 on average
C. Airway obstruction
1. Causes a reduction in ventilation
2. $\dot{V}/\dot{Q}$ is reduced (to 0 in complete airway occlusion).
3. A $\dot{V}/\dot{Q}$ of 0 is considered a shunt and no gas exchange will occur (areas are perfused, but not ventilated).
D. Blood flow obstruction
1. Blockage of a pulmonary artery or smaller vessel causes a reduction in perfusion.
2. A perfusion value of 0 yields an infinite $\dot{V}/\dot{Q}$ ratio.
3. A $\dot{V}/\dot{Q}$ of infinity is considered **physiologic dead space.**
E. Pulmonary embolism results in increased $\dot{V}/\dot{Q}$ ratio.
F. Blood flow and ventilation vary over the regions of the lung (Figure 4-5).

Allergies and allergic asthma release histamine, which is a powerful constrictor of airway smooth muscle and causes increased airway resistance.

SRS-A is a combination of the leukotrienes C_4 and D_4 (LTC_4 and LTD_4). In the treatment of asthma, zileuton blocks production of leukotrienes by inhibiting the lipoxygenase enzyme, whereas zafirlukast blocks leukotriene receptors. Leukotriene A_4 (LTA_4) is a precursor to leukotriene B_4 (LTB_4), LTC_4, and LTD_4. LTB_4 is responsible for chemotaxis of neutrophils and adhesion of white blood cells.

Anatomic shunts are passageways of blood flow that go from the venous circulation to the arterial circulation without passing through the lungs. Normally about 2% of the cardiac output is shunted. However, it can be as much as 50% in certain congenital malformations (e.g., tetralogy of Fallot produces a right to left shunt).

There are two types of dead space:
(1) **Anatomic dead space,** measured by the **Fowler method,** is usually about 150 mL.
(2) **Physiologic dead space,** measured by the **Bohr method,** is considered to be the volume of the lung that does not eliminate CO_2.

THE RESPIRATORY SYSTEM

During exercise, pulmonary vascular resistance decreases as a result of dilation of the lung arterioles by metabolic products. The $\dot{V}/\dot{Q}$ ratio becomes uniform over the entire lung. Conversely, during hypoxia, lack of oxygen constricts local lung vasculature, thus increasing pulmonary vascular resistance; this is opposite of what takes place in the systemic circulation, where lack of oxygen results in vasodilation.

FIGURE 4-5 Pulmonary circulation

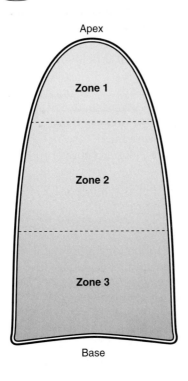

Zone 1
- Lowest blood flow
- Alveolar pressure > Arterial pressure > Venous pressure
- Capillaries collapse due to high alveolar pressure
- Ventilation ($\dot{V}$) is decreased less than blood flow [also called perfusion ($\dot{Q}$)]

so: $\dfrac{\dot{V}}{\dot{Q}} = \dfrac{\downarrow}{\downarrow\downarrow} = \uparrow$ (Ventilation in excess of perfusion)

Zone 2
- Blood flow is higher than Zone 1, but lower than Zone 3
- Arterial pressure > Alveolar pressure > Venous pressure
- Capillaries remain open because arterial pressure is greater than alveolar pressure
- Ventilation ($\dot{V}$) is approximately equivalent to perfusion ($\dot{Q}$)

so: $\dfrac{\dot{V}}{\dot{Q}} \approx 1$

Zone 3
- Highest blood flow
- Arterial pressure > Venous pressure > Alveolar pressure
- Capillaries remain open because arterial pressure is higher than both alveolar and venous pressure
- Ventilation ($\dot{V}$) is increased less than perfusion ($\dot{Q}$)

so: $\dfrac{\dot{V}}{\dot{Q}} = \dfrac{\uparrow}{\uparrow\uparrow} = \downarrow$ (Perfusion in excess of ventilation)

CONTROL OF BREATHING

I. Medulla
A. Mediates inspiration and expiration
B. Generates the basic breathing rhythm
C. Receives input via the vagus and glossopharyngeal nerves
D. Sends output via the **phrenic** nerve to the diaphragm and via the spinal nerve to the intercostals and abdominal wall
E. The cerebral cortex can override the medulla and provide voluntary control of breathing if desired.

II. The central nervous system seeks to keep PaO₂ (partial pressure of arterial oxygen) and PaCO₂ (partial pressure of arterial CO₂) within a narrow range.

III. Depth and rate of respiration control these variables.
A. **Central control**
1. Chemoreceptors in the **medulla** sense the pH of the cerebrospinal fluid.
2. CO_2 crosses the blood–brain barrier and increases the **H⁺ concentration** (which decreases the pH).
3. Increases in [H⁺] directly stimulate the central chemoreceptors, which stimulate breathing.
4. Decreases in [H⁺] reduce stimulation of the receptors and slow respiration.
B. **Peripheral control**
1. Chemoreceptors in the **carotid bodies** and at the aortic arch bifurcation sense changes in Pa_{O_2}, Pa_{CO_2}, and [H⁺].
2. Decreases in **Pao₂** below 60 mm Hg stimulate the peripheral chemoreceptors to increase rate and depth of breathing (in the absence of lung disease, decreased Pa_{O_2} is rarely the driving force for respiration).

3. Increases in **Paco$_2$** potentiate peripheral chemoreceptor response to Pao$_2$ (major direct effect of changes in Paco$_2$ is on the central chemoreceptors).

4. Increases in arterial [H$^+$] directly stimulate the chemoreceptors, independent of the Paco$_2$ (causes increased respiration in metabolic acidosis).

5. Stimulation of irritant receptors in large airways and stretch receptors in small airways inhibits inspiration.

C. **Abnormal breathing**

1. **Cheyne-Stokes breathing**
   a. Tidal volumes variably increase and decrease and are separated by a period of apnea.
   b. This breathing abnormality is associated with drug overdose, hypoxia, and CNS depression.

2. **Kussmaul's breathing**
   a. Rate and depth of respiration are **increased.**
   b. This abnormality is associated with diabetic ketoacidosis (DKA) and other forms of metabolic acidosis.

3. **Sleep apnea**
   a. **Obstructive sleep apnea**
      (1) Risk factors
         (a) Middle age
         (b) Male
         (c) Obesity
         (d) Smoker
         (e) History of hypertension
         (f) History of pharyngeal malformations
         (g) Use of alcohol and other drugs
      (2) **Characteristics**
         (a) Ventilatory effort exists.
         (b) Airway is obstructed.
         (c) Apnea is terminated by self-arousal.
         (d) Apnea usually occurs in the nasopharynx or oropharynx when muscles relax during rapid eye movement (REM) sleep.

   b. **Central sleep apnea**
      (1) Ventilatory effort does not exist.
      (2) Airway is not obstructed.
      (3) Patient does not arouse self.
      (4) Central sleep apnea, like obstructive sleep apnea, occurs in the REM stage of sleep.
      (5) It is carbon dioxide threshold dependent—there is decreased chemoreceptor sensitivity to O$_2$ and CO$_2$ concentrations.

   c. **Therapy** includes weight loss (for obstructive sleep apnea), continuous positive airway pressure (CPAP), and, in some cases, tricyclic antidepressants.

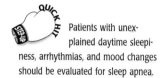

Patients with unexplained daytime sleepiness, arrhythmias, and mood changes should be evaluated for sleep apnea.

IV. Gas exchange

A. Diffusion of gas depends on the **partial pressure difference** between the gas in the alveolus and the gas in the blood (i.e., the difference in pressure across the blood–air barrier).

B. Partial pressure

1. The alveolar partial pressure of oxygen (Pao$_2$) can be calculated as follows:

$$\text{Pao}_2 = (760 \text{ mm Hg} - 47 \text{ mm Hg}) \text{ Fio}_2 - (\text{Paco}_2/0.8)$$

where 760 mm Hg = total atmospheric pressure (at sea level)
47 mm Hg = partial pressure of completely humidified air as found in the alveoli

The blood–air barrier is made up of:
(1) Membrane and cytoplasm of type I pneumocytes
(2) Fused basement membrane of type I pneumocytes and endothelial cells
(3) Membrane and cytoplasm of endothelial cells.

F_{IO_2} = percent of air that is oxygen (normally 0.21 at sea level)

PA_{CO_2} = partial pressure of CO_2 in the alveoli (normally 40)

and 0.8 = ratio of volume of CO_2 produced to the volume of O_2 consumed

2. For O_2, higher pressures will force more oxygen into the blood and allow it to equilibrate more readily.
3. For CO_2, higher partial pressures in the blood (or lower in the alveoli) will force more CO_2 out of the blood and into the lungs, where it can be expired.
4. The amount of O_2 delivered to the tissues are also determined by hemoglobin concentration and red blood cell number (hematocrit) (see System 10, "Hematopoietic and Lymphoreticular System").

C. Disease affects diffusion capacity of the lung.
1. Fibrosis causes a thickening of the interstitium, which hinders diffusion across the blood–air barrier.
2. Emphysema destroys the alveolar walls and decreases the area available for gas exchange.

LUNG DEFENSES

I. Anatomic barriers

A. Impaction
1. Large particles **greater than 10 μm** fail to turn the corners of respiratory tract.
2. Common site: **nasopharynx**

B. Sedimentation
1. Medium particles between **2 and 10 μm** settle as a result of weight.
2. Common site: **small airways**

C. Diffusion
1. Small particles between **0.5 and 2 μm** are engulfed by alveolar macrophages (dust cells).
2. Common site: **alveoli**

D. Suspension: particles **less than 0.5 μm** remain suspended in air.

II. Nonspecific

A. **Mucociliary escalator**
1. Particles are trapped in gel layer of upper airway.
2. Ciliary motion removes particles.

B. **Cough**
1. Cough is a bronchoconstriction that occurs to prevent penetration of particles.
2. It is also defined as deep inspiration followed by forced expiration.
3. The cough reflex can be suppressed by antitussive agents such as opioids (see Chapter 8, "Musculoskeletal System").
4. Specific mechanisms include **secretory IgA** and complement.

The right main bronchus is more vertically oriented than the left main bronchus, and is therefore more commonly the path taken by aspirated particles.

Slow, deep breaths increase the deposition of dust by sedimentation and diffusion, whereas exercise results in higher rates of airflow and increased deposition by impaction.

ADULT RESPIRATORY DISTRESS SYNDROME AND NEONATAL RESPIRATORY DISTRESS SYNDROME

This group of diseases often leads to respiratory failure and death (Table 4-1).

TABLE 4-1	Adult Respiratory Distress Syndrome (ARDS) and Neonatal Respiratory Distress Syndrome (NRDS)	
	ARDS **(Diffuse Alveolar Damage)**	**NRDS** **(Hyaline Membrane Disease)**
Age group	*Adults*	*Premature infants*
Causes	**Shock, infection, trauma,** oxygen toxicity (free radical damage), or aspiration	**Lack of surfactant** production
Pathophysiology	Impaired gas exchange caused by pulmonary hemorrhage, pulmonary edema, or atelectasis	Increased work to expand lungs; infant can clear lungs of fluids, but cannot fill lungs with air; atelectasis
Features	Respiratory insufficiency; cyanosis; hypoxemia; heavy, wet lungs; diffuse pulmonary infiltrates on radiograph; hyaline membranes in alveoli; pneumothorax may result—may be rapid and fatal	Respiratory insufficiency; cyanosis; hypoxemia; heavy, wet lungs; diffuse pulmonary infiltrates on radiograph; hyaline membranes in alveoli

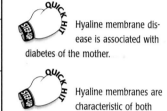

Hyaline membrane disease is associated with diabetes of the mother.

Hyaline membranes are characteristic of both ARDS and NRDS but are caused by distinctly different pathologic mechanisms.

PNEUMOTHORAX

I. Simple pneumothorax
A. May be caused by **spontaneous** rupture of a bleb (congenital or secondary to paraseptal emphysema) or penetrating trauma
B. Is most commonly seen in **men 20–40 years of age**
C. Presents as sudden chest pain, shortness of breath, **cough,** and no breath sounds over the affected lung
D. Has a 50% recurrence rate
E. Treatment includes monitoring small defects and chest tube with vacuum for larger defects.

II. Tension pneumothorax
A. A flap of tissue allows air to enter pleural space but not to escape.
B. Pressure builds, the mediastinum is displaced, the **trachea deviates away from the lesion,** jugular venous distention (JVD) occurs, and breath sounds are uneven.
C. Cardiovascular and respiratory compromise may be rapidly **fatal.**

III. Open sucking chest wound
A. Penetrating trauma to the chest wall and pleura can cause this condition.
B. If the diameter of the lesion approaches the diameter of the trachea, air will preferentially enter through the defect.

Flail chest is caused by multiple fractures of four or more consecutive ribs and leads to paradoxical movement of the injured area of the chest wall with respiration.

PULMONARY VASCULAR DISEASES

There are a variety of diseases that primarily affect the vasculature of the lungs (Table 4-2).

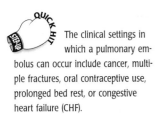

The clinical settings in which a pulmonary embolus can occur include cancer, multiple fractures, oral contraceptive use, prolonged bed rest, or congestive heart failure (CHF).

Fat emboli are often caused by crush injury with fracture of the long bones and orthopedic surgery.

TABLE 4-2 Pulmonary Vascular Diseases

Disease	Etiology	Features	Complications
Pulmonary hypertension	Primary—unknown etiology Secondary—owing to COPD or increased pulmonary blood flow (as seen with a left to right shunt)	Loud **S2** **Right ventricular hypertrophy** Heart-failure cells	Leads to **cor pulmonale**
Pulmonary embolism	Commonly from proximal **deep vein thrombosis** (usually lower limb) as a result of **Virchow's triad:** blood stasis, endothelial damage (fat, infection, trauma), and hypercoagulable states	**Hemorrhagic,** red, wedge-shaped infarct Acute-onset dyspnea, chest pain, tachycardia, hypotension $\dot{V}/\dot{Q}$ ratio approaches infinity Saddle embolus—an embolus lodged at the pulmonary artery bifurcation, often fatal	Can lead to cardio-vascular collapse and sudden death
Pulmonary edema	Obliteration of alveoli as a result of intra-alveolar accumulation of fluid	Heart failure or overload leads to **increased hydrostatic pressure** Inflammatory alveolar reactions (owing to drugs, pneumonia, sepsis, and uremia) leads to **increased capillary permeability**	Hypoxia
Wegener's granulomatosus	Etiology is unknown but thought to be autoimmune in nature	Focal necrotizing **vasculitis** affecting small- to medium-sized vessels Acute necrotizing **granulomas of upper and lower respiratory tract** Bilateral nodular and cavitary infiltrates seen on chest radiograph Mucosal ulceration of nasopharynx seen on examination Associated with c-ANCA	Untreated disease is fatal within several years

c-ANCA=cytoplasmic antineutrophil cytoplasmic antibody.

CHRONIC OBSTRUCTIVE PULMONARY DISEASE (COPD)

I. Types of COPD (Table 4-3)

TABLE 4-3 Types of Chronic Obstructive Pulmonary Disease (COPD)		
Disease	**Pathophysiology**	**Clinical Features and Management**
Asthma	**Increased sensitivity** of bronchioles; muscle hypertrophy; airway mucus plugs and **Charcot-Leyden crystals**	**Wheezing;** shortness of breath; common treatment options include inhaled steroids and β_2-agonists
Bronchitis	Caused by persistent irritants and infections; hyperplasia of goblet cells and submucosal glands **(increased Reid index); excess mucus;** possible cor pulmonale	"Blue bloater"; defined as a **productive cough** for 3 consecutive months over 2 consecutive years; patients must quit **smoking** *→ peripheral*
Emphysema	Dilated alveoli; damaged alveolar walls; **decreased elastic recoil;** centrilobular, panacinar (α_1-antitrypsin deficiency), paraseptal, and irregular forms	"Pink puffer"; paraseptal type may lead to pneumothorax; patients must quit **smoking**
Bronchiectasis	**Irreversible,** pathologic bronchial dilation; chronic infection; destruction of bronchial wall; commonly caused by bronchial **obstruction** (e.g., tumor)	Purulent sputum; hemoptysis; possible lung abscess; associated with cystic fibrosis and Kartagener's syndrome

COPD is characterized by **airflow obstruction.** This is in contrast to restrictive pulmonary diseases, which demonstrate **defective lung expansion.** Obstructive disorders have increased TLC, decreased FEV$_1$, and decreased FEV$_1$/FVC. Restrictive disorders show reduced lung volumes and normal or increased FEV$_1$/FVC.

Status asthmaticus is a prolonged asthmatic attack that does not respond to therapy and can be fatal.

There are many types of asthma: extrinsic (children), intrinsic (adults), exercise-induced, or cold air–induced.

Emphysema and bronchitis often coexist in the same patient.

II. Therapeutic agents used in asthma

A. Inhaled agents

1. β_2-Agonists

   a. β_2-Agonists are useful for treatment for an acute asthma attack characterized by shortness of breath, chest tightness, wheezing, and cough as a result of bronchoconstriction.

      (1) The β_2-agonists stimulate adenylyl cyclase resulting in the conversion of ATP to cAMP; the increased levels of cAMP result in a myriad of effects depending on the cell type in question.

      (2) β_2-Agonists are potent dilators of the bronchi. They act by relaxing smooth muscle in the airways.

      (3) Systemic activation of β_2-specific receptors (which is minimal with inhaled β_2-agonists) may result in vasodilation, a slight decrease in peripheral resistance, bronchodilation, increased glycogenolysis in muscle and in the liver, increased release of glucagon, and relaxation of uterine smooth muscle.

   b. Side effects include tachycardia, hyperglycemia, hypokalemia, and hypomagnesemia.

   c. β_2-Agonists have no effect on the inflammation associated with asthma.

   d. Selected β_2-agonists

      (1) **Albuterol** or **terbutaline** provides immediate relief of acute attacks without α_1-adrenoceptor or β_1-adrenoceptor stimulation.

      (2) **Salmeterol** has a longer duration of action and a slower onset of action.

2. Corticosteroids

   a. In cases of moderate asthma, corticosteroids (inhaled or systemic) can be used to decrease the associated inflammation.

b. Inhaled corticosteroids such as beclomethasone, triamcinolone, and flunisolide decrease the effect that inflammatory cells (mast cells, eosinophils, macrophages) have on the airway.

c. In cases of severe asthma, intravenous methylprednisolone or oral prednisone may be necessary for a short period.

d. The side effects of inhaled steroids are minimal when compared with systemic steroid use. However, adverse reactions can occur and include oral candidiasis, and, with long-term use, osteoporosis.

B. Other asthma medications
   1. **Cromolyn,** a prophylactic anti-inflammatory agent
   2. **Ipratropium,** a derivative of atropine that blocks the vagal aspect of airway smooth muscle contraction and mucous secretion
   3. **Theophylline,** a bronchodilator, which may result in seizures and arrhythmias
   4. Newer agents
      a. **Zileuton,** a 5-lipoxygenase inhibitor, blocks the conversion of arachidonic acid into leukotrienes, which are responsible for chemotaxis, increased secretion, and bronchospasm.
      b. **Zafirlukast** prevents the chemotactic and bronchospastic effects of leukotriene D_4 (LTD$_4$) by blocking its receptor.

INTERSTITIAL LUNG DISEASE (ILD) (Table 4-4)

ILD is a noninfectious, nonmalignant condition characterized by inflammation and pathologic changes of the alveolar wall. Differentiation and diagnosis often require histologic evaluation of the lung.

Order of β-agonist potency (most potent to least potent): isoproterenol, epinephrine, norepinephrine. Order of α-agonist potency: epinephrine, norepinephrine, isoproterenol.

β$_2$-Selective agents such as terbutaline can be used in premature labor to prevent contractions.

Interstitial lung disease can be a side effect of bleomycin, methotrexate, and amiodarone.

Interstitial lung diseases demonstrate alveolar wall fibrosis.

Eosinophilic granuloma, Letterer-Siwe, and Hand-Schüller-Christian are all subsets of histiocytosis X.

Sarcoidosis patients often demonstrate **anergy** when challenged with the tuberculin skin test, despite a polyclonal hyperglobulinemia.

TABLE 4-4   Interstitial Lung Disease

Disease	Pathophysiology	Population Most at Risk	Clinical Features
Eosinophilic granuloma	Presence of Langerhans-like cells and **Birbeck granules;** subset of histiocytosis X	Former **smokers**	Lesions in lung or ribs; pneumothorax
Goodpasture's syndrome	Pulmonary hemorrhage; anemia; glomerulonephritis; **anti-basement membrane antibodies**	Males; middle-aged people	**Hemoptysis;** hematuria
Idiopathic pulmonary fibrosis	Chronic **inflammation of alveolar wall;** fibrosis; cystic spaces	Sixth decade of life	**Honeycomb lung;** fatal within years
Sarcoidosis	Interstitial fibrosis; diagnosis based on biopsy showing **noncaseating granulomatous lesions;** uveitis; polyarthritis	**Young black females**	Dyspnea on exertion, dry cough, fever, fatigue, and bilateral hilar lymphadenopathy
Hypersensitivity pneumonitis (farmer's lung)	Prolonged exposure to organic antigens in atopic individuals; interstitial inflammation; alveolar damage leads to chronic, fibrotic lung	People with an occupational history of farming or bird-keeping	**Dry cough, chest tightness,** general malaise, and fever

THE RESPIRATORY SYSTEM

ENVIRONMENTAL LUNG DISEASES (PNEUMOCONIOSIS) (Table 4-5)

This group of diseases is often caused by workplace exposure to various organic and chemical irritants. A careful history and pulmonary function testing are often important for diagnosis.

TABLE 4-5	Environmental Lung Diseases (Pneumoconiosis)	
Disease	**Pathophysiology**	**Clinical Features**
Anthracosis	Carbon dust ingested by alveolar macrophages; visible **black deposits**	Usually asymptomatic
Asbestosis	Asbestos fibers ingested by alveolar macrophages; fibroblast proliferation; interstitial fibrosis (lower lobes); **asbestos bodies and ferruginous bodies;** pleural plaques and effusions	Increased risk of bronchogenic carcinoma and **malignant mesothelioma;** synergistic effect of asbestos and tobacco
Coal worker's pneumoconiosis	Carbon dust ingested by alveolar macrophages forms bronchiolar **macules;** may progress to fibrosis	Plaques are asymptomatic; often benign, may progress to fibrosis; may be fatal owing to pulmonary hypertension and **cor pulmonale**
Silicosis	Silica dust ingested by alveolar macrophages causing release of harmful enzymes; **silicotic nodules**	Nodules may obstruct air or blood flow; concurrent tuberculosis common **(silicotuberculosis)**
Berylliosis	Induction of cell-mediated immunity leads to noncaseating granulomas; several organ systems affected; histologically identical to sarcoidosis	Increases lung cancer

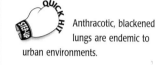

Anthracotic, blackened lungs are endemic to urban environments.

Silicosis is an **occupational** disease seen in individuals involved in mining, stonecutting, and glass production.

RESPIRATORY INFECTIONS

I. Pneumonia

A. Pathogenesis
1. Most commonly, pneumonia is caused by **aspiration** from the oropharynx.
2. Alcoholism, nasogastric tubes, and obtunded states increase risk of contracting pneumonia.
3. Normal flora consists of Gram-positive cocci.
4. Hospitalized patients are colonized by Gram-negative rods (nosocomial infections).
5. Other portals of entry include respiratory droplets, contiguous spread, or traumatic inoculation.

B. **Clinical manifestations**
1. **Typical pneumonia** presents with acute fever, purulent sputum, pleuritic pain, and lobar "whited out" infiltrate on chest radiograph (e.g., *Streptococcus pneumoniae*).
2. **Atypical pneumonia** is characterized by slow onset of nonproductive cough, headache, gastrointestinal (GI) symptoms, and diffuse patchy infiltrate on chest radiograph (e.g., *Mycoplasma pneumoniae*).

C. Location of pathology and typical organisms
1. **Lobar** (intra-alveolar infiltrate): *S. pneumoniae*
2. **Bronchopneumonia** (bronchiolar infiltrate): *Staphylococcus aureus, Haemophilus influenza*
3. **Interstitial** (diffuse infiltrate in alveolar wall): *M. pneumoniae*

D. Etiology
  1. Bacterial and *Mycoplasma* pneumonias (Table 4-6)
  2. Viral pneumonia (Table 4-7)
  3. Fungal pneumonia (Table 4-8)
E. Clinical diagnosis of pneumonia (Table 4-9 and Table 4-10)

TABLE 4-6   Bacterial and Mycoplasma Pneumonia

Bacteria	Presentation	Population Most at Risk	Clinical Features
Streptococcus pneumoniae	Typical	**Adults**	Most common cause of pneumonia
Haemophilus influenzae	Typical	Elderly	Complicates viral infection; chronic respiratory disease
Staphylococcus aureus	Typical	Can cause typical community-acquired pneumonia but also infects immunocompromised and hospitalized patients	Abscesses; complicates viral infection
Streptococcus agalactiae	Typical	**Neonates** (along with *Escherichia coli*)	Similar to *S. pneumoniae*
Mycoplasma pneumoniae	Atypical	**Young adults**	Most common cause of atypical pneumonia; positive cold-agglutinin test
Legionella pneumophila	Atypical	Immunocompromised patients	Found in drinking water and air conditioners
Klebsiella pneumoniae	Atypical	Patients with alcoholism	Aspiration of gastric contents
Chlamydia psittaci	Atypical	**Pet bird** owners	Bradycardia; splenomegaly
Chlamydia trachomatis	Atypical	Neonates	Most common cause of preventable blindness (trachoma)
Chlamydia pneumoniae	Atypical	Young adults	Upper and lower pulmonary tract infection
Coxiella burnetii	Atypical	Dairy workers (via inhalation)	Fever
Francisella tularensis	Atypical	Hunters, veterinarians, livestock workers	Granulomatous nodules

TABLE 4-7   Viral Pneumonia

Virus	Pathophysiology	Clinical Features
Respiratory syncytial virus (types 1 and 2)	Atypical	Also causes bronchiolitis; more common in winter months; can cause serious respiratory distress in infants
Influenza	Atypical	**Often complicated by secondary bacterial infection**

QUICK HIT

Aspirin therapy for the fever of influenza and varicella zoster infections in children is contraindicated as it may cause Reye's syndrome. Clinical manifestations of Reye's syndrome include encephalopathy and potentially fatal liver damage.

TABLE 4-8 **Fungal Pneumonia**

Etiology	Pathophysiology	Clinical Features
Histoplasma capsulatum	Atypical	Most infections are subclinical; organisms in macrophages
Coccidioides immitis	Atypical	Most infections are subclinical; "valley fever"
Pneumocystis carinii	Atypical	Often fatal common opportunistic infection in immunocompromised patients (such as HIV patients)

QUICK HIT

Other less common sources of fungal lung infection include *Cryptococcus neoformans* and *Aspergillus* (resulting in a **fungus ball**) in immunocompromised individuals.

QUICK HIT

Pneumocystis carinii is sometimes classified as a parasite.

TABLE 4-9 **Clinical Diagnosis of Pneumonia**

	Bacterial	Viral	Mycoplasma
Age	Any; often under 2 years	Any	Young adults
Fever	>39°C	<39°C	<39°C
Onset	Abrupt	Gradual	Gradual fever; gradual cough
Relatives	Healthy	Sick (concurrent)	Sick (2–3 weeks previous)
Cough	Productive	Dry	Paroxysmal
Pleuritic chest pain	Yes (splinting)	No	No
Physical examination	Tubular breath sounds; dull to percussion	Bilateral, diffuse rales	Rales in one or two segments
Radiographic findings	Consolidated "whited out" lobe	Diffuse; patchy; bilateral	Patchy; one or two lobes; no consolidation

TABLE 4-10 **Most Common Causative Agents of Pneumonia by Age**

	Children (birth–20 years of age)	Young Adults (20–40 years of age)	Adults (40–60 years of age)	Elderly (60 years of age and older)
Causative agents in each age group	RSV *M. pneumoniae* *Chlamydia pneumoniae* *S. pneumoniae*	*M. pneumoniae* *S. pneumoniae*	*S. pneumoniae* *M. pneumoniae* *H. influenzae*	*S. pneumoniae* Anaerobes *H. influenzae* RSV

RSV=respiratory syncytial virus.

II. Tuberculosis and its treatment (Figure 4-6)

FIGURE
4-6 **Tuberculosis**

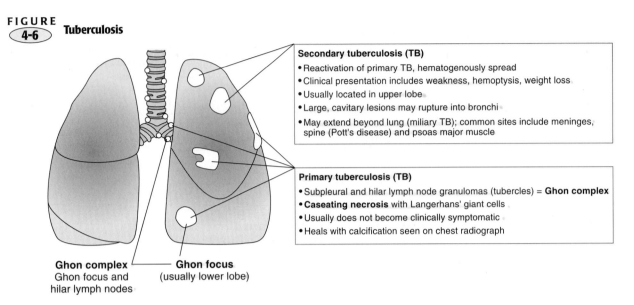

Secondary tuberculosis (TB)
- Reactivation of primary TB, hematogenously spread
- Clinical presentation includes weakness, hemoptysis, weight loss
- Usually located in upper lobe
- Large, cavitary lesions may rupture into bronchi
- May extend beyond lung (miliary TB); common sites include meninges, spine (Pott's disease) and psoas major muscle

Primary tuberculosis (TB)
- Subpleural and hilar lymph node granulomas (tubercles) = **Ghon complex**
- **Caseating necrosis** with Langerhans' giant cells
- Usually does not become clinically symptomatic
- Heals with calcification seen on chest radiograph

Ghon complex
Ghon focus and
hilar lymph nodes

Ghon focus
(usually lower lobe)

A. **Multiple drug therapy** is used for the treatment of tuberculosis in an effort to combat drug resistance.

B. One of the most common therapeutic regimens includes **isoniazid, rifampin,** and **pyrazinamide** for a period of 2 to 3 months, followed by isoniazid and rifampin for a period of 4 to 6 months.

C. Ethambutol may be added to the regimen to prevent development of resistance and increase the effectiveness of treatment.

1. Isoniazid (INH)
   a. INH, which diffuses into all body fluids, including breast milk, targets the outer layer of the mycobacteria.
   b. One of the most common side effects of INH therapy is paresthesias, which can be corrected by the administration of **pyridoxine** (vitamin B$_6$).

2. Rifampin
   a. Rifampin inhibits RNA synthesis by blocking the β subunit of bacterial DNA-dependent RNA polymerase.
   b. This agent also induces **cytochrome P-450** enzymes in the liver and can decrease the half-lives of other agents in this way.
   c. One of the side effects of rifampin is **orange-red color** of the stool or urine.

III. Upper respiratory infections

A. Sinusitis
   1. Results from obstructed drainage outlets of the sinuses
   2. Caused by *S. pneumoniae, H. influenzae, Moraxella*

B. Rhinitis
   1. Viral rhinitis
      a. Most commonly caused by **rhinoviruses and coronaviruses,** also by adenoviruses and parainfluenza viruses
      b. Common cold
   2. Bacterial rhinitis
      a. Often secondary to viral infection
      b. Commonly caused by *Streptococcus, Staphylococcus, H. influenzae*
   3. Allergic rhinitis
      a. Type 1 hypersensitivity reactions
      b. Characterized by eosinophilia

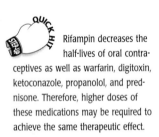

Rifampin decreases the half-lives of oral contraceptives as well as warfarin, digitoxin, ketoconazole, propanolol, and prednisone. Therefore, higher doses of these medications may be required to achieve the same therapeutic effect.

Sudden infant death syndrome (SIDS) is the death of a child under 1 year of age from unexplained causes (even after autopsy). The infant is usually asleep in the prone position and has a history of an **upper respiratory infection.**

THE RESPIRATORY SYSTEM

C. Laryngitis
1. Characterized by edema and inflammation of the vocal cords
2. Caused by infection (*M. pneumoniae*, parainfluenza virus) or overuse
D. Croup versus epiglottitis (Table 4-11)

TABLE 4-11	**Croup Versus Epiglottitis**	
	Croup	**Epiglottitis**
Organism	Parainfluenza type 2 virus	*H. influenzae*
Pathology	Inflammation of subglottic trachea	Inflamed epiglottis
Age	6 months to 2 years	1 to 5 years
Fever	<39°C	>39°C
Onset	Gradual (barking cough to **stridor**)	Abrupt; **stridor**
Associated symptoms	Rhinorrhea; hoarseness; conjunctivitis	None
Degree of illness	Not toxic; degree of symptoms greater than degree of illness	Toxic
Physical examination	Writhing; anxious; subglottic edema on radiograph	Quiet; **"sniffing position"**; drooling; "thumb-print" epiglottis on radiograph
Outcome	Self-limiting	Medical emergency; 90% of patients require surgery to reestablish airway

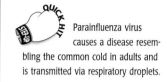

Parainfluenza virus causes a disease resembling the common cold in adults and is transmitted via respiratory droplets.

CYSTIC FIBROSIS (CF)

I. CF is the **most common lethal genetic disease in whites.**

II. Autosomal recessive mutation occurs on chromosome 7, the cystic fibrosis **transmembrane conductance regulator (CFTR) gene. This leads to**
A. Altered **chloride** and water transport in cells
B. Deletion of phenylalanine at position 508 (**ΔF508**)
C. High sodium and chloride concentrations on sweat test
D. Malfunction of exocrine glands increases mucus viscosity, which leads to organ malfunction

III. Chronic pulmonary disease
A. Most serious complication and **leading cause of death** in patients with CF.
B. *Pseudomonas aeruginosa* infections are common.
C. Increased residual volume (RV) and increased total lung capacity (TLC) are characteristic of chronic pulmonary disease.
D. Atelectasis
E. Bronchiectasis

IV. Pancreatic insufficiency
A. Nutritional deficiencies (especially of fat-soluble vitamins A, D, E, and K)
B. **Steatorrhea**

V. Meconium ileus

VI. Treatment of cystic fibrosis includes symptomatic treatment and gene therapy.

Superior sulcus tumors (**Pancoast's**) involve the apex of the lung and result in **Horner's syndrome** (ptosis, miosis, anhydrosis). **Superior vena cava syndrome** occurs when the superior vena cava is obstructed, resulting in facial cyanosis and swelling.

Nasopharyngeal carcinoma, common in Southeast Asia and East Africa, is caused by the Epstein-Barr virus.

Paraneoplastic syndrome is a clinical and biochemical disturbance caused by a neoplasm that is not directly related to the primary tumor or metastases. Secretion of parathyroid hormone (PTH)-like hormone results in hypercalcemia. Ectopic antidiuretic hormone (ADH) production leads to syndrome of inappropriate antidiuretic hormone (SIADH) with urinary retention and high urine osmolality. Adrenocorticotropic hormone (ACTH)-producing tumors lead to Cushing's syndrome.

LUNG NEOPLASMS (Table 4-12)

I. **Lung neoplasms** are the **leading cause of cancer death for both men and women in the United States.**

II. Lung is the **second most common type** of cancer (with the first being prostate cancer in men and breast cancer in women).

III. **Lung cancer deaths among women are rising rapidly as a result of increased smoking in this population.**

IV. **Symptoms include cough, hemoptysis, airway obstruction, weight loss, and paraneoplastic syndromes.**

TABLE 4-12 Lung Neoplasms

Tumor	Location and Histology	Clinical Features
Adenocarcinoma	**Peripheral;** subpleural; usually on preexisting **scars;** glandular	**Most common type;** may be related to smoking; CEA positive; K-ras oncogenes
Bronchioalveolar	**Peripheral;** subtype of adenocarcinoma; tumor cells line alveolar walls	**Less strongly associated with smoking;** autoantibodies to surfactant may exist
Carcinoid	Major bronchi; spread by direct extension	Increased secretion of **5-HT;** flushing; wheezing; heart disease; low malignancy
Large cell	**Peripheral;** undifferentiated; giant cells with pleomorphism	Poor prognosis; metastasis to the brain; smoking
Metastasis	**Cannonball** lesions	**Higher incidence than primary lung cancer**
Small cell (oat cell)	**Central;** undifferentiated; **most aggressive;** small, dark blue cells	Poor prognosis; increased in smokers; ectopic ACTH and ADH secretion
Squamous cell	**Central;** mass from bronchus; keratin pearls; cavitation	Increased in smokers; secretion of **PTH-like peptide**

ACTH=adrenocorticotropic hormone; *ADH*=antidiuretic hormone; *CEA*=carcinoembryonic antigen; *5-HT*=serotonin; *PTH*=parathyroid hormone.

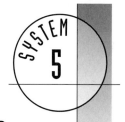

The Gastrointestinal System

INNERVATION AND BLOOD SUPPLY OF THE GASTROINTESTINAL TRACT (Figure 5-1)

 The boundaries of the epiploic foramen of Winslow (opening of the lesser sac) are the hepatoduodenal ligament (containing the common bile duct, the proper hepatic artery, and the portal vein) located anteriorly, the caudate lobe of the liver located superiorly, the duodenum located inferiorly, and the inferior vena cava located posteriorly.

FIGURE 5-1 Innervation and blood supply of the gastrointestinal tract

▢ Foregut ▢ Midgut ▢ Hindgut

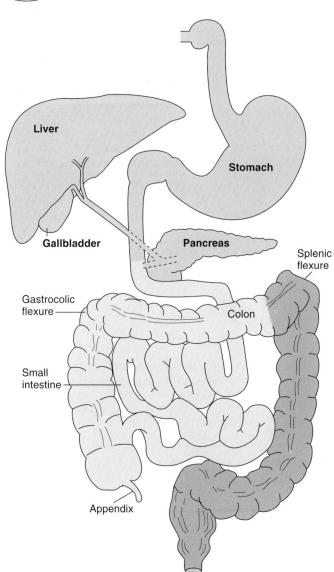

1) Foregut
- Derivatives
  - Esophagus
  - Stomach
  - First part of duodenum
  - Liver
  - Gallbladder
  - Pancreas
  (formed from fusion of dorsal and ventral buds)
- Supplied by celiac trunk
- Vagal parasympathetic nerve, thoracic nerve, and splanchnic sympathetic nerve

2) Midgut
- Derivatives
  - Second, third, and fourth parts of duodenum
  - Jejunum
  - Ileum
  - Appendix
  - Proximal two thirds of colon (up to splenic flexure)
- Supplied by superior mesenteric artery
- Vagal parasympathetic nerve, thoracic splanchnic sympathetic nerve

3) Hindgut
- Derivatives
  - Distal one third of colon including sigmoid colon and rectum to pectinate line
- Supplied by inferior mesenteric artery
- Pelvic splanchnic (S2-S4) parasympathetic nerve, and lumbar splanchnic sympathetic nerve

4) Ectoderm
- Derivatives
  - Oropharynx (anterior two thirds of tongue, lips, parotid glands, tooth enamel)
  - Anus, distal rectum (from pectinate line outward)

HORMONES OF THE GASTROINTESTINAL SYSTEM (Figure 5-2)

FIGURE 5-2 Hormones of the gastrointestinal system

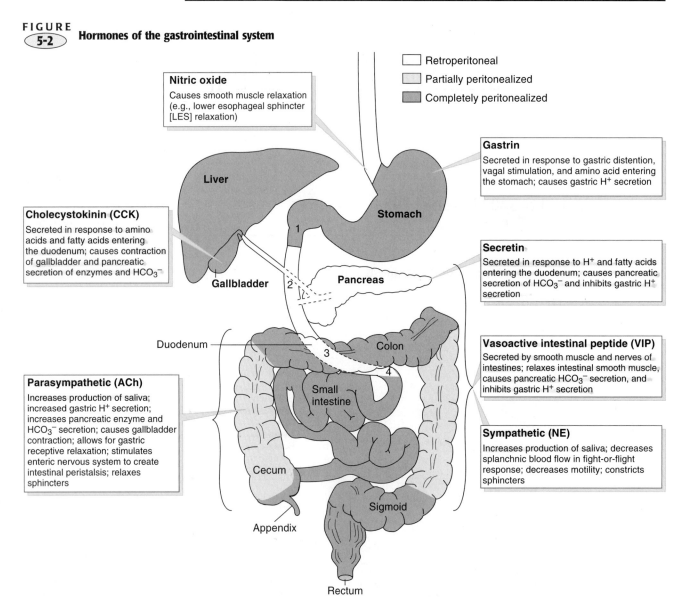

Nitric oxide
Causes smooth muscle relaxation (e.g., lower esophageal sphincter [LES] relaxation)

☐ Retroperitoneal
◻ Partially peritonealized
■ Completely peritonealized

Gastrin
Secreted in response to gastric distention, vagal stimulation, and amino acid entering the stomach; causes gastric H$^+$ secretion

Cholecystokinin (CCK)
Secreted in response to amino acids and fatty acids entering the duodenum; causes contraction of gallbladder and pancreatic secretion of enzymes and HCO$_3^-$

Secretin
Secreted in response to H$^+$ and fatty acids entering the duodenum; causes pancreatic secretion of HCO$_3^-$ and inhibits gastric H$^+$ secretion

Vasoactive intestinal peptide (VIP)
Secreted by smooth muscle and nerves of intestines; relaxes intestinal smooth muscle, causes pancreatic HCO$_3^-$ secretion, and inhibits gastric H$^+$ secretion

Parasympathetic (ACh)
Increases production of saliva; increased gastric H$^+$ secretion; increases pancreatic enzyme and HCO$_3^-$ secretion; causes gallbladder contraction; allows for gastric receptive relaxation; stimulates enteric nervous system to create intestinal peristalsis; relaxes sphincters

Sympathetic (NE)
Increases production of saliva; decreases splanchnic blood flow in fight-or-flight response; decreases motility; constricts sphincters

Liver
Stomach
Gallbladder
Pancreas
Duodenum
Colon
Small intestine
Cecum
Sigmoid
Appendix
Rectum

Ach=acetylcholine; *H$^+$*=hydrogen; *HCO$_3^-$*=bicarbonate; *NE*=norepinephrine.

With the exception of a Meckel's diverticulum, which can remain asymptomatic throughout life, congenital malformations of the gastrointestinal (GI) tract will manifest themselves during the neonatal period.

IMPORTANT CONGENITAL MALFORMATIONS OF THE GASTROINTESTINAL SYSTEM (Table 5-1)

TABLE 5-1 Important Congenital Malformations of the Gastrointestinal System	
Malformation	**Clinical Features**
Hypertrophic pyloric stenosis	Thickening of the pylorus musculature **Projectile vomiting** Palpable knot "olive" in the pyloric region
Extrahepatic biliary atresia	Incomplete recanalization of bile duct during development Presents shortly after birth Dark urine Clay-colored stool Jaundice
Annular pancreas	Abnormal fusion of ventral and dorsal pancreatic buds forming a constricting ring around the duodenum Duodenal obstruction presents shortly after birth
Meckel's diverticulum	Persistent remnant of the vitelline duct Forms an outpouching (true diverticulum) in the ileum Ulceration and bleeding 50% contain either gastric or pancreatic tissue
Malrotation of the midgut	Normal 270° rotation is not completed Cecum and appendix lie in upper abdomen Associated with **volvulus** (twisting of intestine) causing an obstruction
Intestinal stenosis or atresia	Results from failure of the normal recanalization of the lumen May produce failure to thrive
Hirschsprung's disease (congenital or toxic megacolon)	Failure of **neural crest cells** to migrate to colon No peristalsis Constipation and abdominal distention in newborn **Bowel movement precipitated by digital rectal examination**
Anal agenesis	Lack of anal opening as a result of improper formation of the urorectal septum May cause rectovesical (anus to bladder), rectovaginal, or rectourethral fistula

Rule of 2's for Meckel's diverticulum: 2 feet from ileocecal junction; 2 inches long; 2%; of the population affected; two types of ectopic tissue involved (gastric or pancreatic).

Duodenal atresia is associated with Down's syndrome and demonstrates a characteristic "**double-bubble**" sign on radiograph and ultrasound.

THE OROPHARYNX, ESOPHAGUS, AND STOMACH

I. The digestion of food begins in the oral cavity with salivary enzymes.

II. The esophagus transports food to the stomach.
   A. **The upper third** of the esophagus is **skeletal muscle.**
   B. **The middle third** is **both** skeletal and smooth muscle.
   C. **The lower third** is **smooth muscle.**
   D. The lower esophageal sphincter relaxes in preparation for the passage of food into the stomach.

III. The stomach receives and stores food.
   A. **Receptive relaxation**—the stomach relaxes to accommodate entering food (a vagovagal reflex)
   B. Three phases of gastric secretion
     1. **Cephalic phase**—the sight, smell, taste, or thought of food stimulates secretion

In achalasia, the lower esophageal sphincter is unable to relax, there is dysmotility of the esophagus, and food cannot enter the stomach. Achalasia has a characteristic "**bird beak**" appearance on a barium swallow radiograph.

2. **Gastric phase**—secretion is caused by the entry of food into the stomach
3. **Intestinal phase**—food entering the intestine causes a feedback stimulation of gastric secretion

C. Important gastric secretions
   1. **Hydrochloric acid** is secreted by parietal cells of the fundus.
      a. Stimulated by gastrin, histamine, and vagal stimulation
      b. Inhibited by **omeprazole** (proton-pump inhibitor), **cimetidine** (H_2 blocker), chyme in small intestine via gastric inhibitory peptide (GIP) and secretin
   2. **Intrinsic factor** is secreted by parietal cells of the fundus.
      a. Binds to vitamin B_{12} (extrinsic factor)
      b. **Vitamin B_{12}-intrinsic factor** complex absorbed in **terminal ileum**
   3. **Pepsinogen** is secreted by chief cells.
      a. Pepsinogen is converted to pepsin by the low pH of the stomach.
      b. Pepsin begins digestion of protein.
   4. **Gastrin** secreted by the G cells of the antrum and pylorus stimulates the release of hydrochloric acid (HCl) from parietal cells.
   5. Somatostatin is secreted by a variety of cells throughout the GI tract and has a global inhibitory effect.

D. The stomach grinds food into small particles and forces it into the duodenum.
   1. Grinding (trituration) takes place in peristaltic waves occurring at a rate of 3 to 5 waves per minute.
   2. **Migrating motor complexes** (MMC), stimulated by motilin, occur in the interdigestive period and serve to flush undigested food through the GI system.

IV. Nonneoplastic disorders of the oropharynx, esophagus, and stomach (Table 5-2)

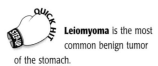

Leiomyoma is the most common benign tumor of the stomach.

TABLE 5-2 Nonneoplastic Disorders of the Oropharynx, Esophagus, and Stomach

Disorder	Etiology and Pathology	Clinical Features	Notes
Sialolithiasis	Blockage of salivary gland duct preventing release of saliva; follows chronic sialadenitis (inflammation of the salivary glands)	Acute pain; usually in submandibular gland or Stensen's duct of the parotid gland	Passage of stone can be induced by stimulating secretion of saliva (e.g., by sucking on a lemon)
Pleomorphic adenoma	Increased risk with radiation exposure	Benign, recurring, mixed cell tumor of the parotid; may lead to facial nerve injury	Most frequent salivary gland tumor; more common in women 20–40 years of age
Esophageal variceal bleeding	Bleeding from esophageal varices owing to portal hypertension	Hematemesis; signs of portal hypertension (i.e., caput medusae, ascites)	Usually treated with vasoconstrictors (vasopressin); endoscopy required for diagnosis (to rule out bleeding ulcers)
Boerhaave's syndrome	Complete rupture of the esophagus (all layers); caused by severe retching	Often presents as left pneumothorax; surgical correction necessary	Esophageal reflux disease predisposes to this condition

(continued)

TABLE 5-2 Nonneoplastic Disorders of the Oropharynx, Esophagus, and Stomach *(Continued)*

Disorder	Etiology and Pathology	Clinical Features	Notes
Mallory-Weiss tear	Laceration of the gastroesophageal junction; usually caused by severe retching	Poststretching hematemesis	Alcoholics at increased risk
Acute gastritis	NSAIDs; smoking; alcohol; aspirin; steroids; burn injury (Curling's ulcer); brain injury (Cushing's ulcer)	Erosive; acute inflammation; necrosis; hemorrhage; **"coffee-ground" vomitus**	Blood in the nasogastric tube
Chronic gastritis	Type A (fundal): autoimmune pernicious anemia, aging; Type B (antral): *Helicobacter pylori*	Nonerosive; mucosal inflammation and atrophy of mucosa	Risk factor for gastric carcinoma
Gastric ulcers	***H. pylori*** (70% of cases); bile-induced gastritis; increased permeability of gastric mucosa; associated with use of aspirin and NSAIDs	Postprandial pain; bleeding; perforation; obstruction	Usually near lesser curvature; not dependent on increased gastric acid secretion; not precancerous
Dumping syndrome	Postvagotomy; unimpeded passage of hypertonic food to the small intestine causing distention as a result of osmotic flow of water into the lumen	Nausea; diarrhea; palpitations; sweating; lightheadedness; reactive hypoglycemia	Can be prevented by eating only small meals and ingesting solids and liquids separately

NSAIDs=nonsteroidal anti-inflammatory drugs

QUICK HIT

GERD (gastro-esophageal reflux disease), a common gastroesophageal disorder, is usually treated with H_2 blockers such as cimetidine or ranitidine, or in more severe cases with proton-pump inhibitors such as omeprazole or lansoprazole.

QUICK HIT

Cyclo-oxygenase-2 (COX-2) inhibitors such as celecoxib and rofecoxib not only reduce the adverse GI side effects and ulcers of normal nonsteroidal anti-inflammatory drugs (NSAIDs) but also do not inhibit platelet function.

V. Neoplastic disorders of the oropharynx, esophagus, and stomach (Table 5-3)

TABLE 5-3 Neoplastic Disorders of the Oropharynx, Esophagus, and Stomach

Disorder	Etiology and Pathology	Clinical Features	Notes
Oral cancer	**Smoking;** chewing tobacco; alcohol	Squamous cell carcinoma; may involve tongue	Leukoplakia (white patch on the mucus membrane that cannot be wiped off) is a common precursor lesion
Esophageal adenocarcinoma	**Barrett's esophagus;** complication of gastroesophageal reflux disease	**Columnar metaplasia of esophageal squamous epithelium;** distal third of the esophagus	More common in whites

(continued)

THE GASTROINTESTINAL SYSTEM

TABLE 5-3	Neoplastic Disorders of the Oropharynx, Esophagus, and Stomach *(Continued)*		
Disorder	**Etiology and Pathology**	**Clinical Features**	**Notes**
Esophageal squamous cell carcinoma	Alcohol and tobacco use; esophagitis	Dysphagia; anorexia; pain	More common in blacks
Gastric carcinoma	***H. pylori;*** gastritis; low-fiber diet, nitrosamines; blood group A; high-salt diet; increased incidence in Japan owing to greater consumption of smoked foods	Aggressive spread from antrum to nodes and liver; **Virchow's node** (enlarged left-sided supraclavicular lymph node); **Krukenberg tumor** (metastatic disease to the ovaries from the stomach characterized by mucinous, signet ring cells)	More common in men over 50 years of age; infiltration of stomach walls with tumor cells and subsequent fibrosis leads to linitis plastica (leather-bottle stomach)

Nonneoplastic and neoplastic disorders originating proximal to the pyloric sphincter often present with hematemesis and dysphagia as a result of alcohol and tobacco abuse.

THE SMALL INTESTINE, LARGE INTESTINE, AND RECTUM

I. Muscular layers of the GI tract (Figure 5-3)

FIGURE
5-3 Picture of muscular layer of the GI tract

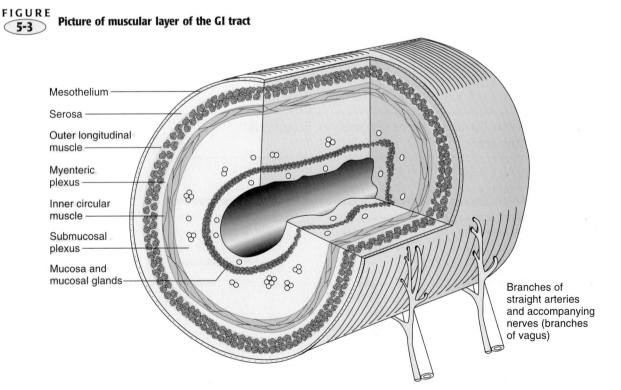

Mesothelium

Serosa

Outer longitudinal muscle

Myenteric plexus

Inner circular muscle

Submucosal plexus

Mucosa and mucosal glands

Branches of straight arteries and accompanying nerves (branches of vagus)

II. The **small intestine** digests and absorbs food.

A. Digestion is mediated by a variety of GI hormones including cholecystokinin (CCK), secretin, somatostatin, and others (see Figure 5-2).

B. Carbohydrates

1. Pancreatic amylase hydrolyzes glycogen, starch, and most other complex carbohydrates to disaccharides.
2. Disaccharides are broken down to monosaccharides by intestinal brush border enzymes and absorbed.
3. Monosaccharides are absorbed by a variety of mechanisms.
   a. Glucose and galactose are absorbed by sodium (Na^+)-dependent transport.
   b. Fructose is absorbed by facilitated diffusion.

C. **Protein**

1. Degraded to amino acids, dipeptides, and tripeptides by proteases produced by the pancreas
   a. Activation of **trypsinogen to trypsin**
      (1) Autoactivated
      (2) Activated by intestinal brush border enterokinases
   b. Trypsin degrades the peptide bonds of arginine or lysine.
   c. Trypsin also **activates the other proteolytic pancreatic enzymes.**
2. Proteins are absorbed by an Na^+-dependent transport.
   a. Separate carriers for acidic, basic, and neutral amino acids
   b. Dipeptides and tripeptides are absorbed faster than single amino acids.

D. **Fats**

1. Lipids are broken into droplets by the mixing action of the stomach.
2. **Pancreatic lipase** (and to a lesser extent salivary lipase) **hydrolyzes triacylglycerol to fatty acids and 2-monoacylglycerol.**
3. Bile salts (amphipathic molecules) emulsify the hydrolyzed products and form micelles.
4. **Micelles** allow for fat absorption (Figure 5-4).

 Lactose intolerance is caused by a genetic absence or decrease in lactase. Lactose cannot be broken down; it remains in the lumen of the gut and causes osmotic diarrhea.

 Often the amino acid transporter found in the intestines is identical to the amino acid transporter found in the renal tubules. As such, diseases that affect these transporters have multiorgan system effects. One of these diseases is Hartnup's, which is a defect in the intestinal and renal tubular absorption of neutral amino acids leading to excretion of tryptophan derivatives and causing pellagra-like symptoms.

THE GASTROINTESTINAL SYSTEM

FIGURE 5-4 Absorption and digestion of fats (lipid metabolism)

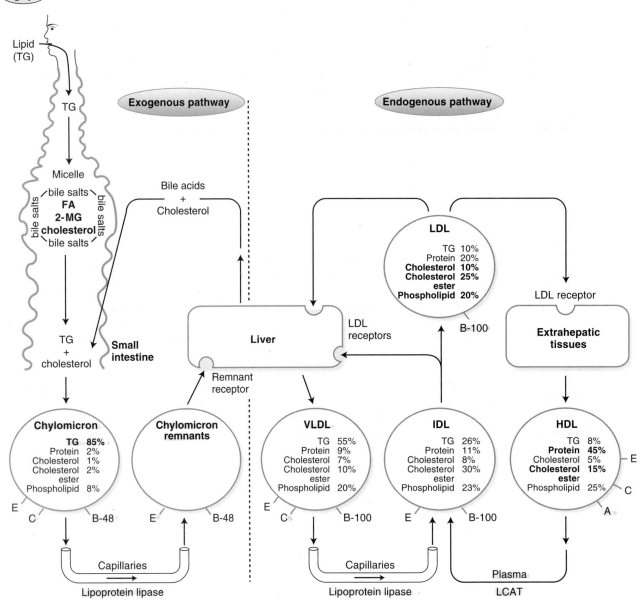

A, B, C, and E=lipoproteins involved with lipid metabolism; *FA*=fatty acid; *HDL*=high-density lipoprotein; *IDL*=intermediate-density lipoprotein; *LCAT*=lecithin-cholesterol acyltransferase; *LDL*=low-density lipoprotein; *MG*=monoglyceride; *TG*=triglyceride; *VLDL*=very low-density lipoprotein. (Adapted from Goldstein J, Kita T, and Brown M: Defective lipoprotein receptors and atherosclerosis. N Engl J Med 1983;309:288.)

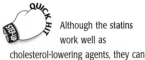

Although the statins work well as cholesterol-lowering agents, they can be **hepatotoxic.** Therefore, patients who take them should undergo routine liver function tests.

5. A variety of familial and acquired disorders may disrupt lipid metabolism, resulting in **hyperlipidemia.**
   a. Hyperlipidemia, especially high levels of LDL's, is associated with coronary artery disease.
   b. Typically, treatment first involves dietary intervention and then drug therapy, regardless of the cause of the hyperlipidemia.
      (1) **3-Hydroxy-3-methylglutaryl coenzyme A (HMG-CoA) reductase inhibitors,** also known as **"statins,"** such as atorvastatin, lovastatin, and pravastatin, are an effective and widely used means of lowering LDL.
      (2) **Bile acid-binding resins** such as cholestyramine and colestipol work by binding bile acids in the intestine and promoting their subsequent loss in the stool, which ultimately lowers LDL levels.

(3) **Nicotinic acid (niacin)** inhibits release of lipoproteins from the liver, lowering very low-density lipoproteins (VLDL) and LDL.

III. The **large intestine** stores and excretes nondigestible material.

A. Absorbs 2–3 L/day of water

B. **Secretes potassium (K^+)**

C. Mediates defecation of undigested material through both voluntary and involuntary (rectosphincteric reflex) mechanisms

LOCATION OF ABSORPTION OF VITAMINS, MINERALS, AND NUTRIENTS (Figure 5-5)

FIGURE 5-5 Location of absorption of vitamins, minerals, and nutrients

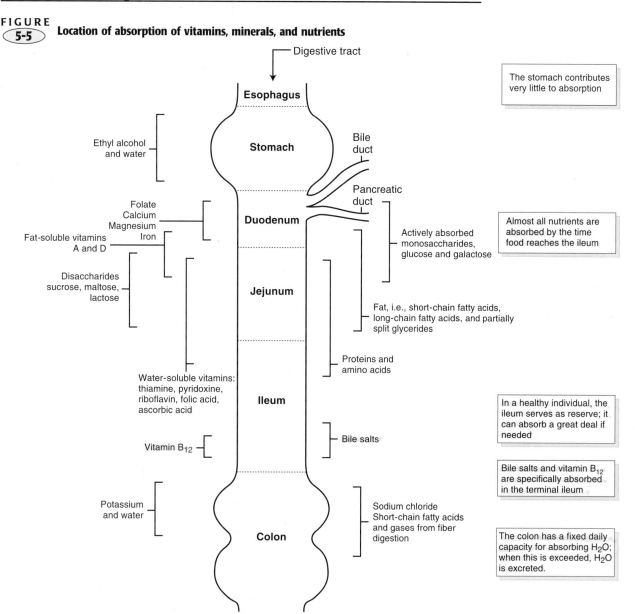

H_2O=water. (Adapted from James P. Ryan, PhD, Physiology, 1997.)

Common clinical disorders of the gastrointestinal tract, distal to the pyloric sphincter, will usually present as vague abdominal pain as a result of stimulation of the visceral afferent nerves. If the parietal peritoneum (the abdominal wall), innervated by the somatic afferent nerves, is irritated owing to the lesion, the pain will become more localized (as is seen in acute appendicitis).

COMMON CLINICAL DISORDERS OF THE SMALL INTESTINE, LARGE INTESTINE, AND RECTUM (Table 5-4)

THE GASTROINTESTINAL SYSTEM

> **QUICK HIT**
> Posterior duodenal ulcers are associated with erosion of the gastroduodenal artery and subsequent hemorrhage.

> **QUICK HIT**
> *Helicobacter pylori* infection is pharmacologically treated with "**triple therapy.**" The therapeutic regimen typically includes a proton-pump inhibitor (omeprazole) and two of the following antibiotics: clarithromycin, amoxicillin, and metronidazole.

> **QUICK HIT**
> Small bowel obstructions are usually caused by adhesions, whereas large bowel obstructions are most commonly a result of neoplasms. Ileus, a common cause of temporary small bowel paralysis, commonly occurs postoperatively.

> **QUICK HIT**
> Diverticulosis, the most common cause of bleeding from the lower GI tract, can be differentiated from diverticulitis because, typically, diverticulitis does not cause bleeding but is painful, whereas diverticulosis does cause bleeding but is typically painless.

TABLE 5-4 Common Clinical Disorders of the Small Intestine, Large Intestine, and Rectum

Disorder	Etiology and Pathology	Clinical Features	Notes
Hiatal hernia	Saclike herniation of stomach through diaphragm; smoking; obesity	Retrosternal pain (worse in supine position); can lead to **gastroesophageal reflux disease**	Usually occurs in the sliding (vs. rolling) form
Duodenal ulcers	***H. pylori*** (in 90% of cases); hypersecretion of acid; smokers; Zollinger-Ellison syndrome; blood group O; associated with NSAID use	Coffee-ground vomitus; **smooth border;** clean base; black stools; pain at night or 2 hours postprandial; perforation may result in acute pancreatitis	Not precancerous
Ischemic bowel disease	Atherosclerosis of celiac artery or mesenteric artery	Abdominal pain; nausea; vomiting; stool positive for blood test	Usually affects watershed areas (splenic flexure or rectosigmoid junction)
Diverticulitis	Outpouchings of the colon obstructed with fecalith leading to inflammation or infection; low-fiber diet	Usually involves the **sigmoid colon;** fever; leukocytosis; colicky pain; usually multiple in number and cause increased risk of perforation	False diverticula: pockets of mucosa and submucosa herniated through muscular layer
Appendicitis	Obstruction (usually fecalith or lymphoid hyperplasia); bacterial proliferation and mucosal invasion	Nausea; vomiting; anorexia; abdominal pain that migrates from epigastrium to right lower quadrant (RLQ); pain at **McBurney's point;** psoas sign or obturator sign; increased WBCs in blood	Differential diagnosis in females includes ectopic pregnancy, ovarian torsion, ruptured ovarian cyst, and pelvic inflammatory disease
Adenocarcinoma	Chronic inflammatory bowel disease; low-fiber diet; older age; hereditary polyposis or adenomatous disorders	**Increased CEA** (not diagnostic, used to assess treatment); rectosigmoid tumors present in an **annular manner** producing early obstruction and constipation; **left-sided tumors present with blood in the stool, whereas right-sided tumors typically present with anemia, as a result of occult blood loss**	Screen for occult blood in stool and flexible sigmoidoscopy; screening colonoscopy with a positive family history; third most common cause of cancer death (after lung and prostate/breast)
Carcinoid tumor	Arise from **neuroendocrine cells** (Kulchitsky's cells); release vasoactive peptides such as histamine, serotonin, and prostaglandins	**Increased 5-HIAA in urine;** diarrhea; **flushing;** right-sided heart valve lesions; hypotension; bronchospasm	Most common tumor of the appendix, but also found in the ileum, rectum, and bronchus

CEA=carcinoembryonic antigen; *5-HIAA*=5-hydroxyindoleacetic acid; *NSAID*=nonsteroidal anti-inflammatory drug; *WBC*=white blood cell

Diarrhea, the passage of abnormal amounts of fluid or semisolid fecal matter, can be mediated by a number of mechanisms. Osmotic diarrhea results when unabsorbed solutes increase intraluminal oncotic pressure, causing an outpouring of water. Surgical resection can lead to an inadequate surface for absorption of nutrients, resulting in a form of **osmotic diarrhea.** Active ion secretion causing obligatory water loss is termed **secretory diarrhea.** Altered intestinal motility, in which there is an alteration of the normally coordinated control of intestinal propulsion, may also result in diarrhea (often alternating with constipation). Finally, sloughing of colonic mucosa, caused by inflammation and necrosis, often as a result of infection, causes an **exudative form of diarrhea.**

● **Bacterial Causes of Diarrhea** (Table 5-5)

TABLE 5-5	Bacterial Causes of Diarrhea		
Infectious Agent	**Clinical Features**	**Treatment**	**Notes**
Shigella	**Shiga-toxin** causes **bloody** diarrhea, mild to severe, 1–2 weeks in duration; fever for 3–4 days	Bismuth, ampicillin, ciprofloxacin, or trimethoprim-sulfamethoxazole	Fecal leukocytes and stool culture necessary for diagnosis
Salmonella	**Bloody** diarrhea; fever; cramps; nausea	Supportive therapy only; no opiates, tetracycline may be used if needed	Commonly acquired from **eggs** or **poultry, or turtles;** diagnosis based on stool culture; increased susceptibility in immuno-compromised patients
Campylobacter jejuni	**Bloody** diarrhea; fever; crampy abdominal pain; self-limited, but may persist for 3–4 weeks	Supportive therapy or possibly erythromycin	**Leading cause of food-borne diarrhea** in United States
Vibrio cholerae	**Watery** diarrhea **(rice-water stools),** vomiting, and dehydration occur after 12–48 hours of incubation	Supportive therapy only; no opiates	Caused by **toxin;** most often occurs in underdeveloped nations; commonly associated with consumption of raw oysters
Clostridium difficile	**Watery** diarrhea caused by antibiotic-induced suppression of normal colonic flora and *C. difficile* overgrowth; **pseudomembranes** on the colonic mucosa	Metronidazole, oral vancomycin	Exotoxin-mediated; termed pseudomembranous colitis because of the false membranes created on the colon by the bacterial infection
Enterotoxigenic *Escherichia coli* (traveler's diarrhea)	**Watery** diarrhea; 3–6 days duration; occasional fever and vomiting	Bismuth, trimethoprim-sulfamethoxazole, doxycycline, ciprofloxacin	Antibiotics reduce duration of infection to 1–2 days
Enterohemorrhagic *E. coli* (O157:H7)	**Shiga-like toxin** causes **bloody** diarrhea	Supportive therapy	Typically, food-borne transmission (e.g., **uncooked hamburger**); diagnosis made by stool culture
Yersinia enterocolitica	**Bloody** diarrhea; fever; cramps; nausea	Supportive therapy only; no opiates	Transmitted by food or contaminated domestic animal feces; clinically indistinguishable from *Salmonella* or *Shigella*

Salmonella requires at least 100,000 organisms to be infectious. *Shigella*, however, requires only 100.

Vibrio cholerae produces an exotoxin that activates adenylate cyclase in the crypt cells. The increase in cAMP activates Cl⁻ secretory channels. Consequently, sodium and water accompany Cl⁻ into the lumen, which results in an osmotic diarrhea.

THE GASTROINTESTINAL SYSTEM

● **Viral Causes of Diarrhea** (Table 5-6)

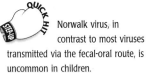

QUICK HIT

Norwalk virus, in contrast to most viruses transmitted via the fecal-oral route, is uncommon in children.

TABLE 5-6	Viral Causes of Diarrhea		
Infectious Agent	**Clinical Features**	**Treatment**	**Notes**
Rotavirus	Severe, dehydrating diarrhea; vomiting; low-grade fever	Supportive therapy only	**Most common cause of diarrhea in infants;** usually occurs during **winter** months
Norwalk virus	Mild diarrhea and vomiting	Supportive therapy only	Epidemics in underdeveloped countries; **affects older children and adults**
Adenovirus (serotypes 40 & 41)	Diarrhea and moderate vomiting	Supportive therapy only	Second to rotavirus as cause of gastroenteritis in children

● **Protozoal Causes of Diarrhea** (Table 5-7)

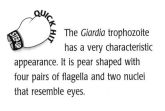

QUICK HIT

The *Giardia* trophozoite has a very characteristic appearance. It is pear shaped with four pairs of flagella and two nuclei that resemble eyes.

TABLE 5-7	Protozoal Causes of Diarrhea		
Infectious Agent	**Clinical Features**	**Treatment**	**Notes**
Entamoeba histolytica	**Bloody** diarrhea; lower abdominal pain; may lead to dysentery with 10–12 bloody and mucous stools per day	Metronidazole	Caused by ingestion of viable cysts via fecal-oral route
Giardia lamblia	**Watery,** foul-smelling diarrhea; nausea; anorexia; cramps lasting weeks to months	Metronidazole	Fecal-oral transmission; often contracted while **camping**
Cryptosporidium	**Watery** diarrhea with large fluid loss; symptoms persist in immunocompromised patients; is self-limited in healthy individuals	Supportive therapy	Immunocompromised patients (especially **AIDS patients**); fecal-oral transmission of oocysts

● **Inflammatory Bowel Conditions** (Table 5-8)

It has been speculated that the pathogenesis of inflammatory bowel disease (IBD) is related to activation of the immune system and consequent release of cytokines and inflammatory mediators. The cause of IBD has yet to be discovered; however, there is some suggestion of a genetic component.

TABLE 5-8	Comparison of Inflammatory Bowel Conditions	
	Crohn's Disease	**Ulcerative Colitis**
Typical patient	• Young person of Jewish descent • Bimodal age distribution: 25–40 years of age and 50–65 years of age • Female > male	• Person of Jewish descent • Recently quit smoking • Bimodal age distribution: 20–35 years of age and 65+ years of age • Male > female
Clinical findings	• Diarrhea • Abdominal pain • Fever • Malabsorption • Obstruction	• Bloody, mucous diarrhea • Abdominal pain • Fever • Weight loss • Toxic megacolon

(continued)

TABLE 5-8 **Comparison of Inflammatory Bowel Conditions (Continued)**

	Crohn's Disease	Ulcerative Colitis
Location	• Small Intestine • Colon • "Mouth to anus"	• Colon • Rectum
Histologic findings	• Full-thickness inflammation • **Granulomas**	• Mucosal inflammation • **Crypt abscesses**
Gross findings	• **Cobblestone appearance** • Wall thickening with narrowed lumen • **Skipped areas** • **Fistulas**	• Pseudopolyps • Widened lumen • Toxic megacolon
Diagnostic evaluation	• Colonoscopy • Barium enema • Upper GI series with small-bowel followthrough	• Colonoscopy • Barium enema • Upper GI series with small-bowel followthrough
Risk of malignancy	• Small increase	• Large increase
Associated systemic manifestations	• Arthritis • Eye lesions • Erythema nodosum • Pyoderma gangrenosum • Aphthous ulcers	• Arthritis • Eye lesions • Erythema nodosum • Pyoderma gangrenosum • Sclerosing cholangitis
Medical treatment	• Sulfasalazine • Steroids • Metronidazole	• Sulfasalazine • Steroids • Metronidazole
Indications for surgery	• Obstruction • Massive bleeding • Perforation • Refractory to medical treatment • Cancer • Toxic megacolon	• Toxic megacolon • Cancer • Massive bleeding • Failure to mature • Refractory to medical treatment

GI=gastrointestinal

MALABSORPTION SYNDROMES OF THE SMALL INTESTINE (Table 5-9)

Malabsorption may produce a variety of symptoms ranging from diarrhea to steatorrhea to specific nutrient deficiencies. For example, iron, vitamin B_{12}, fat-soluble vitamins (A, D, E, and K), or protein may be poorly absorbed and lead to systemic manifestations.

TABLE 5-9 **Malabsorption Syndromes of the Small Intestine**

Syndrome	Pathology	Clinical Features	Notes
Abetalipoproteinemia	Lack of apoprotein B; defective chylomicron assembly; enterocytes congested with lipid	Acanthocytes ("burr" cells) in blood; **no chylomicrons, VLDL, or LDL in blood**	Autosomal recessive
Celiac disease (nontropical sprue)	Gluten sensitivity	Foul-smelling, pale stool; **villi of small intestine blunted;** stunted growth; symptoms disappear when gluten is removed from diet	Associated with HLA-B8 and DQW2; predisposes to T-cell lymphoma, and GI and breast cancer

(continued)

TABLE 5-9 **Malabsorption Syndromes of the Small Intestine** *(Continued)*

Syndrome	Pathology	Clinical Features	Notes
Disaccharidase deficiency	Enzyme deficiency; bacterial digestion of unabsorbed disaccharide	Diarrhea; bloating	Most commonly lactase deficiency
Tropical sprue	Etiology unclear	Affects small intestine; may cause vitamin deficiencies and megaloblastic anemia	Possible infectious cause
Whipple's disease	Systemic disease caused by *Tropheryma whippelii*	Diarrhea; weight loss; lymphadenopathy; hyperpigmentation; **macrophages laden with T. whippelii**	Older white males
Bacterial overgrowth	Bacterial overpopulation of small intestine owing to stasis, raised pH, impaired immunity, or **clindamycin** therapy	Inflammatory infiltrate in bowel wall	Treat with antibiotics

GI=gastrointestinal; *HLA-B8*=human leukocyte antigen-B8; *LDL*=low-density lipoprotein; *VLDL*=very low-density lipoprotein

NEOPLASTIC POLYPS (Table 5-10)

Gastrointestinal polyps can be very diverse in their presentation. Individuals can be asymptomatic, as is usually the case with tubular adenomas, or can present with serious systemic manifestations such as anemia secondary to invasive cancer.

TABLE 5-10 **Neoplastic Polyps**

Tubular Adenoma	Tubulovillous Adenoma	Villous Adenoma
• Usually **benign**	• Greater potential of malignancy than tubular adenoma	• Highly **malignant**
• Multiple	• Morphologically, shares features of both tubular and villous adenomas	• **Sessile** tumors • Fingerlike projections
• **Pedunculated** tumors		
• Greater chance of malignancy if genetically predisposed		
• Most common polyp		

● Comparison of Polyposis Conditions (Table 5-11)

Disease	Inheritance	Clinical Features
Familial adenomatous polyposis	Autosomal dominant	Colon lined with hundreds of polyps; potential for malignancy approaches 100%
Turcot's syndrome	Autosomal dominant	Colonic polyps and **CNS tumors;** potential for malignancy approaches 100%
Gardner's syndrome	Autosomal dominant	Colonic polyps; soft tissue and **bone tumors;** potential for malignancy approaches 100%
Peutz-Jeghers syndrome	Autosomal dominant	Benign hamartomatous polyps of the GI tract (especially the small intestine); **hyperpigmented mouth, hands, and genitalia;** increased incidence of tumors of the uterus, breast, ovaries, lung, stomach, and pancreas; no malignant potential
Familial nonpolyposis syndrome	Autosomal dominant	**Defect in DNA repair** causing large number of colonic lesions (especially proximal); potential for malignancy approaches 50%

TABLE 5-11 Comparison of Polyposis Conditions

CNS=central nervous system; *DNA*=deoxyribonucleic acid; *GI*=gastrointestinal

THE HEPATOBILIARY SYSTEM

I. Microscopic organization of the liver (Figure 5-6)

FIGURE 5-6 Microscopic organization of the liver

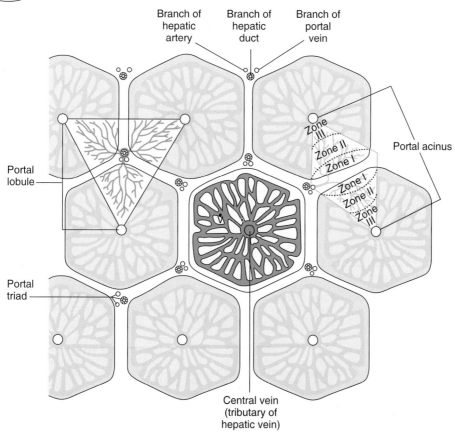

Branch of hepatic artery   Branch of hepatic duct   Branch of portal vein

Zone III
Zone II
Zone I

Portal acinus

Portal lobule

Zone I
Zone II
Zone III

Portal triad

Central vein (tributary of hepatic vein)

II. Enterohepatic cycling and the excretion of bilirubin (Figure 5-7)

FIGURE 5-7 Enterohepatic cycling and the excretion of bilirubin

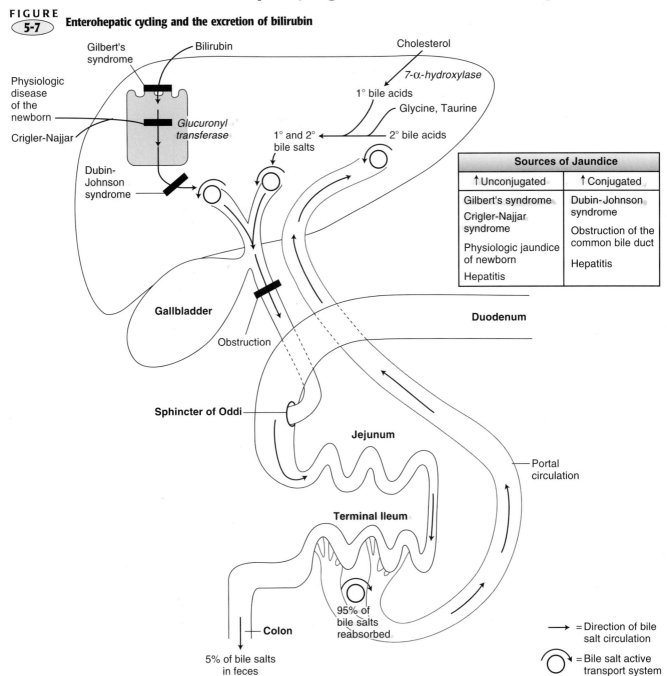

Sources of Jaundice	
↑Unconjugated	↑Conjugated
Gilbert's syndrome	Dubin-Johnson syndrome
Crigler-Najjar syndrome	Obstruction of the common bile duct
Physiologic jaundice of newborn	Hepatitis
Hepatitis	

(Adapted from Bullock J, Boyle J III, Wang MB, eds. NMS Physiology, 3rd ed. Baltimore: Williams & Wilkins, 1995:437.)

Figure 5–8 (opposite). Glycolysis: (1) Hexokinase (and glucokinase in liver). **(2)** Phosphofructokinase-1 (PFK-1): rate-limiting step in glycolysis; induced by insulin; (+) adenosine monophosphate (AMP), fructose 2,6-bisphosphate; (−) adenosine triphosphate (ATP), citrate. **(3)** Pyruvate kinase: irreversible; (+) fructose 1,6-bisphosphate in liver; (−) phosphorylation in response to increase glucagon, alanine. **(4)** Pyruvate dehydrogenase: requires thiamine pyrophosphate (TPP), lipoic acid, flavin adenine dinucleotide (FAD), nicotinamide adenine dinucleotide (NAD), coenzyme A (CoA); irreversible; occurs in mitochondria; (+) pyruvate, insulin; (−) reduced nicotinamide adenine dinucleotide (NADH), acetyl CoA, phosphorylation. **Gluconeogenesis: (5)** Pyruvate carboxylase: requires biotin; (+) citrate; (−) malonyl CoA, phosphorylation. **(6)** Phosphoenolpyruvate carboxykinase (PEPCK): induced by cortisol and glucagon (NOTE: substrate oxaloacetate is transported out of mitochondria as malate and converted back to oxaloacetate before reaction can occur). **(7)** Fructose 1,6-bisphosphatase: induced by glucagon; (−) AMP, fructose 2,6-bisphosphate. **(8)** Glucose 6-phosphatase: induced by glucagon. **(9)** Phosphofructokinase-2: (+) insulin, (−) glucagon; **(9a)** Works in opposite direction when phosphorylated. **Glycogenolysis: (10)** Glycogen phosphorylase and α-1,6-glucosidase: (+) AMP, phosphorylation. **Hexose monophosphate shunt: (11)** Glucose 6-phosphate dehydrogenase. **Tricarboxylic acid (TCA) cycle: (12)** Isocitrate dehydrogenase: rate-limiting step; irreversible; (+) adenosine diphosphate (ADP); (−) ATP, NADH. **(13)** α-Ketoglutarate dehydrogenase: requires TPP, lipoic acid, FAD, CoA; (−) ATP, guanosine triphosphate (GTP), NADH, succinyl CoA. **Urea cycle: (14)** Carbamoyl phosphate synthetase 1. **(15)** Ornithine transcarbamoylase. **(16)** Argininosuccinate synthetase. **(17)** Argininosuccinate lyase. **(18)** Arginase. **Fatty acid synthesis: (19)** Acetyl CoA carboxylase: requires biotin; (+) citrate; (−) malonyl CoA, phosphorylation. ADP=adenosine diphosphate; Ala=alanine; Arg=arginine; Asn=asparagine; ATP=adenosine triphosphate; CoA=coenzyme A; CO_2=carbon dioxide; Cys=cysteine; Gly=glycine; GTP=guanosine triphosphate; His=histidine; Ile=isoleucine; Leu=leucine; Lys=lysine; Met=methionine; NAD=nicotinamide adenine dinucleotide; NADH=reduced nicotinamide adenine dinucleotide; NH_3=ammonia; P=phosphate group; Phe=phenylalanine; Pro=proline; Ser=serine; Thr=threonine; Trp=trytophan; Tyr=tyrosine; UDP=uridine diphosphate; Val=valine.
(Adapted from Champe PC, Harvey RA: Lippincott's Illustrated Reviews: Biochemistry, 2nd edition. Philadelphia, J. B. Lippincott Company, 1994. p. 76)

III. Important biochemical pathways of the liver and digestion (Figure 5-8)

FIGURE
5-8
Important biochemical pathways of the liver and digestion

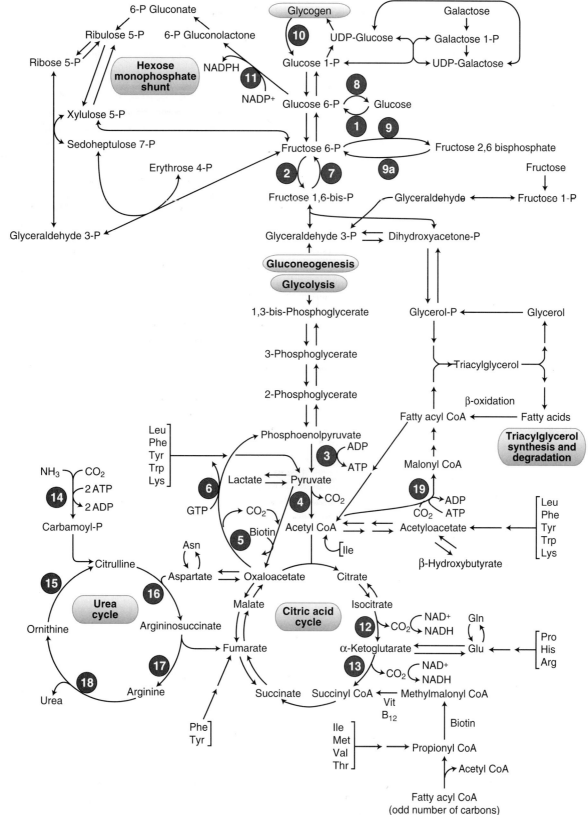

THE GASTROINTESTINAL SYSTEM

IV. Glycolysis versus gluconeogenesis versus glycogenolysis (Table 5-12)

As food is absorbed, the glycolysis pathway is activated and energy is stored as glycogen in the liver. Glycogenolysis provides food for the periods between regular meals. After 30 hours of fasting, all glycogen is depleted and gluconeogenesis becomes the only source of blood glucose.

TABLE 5-12 Glycolysis Versus Gluconeogenesis Versus Glycogenolysis

	Glycolysis	Gluconeogenesis	Glycogenolysis
Description of process	Glucose is broken down to form pyruvate and energy is released	Glucose is formed after 4–6 hours of fasting	**Glucose** is produced from glycogen stores after **2–3 hours of fasting**
Key enzymes and their regulation	Glucokinase (in liver), hexokinase (all tissues); requires ATP; (−) glucose-6-P; see enzyme 1, Figure 5-8 Phosphofructokinase-1 (PFK-1); requires ATP; **rate-limiting step in glycolysis;** (+) AMP, fructose-2-6-bis-P; (−) ATP, citrate; see enzyme 2, Figure 5-8 Pyruvate kinase; produces ATP; (+)fructose-1-6-bis-P; (−)alanine, phosphorylation, ATP; see enzyme 3, Figure 5-8 Pyruvate dehydrogenase; (+)pyruvate, insulin, ADP; (−) NADH, acetyl CoA, phosphorylation; see enzyme 4, Figure 5-8	Pyruvate carboxylase; requires **biotin, CO_2, and ATP;** (+) acetyl CoA; see enzyme 5, Figure 5-8 Phosphoenolpyruvate carboxykinase (PEPCK); requires GTP; (+)cortisol, glucagon; see enzyme 6, Figure 5-8 Fructose-1-6-bisphosphatase; (+) glucagon; (−) AMP, fructose-2-6-bis-P; see enzyme 7, Figure 5-8 Glucose-6-phosphatase; (+) glucagon; see enzyme 8, Figure 5-8	Glycogen phosphorylase; (+) AMP, phosphorylation; see enzyme 10, Figure 5-8 Phosphoglucomutase converts glucose-1-P to glucose-6-P

ADP=adenosine triphosphate; *AMP*=adenosine monophosphate; *ATP*=adenosine triphosphate; *CoA*=coenzyme A; *CO₂*=carbon dioxide; *GTP*=guanosine triphosphate; *NADH*=reduced nicotinamide adenine dinucleotide; *P*=phosphate

V. Defective enzyme diseases (Table 5-13)

With a few exceptions, most defective enzyme diseases are autosomal recessive. Inasmuch as the liver contains a high proportion of metabolic enzymes, it is often affected by these diseases.

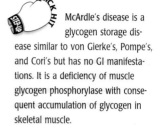

McArdle's disease is a glycogen storage disease similar to von Gierke's, Pompe's, and Cori's but has no GI manifestations. It is a deficiency of muscle glycogen phosphorylase with consequent accumulation of glycogen in skeletal muscle.

TABLE 5-13 Defective Enzyme Diseases

Disease	Defective Enzyme	Clinical Features
Gaucher's disease	Glucocerebrosidase	• Accumulation of **glucocerebroside** • Hepatosplenomegaly • Erosion head of long bones (e.g., femur) • Gaucher's cells (distinctive, **wrinkled paper** appearance) found in liver, spleen, bone marrow
Niemann-Pick disease	Sphingomyelinase	• **"Foamy histiocytes"** in liver, spleen, lymph nodes, and skin • Hepatosplenomegaly • Anemia • Neurologic deterioration
von Gierke's disease	Glucose-6-phosphatase	• Accumulation of glycogen in liver and kidney • Hepatomegaly • Hypoglycemia
Cori's disease	Debranching enzyme	• Accumulation of glycogen in liver and striated muscle • Hepatomegaly • Hypoglycemia • Failure to grow
Pompe's disease	α-1,4-Glucosidase (lysosomal enzyme)	• Accumulation of glycogen in liver and striated muscle • Cardiomegaly • Death owing to cardiac failure before 3 years of age
Galactosemia	Galactose-1-phosphate uridyl transferase	• Accumulation of galactose-1-phosphate in many tissues • **Cataracts** • Cirrhosis • Mental retardation • Failure to thrive
Phenylketonuria	Phenylalanine hydroxylase	• Accumulation of phenylalanine • Cerebral myelin degeneration • **Mental retardation**
Maple syrup urine disease	Branched chain α-ketoacid dehydrogenase	• Inability to metabolize leucine, isoleucine, and valine • Neurologic symptoms • High mortality

VI. Viral hepatitis (Table 5-14)

Viral hepatitis can lead to **direct hyperbilirubinemia,** elevated serum transaminases, icterus, or hepatomegaly, but not ascites. Morphologically, changes range from multifocal hepatocellular necrosis (hepatitis A and hepatitis B) to ballooning degeneration (hepatitis B and hepatitis C) to piecemeal necrosis (hepatitis C).

TABLE 5-14 Viral Hepatitis

	Hepatitis A	Hepatitis B	Hepatitis C	Hepatitis D	Hepatitis E
Virus family	Picornavirus	Hepadnavirus	Flavivirus	Delta agent	Calcivirus
Viral morphology	Single-stranded RNA	Circular, double-stranded DNA	Single-stranded RNA	Incomplete genome of single stranded RNA	Single-stranded RNA
Mode of transmission	Fecal-oral	Sexual and parenteral, transplacental	Parenteral; limited sexual; transplacental	Sexual and parenteral, transplacental	Fecal-oral
Diagnostic test	IgM anti-HAV	HBsAg; anti-HBsAg; HBeAg; HBV DNA; IgM anti-HBcAg	Anti-HCV	Anti-delta Ag	None
Severity	Mild	Moderate	Mild	Severe	Mild
Chronic infection	No	10% of adults 80% to 90% of infants and immuno-compromised	80%–90%	No increase over hepatitis B alone	No
Carrier state	No	Yes	Yes	Yes	No
Hepatocellular carcinoma	No	Yes	Yes	No	No
Prophylaxis and treatment	Immune globulin; vaccine	Hepatitis B immune globulin; vaccine Interferon and nucleoside analogue inhibitors of viral DNA synthesis	Interferon and ribavirin	Hepatitis B immune globulin; vaccine	None
Notes	Incubation period of 14–15 days	**Dane particle:** viral DNA genome, DNA polymerase, HBcAg, HBeAg, HBsAg; ha **reverse transcriptase;** incubation period 60–90 days	**Most frequent cause of transfusion-mediated hepatitis**	Defective in replication; **requires coinfection with hepatitis B**	Hepatitis infection in Third World nations

Ag=antigen; *DNA*=deoxyribonucleic acid; *HAV*=hepatitis A virus; *HBcAg*=hepatitis B core antigen; *HBeAg*=hepatitis B envelope antigen; *HBsAg*=hepatitis B surface antigen; *HCV*=hepatitis C virus; *IgM*=immunoglobulin M; *RNA*=ribonucleic acid

QUICK HIT

Hepatitis B e antigen (HBeAg), an alternative form of the capsid protein, and Hepatitis B surface antigen (HBsAg) are indicators of virus replication. Antibody to hepatitis B surface antigen (HBsAb) is indicative of recovery and immunity. HBsAb is also positive following vaccination. Antibody to hepatitis B capsid antigen (HBcAb) is positive in early infection; in addition HBcAb acts as a marker for hepatitis infection during the "window" period, which is the period during acute infection when HBsAg has become undetectable, but HBsAb has not yet appeared.

VII. Cirrhosis (Table 5-15)

Cirrhosis is a disease of the liver characterized by fibrosis and disorganization of the lobular and vascular structure owing to the destruction and regeneration of hepatocytes.

Cirrhosis often leads to **portal hypertension.** There are three major collateral circulation pathways that allow blood to return to the heart: (1) left gastric to esophageal plexus to azygous to the superior vena cava (SVC) (**esophageal varices**); (2) inferior mesenteric to superior rectal to inferior rectal to inferior vena cava (IVC) (**hemorrhoids**); and (3) ligamentum teres to superficial abdominals to SVC or IVC (**caput medusae**).

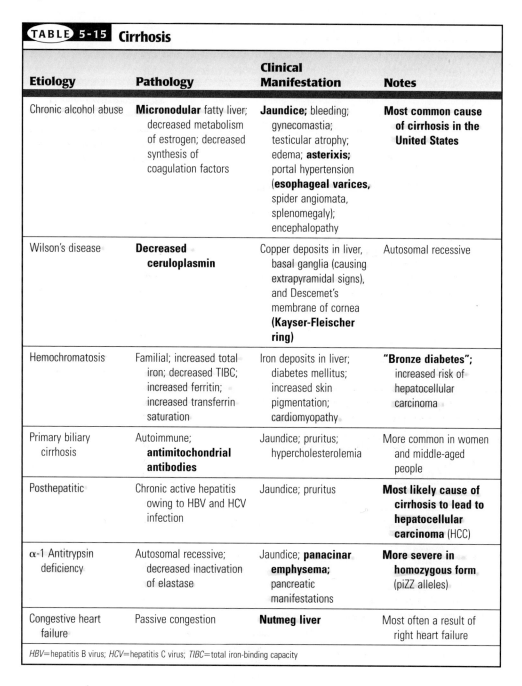

TABLE 5-15	Cirrhosis		
Etiology	**Pathology**	**Clinical Manifestation**	**Notes**
Chronic alcohol abuse	**Micronodular** fatty liver; decreased metabolism of estrogen; decreased synthesis of coagulation factors	**Jaundice;** bleeding; gynecomastia; testicular atrophy; edema; **asterixis;** portal hypertension (**esophageal varices,** spider angiomata, splenomegaly); encephalopathy	**Most common cause of cirrhosis in the United States**
Wilson's disease	**Decreased ceruloplasmin**	Copper deposits in liver, basal ganglia (causing extrapyramidal signs), and Descemet's membrane of cornea (**Kayser-Fleischer ring**)	Autosomal recessive
Hemochromatosis	Familial; increased total iron; decreased TIBC; increased ferritin; increased transferrin saturation	Iron deposits in liver; diabetes mellitus; increased skin pigmentation; cardiomyopathy	**"Bronze diabetes";** increased risk of hepatocellular carcinoma
Primary biliary cirrhosis	Autoimmune; **antimitochondrial antibodies**	Jaundice; pruritus; hypercholesterolemia	More common in women and middle-aged people
Posthepatitic	Chronic active hepatitis owing to HBV and HCV infection	Jaundice; pruritus	**Most likely cause of cirrhosis to lead to hepatocellular carcinoma** (HCC)
α-1 Antitrypsin deficiency	Autosomal recessive; decreased inactivation of elastase	Jaundice; **panacinar emphysema;** pancreatic manifestations	**More severe in homozygous form** (piZZ alleles)
Congestive heart failure	Passive congestion	**Nutmeg liver**	Most often a result of right heart failure

HBV=hepatitis B virus; *HCV*=hepatitis C virus; *TIBC*=total iron-binding capacity

VIII. Common clinical disorders of the hepatobiliary system (Table 5-16)
Hepatobiliary diseases vary in their presentation and etiology. Cholelithiasis is very common and curable with surgery, whereas hepatocellular carcinoma is much less common but usually fatal.

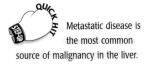 Pigment gallstones occurring in children or young adults with no history of pregnancy may be a result of a congenital hemoglobinopathy (e.g., sickle cell disease or thalassemia).

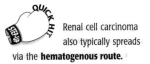 Metastatic disease is the most common source of malignancy in the liver.

Renal cell carcinoma also typically spreads via the **hematogenous route.**

TABLE 5-16 Common Clinical Disorders of the Hepatobiliary System

Disorder	Etiology and Pathology	Clinical Features	Notes
Cholelithiasis (gallstones)	Very common disease; women over 40 years of age; obesity; multiparity	Steatorrhea; nausea; vomiting; bile duct obstruction; jaundice; may lead to cholangitis or cholecystitis; malignancy; positive Murphy's sign	Cholesterol stones (large); pigment stones (seen in hemolytic anemia or excess bilirubin production); mixed stones (majority)
Hepatocellular adenoma (hepatoma)	Benign tumor; women 20–30 years of age taking **oral contraceptives**	Usually found incidentally; may cause pain or hemorrhage	10% may become malignant; oral contraceptive use should be stopped
Adenocarcinoma of the gallbladder	Gallstones	Obstructive jaundice; enlarged gallbladder	**Courvoisier's law:** obstruction of common bile duct enlarges gallbladder while obstructing stones do not; caused by scarring of gallbladder
Hepatocellular carcinoma	Cirrhosis; **hepatitis B; hepatitis C;** aflatoxin B (carcinogen in contaminated peanuts)	Increased α-fetoprotein; jaundice; abdominal distention; ascites	**Hematogenous spread**

THE PANCREAS

● Common Clinical Disorders of the Pancreas (Table 5-17)

In the United States alcohol is the most common cause of pancreatic pathology.

TABLE 5-17 Common Clinical Disorders of the Pancreas

Disorder	Etiology and Pathology	Clinical Features	Notes
Acute pancreatitis	Gallstones (obstructing the ampulla of Vater); alcohol abuse	**Midepigastric pain radiating to back; increased serum amylase** and lipase; hemorrhage may lead to Cullen's or Grey Turner's sign; hypocalcemia	Activation of pancreatic enzymes leads to autodigestion
Chronic pancreatitis	**Alcoholism** in adults; cystic fibrosis in children	**Increased serum amylase** and lipase; **pancreatic calcifications;** epigastric pain; steatorrhea	Irreversible; leads to organ atrophy; may lead to formation of pancreatic pseudocyst

(continued)

TABLE 5-17 **Common Clinical Disorders of the Pancreas (Continued)**

Disorder	Etiology and Pathology	Clinical Features	Notes
Adenocarcinoma of the exocrine pancreas	More common in smokers	Invasive; **Trousseau's syndrome** (migratory thrombophlebitis); radiating abdominal pain; obstructive jaundice; **increased carcinoembryonic antigen** (CEA)	Poor prognosis; over 50% in head of pancreas; more common in blacks, males, patients with diabetes, and people over 60 years of age
Insulinoma (endocrine pancreas)	Originates in β cells	**Whipple's triad:** hypoglycemia, CNS dysfunction, reversal of CNS abnormalities with glucose	Most common islet cell tumor
Gastrinoma (Zollinger-Ellison syndrome)	Gastrin-secreting tumor (most commonly islet cell origin)	Recurrent peptic ulcers	Part of **MEN I**

CNS=central nervous system; *MEN*=multiple endocrine neoplasia

The presence of **C-peptide** in the blood distinguishes endogenous insulin secretions (as in an insulinoma) from exogenous insulin administration (as seen in Munchausen syndrome).

MEN I, also known as Wermer's syndrome, involves neoplasia or hyperplasia of the pancreas, the parathyroid, and the pituitary.

BUGS OF THE GASTROINTESTINAL TRACT

I. Bacterial

Enterobacteriaceae	*Vibrio cholerae*	*Clostridium botulinum*
Salmonella	*Staphylococcus aureus*	*Clostridium difficile*
Shigella	*Campylobacter jejuni*	*Bacillus fragilis*
Escherichia coli	*Helicobacter pylori*	

II. Parasitic

Entamoeba histolytica	*Cryptosporidium*	*Ascaris lumbricoides*
Giardia lamblia	*Trichuris trichiura*	*Strongyloides stercoralis*

III. Viral

Adenovirus	Echovirus	Norwalk agent
Coronavirus	Rotavirus	Reovirus

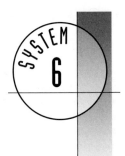

The Renal System

DEVELOPMENT

I. Intermediate mesoderm
A. This forms the **urogenital ridges** on each side of the aorta.
B. The **nephrogenic cord** arises from this urogenital ridge and gives rise wholly or in part to the pronephros, the mesonephros, and the metanephros.

II. Pronephros
A. Forms in the fourth week
B. Quickly regresses by the fifth week
C. Nonfunctional

III. Mesonephros
A. Forms late in the fourth week and is functional until the permanent kidney is able to develop
B. The **mesonephric duct** forms from the mesonephros.
  1. Forms the **ductus deferens, epididymis, ejaculatory duct,** and **seminal vesicle in the male**
  2. Forms the **ureteric bud** from which the **ureter, renal pelvis, calyces,** and **collecting tubules** in both the male and female are derived
  3. No important genital or reproductive derivatives of the mesonephric duct specific to females are formed.

IV. Metanephros
A. Develops into the **adult kidney**
B. Formed during the fifth week from the **ureteric bud** and the metanephric mass (which is induced to form by contact with the ureteric bud) and begins to function in the ninth week
C. Metanephric mesoderm forms the nephrons.
D. "Ascends" from sacral levels to low thoracic levels during its development because of longitudinal growth of the fetus
E. Urogenital sinus forms the **bladder,** which is continuous with allantois. Allantois is equivalent to the median umbilical ligament in the adult.
F. Urethra
  1. Formed from endoderm and urogenital sinus
  2. Distal portion formed from ectoderm

V. Congenital anomalies of the renal system (Table 6-1)

> **QUICK HIT**
> In the adult male, the ureter passes posterior to the ductus deferens; in the adult female, the ureter passes posterior to the uterine artery.

TABLE 6-1	Congenital Anomalies
Anomaly	**Characteristics**
Bilateral renal agenesis (Potter's syndrome)	• Occurs when the ureteric bud does not form • **Oligohydramnios** • Limb deformities • Facial deformities • **Pulmonary hypoplasia** • Bilateral agenesis is not compatible with life
Accessory renal arteries	• Arise from the aorta • Feed a particular section of the kidney • Are end arteries • **Cutting will produce ischemic** infarct in the area they supply
Congenital polycystic kidney disease	• Multiple small and large cysts causing renal insufficiency • Cysts are "closed"—not continuous with collecting system • Enlarged kidneys palpable on newborn examination • Death within days to weeks
Horseshoe kidney	• Inferior poles of the kidneys are fused • Ascent is arrested at the level of the inferior mesenteric artery • Increases probability of Wilms' tumor

 The entire collecting system arises from **the ureteric bud.** The remainder of the renal system arises from the metanephric mesoderm.

 Fanconi's syndrome is a **hereditary** or **acquired** dysfunction of the proximal renal tubules. As a result of impaired glucose, amino acid, phosphate, and bicarbonate reabsorption, it manifests clinically as glycosuria, hyperphosphaturia, aminoaciduria, and acidosis.

GROSS DESCRIPTION OF THE KIDNEY

I. Paired adult kidneys weigh approximately 150 g each.

II. They are located posterior to the peritoneum and at approximately the level of the first lumbar vertebra.

III. The right kidney is slightly lower than the left owing to downward displacement by the liver.

IV. The left renal vein lies posterior to the superior mesenteric artery and anterior to the abdominal aorta.

V. The kidney is highly vascularized; it filters more than 1700 L of blood per day to produce about 1 L of urine.

 The left gonadal (testicular or ovarian) vein drains into the left renal vein; the right gonadal vein drains directly into the inferior vena cava.

THE RENAL SYSTEM

VI. Kidney and urinary tract (Figure 6-1)

FIGURE
6-1   **The kidney and urinary tract**

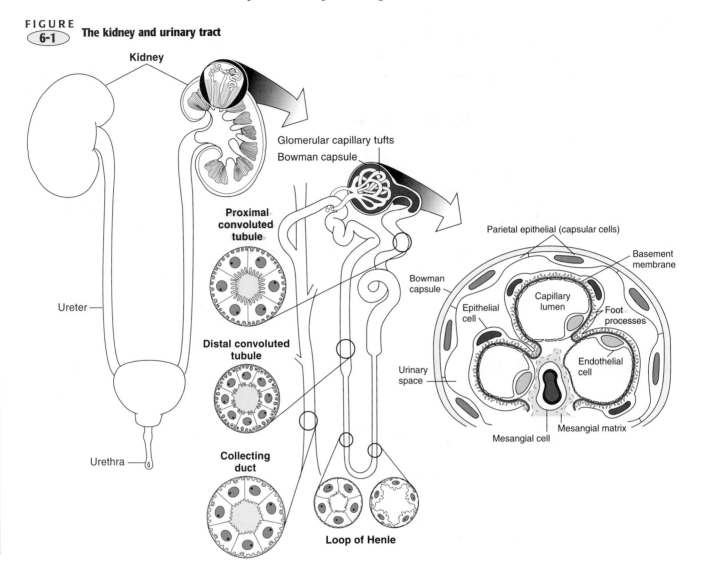

(Adapted from Damjanov I. A Color Atlas and Textbook of Histopathology. Baltimore: Williams & Wilkins, 1996:258–259.)

VII. Distribution of body water (Figure 6-2)

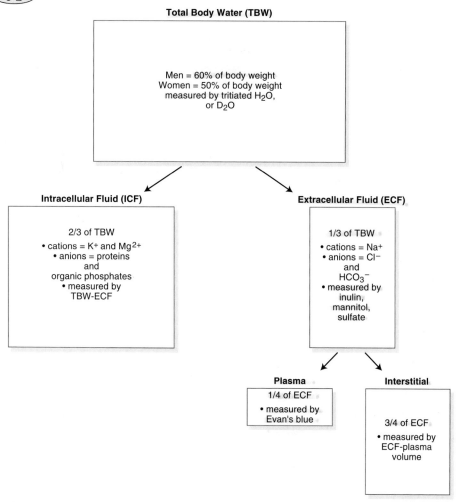

FIGURE 6-2 Distribution of body water

Total Body Water (TBW)

Men = 60% of body weight
Women = 50% of body weight
measured by tritiated H_2O,
or D_2O

Intracellular Fluid (ICF)

2/3 of TBW
• cations = K^+ and Mg^{2+}
• anions = proteins
and
organic phosphates
• measured by
TBW-ECF

Extracellular Fluid (ECF)

1/3 of TBW
• cations = Na^+
• anions = Cl^-
and
HCO_3^-
• measured by
inulin,
mannitol,
sulfate

Plasma

1/4 of ECF
• measured by
Evan's blue

Interstitial

3/4 of ECF
• measured by
ECF-plasma
volume

Cl^-=chloride; D_2O=heavy water; HCO_3^-=bicarbonate; H_2O=water; K^+=potassium; Mg^{2+}=magnesium; Na^+=sodium.

NORMAL KIDNEY FUNCTION

I. Renal blood flow (RBF)
  A. 25% of cardiac output
  B. **RBF = renal plasma flow (RPF)/[1 − hematocrit (Hct)]**
  C. Renal vasculature **autoregulates** RBF, keeping it constant even when arterial pressure varies from 100 to 200 mm Hg.

II. Renal plasma flow (RPF)
  A. Effective RPF is measured by clearance of para-aminohippuric acid (**PAH**), which is filtered and secreted.
  B. This measurement underestimates by 10%.

III. Glomerular filtration rate (GFR)
  A. Normal GFR is 120 mL/min.
  B. It is measured by **inulin** clearance (filtered; not absorbed or secreted).
    1. Decreases in GFR cause a rise in blood urea nitrogen (BUN) and creatinine levels.
    2. GFR decreases with age.

C. GFR is driven by Starling forces (filtration is always favored) (Figure 6-3).

FIGURE 6-3 **Starling forces on the glomerular capillary**

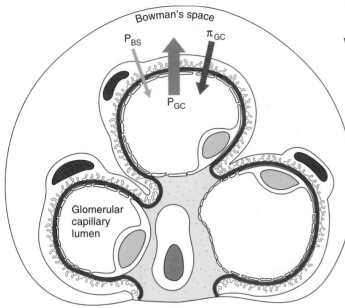

The Starling forces influence the Glomerular Filtration Rate (GFR)

$$GFR = K_F \, [(P_{GC} - P_{BS}) - (\pi_{GC} - \pi_{BS})]$$

Where K_F: the filtration coefficient of the glomerular capillaries

P_{GC}: The hydrostatic pressure exerted by the fluid in the glomerular capillary. A dilated afferent arteriole increases P_{GC}, as does a constricted efferent arteriole.

P_{BS}: The hydrostatic pressure exerted by the fluid in Bowman's space. Blockage or constriction of the ureters increases P_{BS}.

π_{GC}: The oncotic pressure of the glomerular capillary. The value of π_{GC} increases along the length of the capillary because the protein concentration in the capillary increases as water is forced into Bowman's space.

π_{BS}: The oncotic pressure in Bowman's space. This value is usually zero.

D. Renal clearance
1. Removal of a substance from the blood by renal excretion
2. Determined by the following equation:

Clearance = U × V / P (in mL/min)
where   U = concentration of substance in urine in mg/mL
V = urine volume (urine flow rate) in mL/min
P = concentration of substance in mg/mL

3. Factors that determine clearance
   a. Highly cleared substances (e.g., PAH) are those that are filtered and secreted.
   b. Poorly cleared substances are those that are either not filtered (e.g., protein) or completely reabsorbed (e.g., glucose).
   c. Reabsorption
      (1) Limited by the number of transporters for certain compounds (e.g., glucose)
      (2) Transport maximum (T_m) is the maximum rate of reabsorption, at which the transporters are saturated.
      (3) At concentrations above T_m, excess is excreted.

QUICK HIT

The T_m for glucose is reached at approximately 350 mg/dL. Concentrations above this result in an osmotic diuresis, such as that seen in diabetics with hyperglycemia.

IV. Filtration fraction
A. **Filtration fraction (FF) = GFR/RPF**
B. The normal filtration fraction is 20%.

V. Innervation and hormones
A. Juxtaglomerular apparatus (JGA) produces renin and is stimulated by the β-sympathetic adrenergics in the kidney.
B. **Renin** cleaves angiotensinogen to **angiotensin I.**

C. Angiotensin I is cleaved to **angiotensin II** by angiotensin-converting enzyme (**ACE**) in the lung.
  1. Functions of angiotensin II
    a. Stimulates aldosterone release from the zona glomerulosa
    b. Stimulates secretion of antidiuretic hormone (ADH) and adrenocorticotropic hormone (ACTH)
    c. Acts as a potent local vasoconstrictor of the renal arterioles at low plasma levels
    d. Acts as a general systemic vasoconstrictor at high plasma levels
    e. Stimulates thirst
    f. Stimulates epinephrine and norepinephrine release from adrenal medulla
  2. Angiotensin II is inactivated to angiotensin III, a potent stimulator of aldosterone secretion but not an effective vasoconstrictor.

ACE inhibitors **captopril** and **enalapril** reduce hypertension by inhibiting the conversion of angiotensin I to angiotensin II, thereby decreasing the release of aldosterone. The angiotensin II receptor blocker, **losartan**, prevents angiotensin II from interacting with its receptor. This prevents angiotensin II from causing constriction of efferent arterioles.

VI. Hormones and the nephron (Figure 6-4)

FIGURE 6-4 Hormones and the nephron

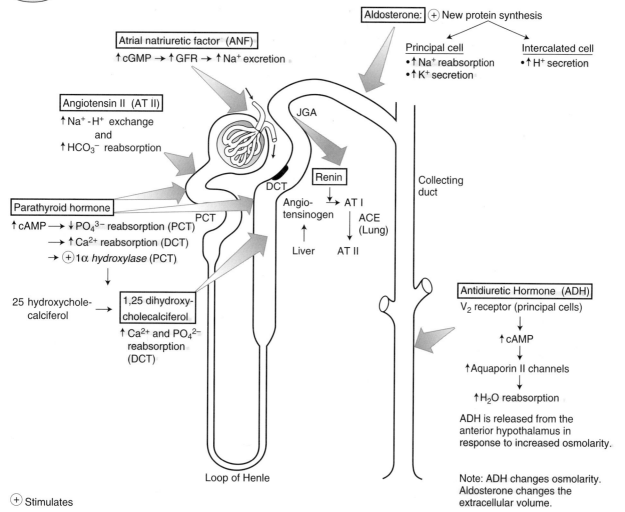

ACE=angiotensin-converting enzyme; AT I=angiotensin I; Ca^{2+}=calcium; cAMP=cyclic adenosine monophosphate; cGMP=cyclic guanosine monophosphate; DCT=distal convoluted tubule; GFR=glomerular filtration rate; H^+=hydrogen ion; HCO_3^-=bicarbonate; H_2O=water; JGA=juxtaglomerular apparatus; K^+=potassium; Na^+=sodium; PCT=proximal convoluted tubule; PO_4^{3-}=phosphate; V_2=vasopressin receptor, type 2.

VII. Effects of volume change on fluid levels (Table 6-2)

A variety of hormones, such as ADH, aldosterone, and atrial natriuretic factor, regulate extracellular and intracellular volumes. Intake and output, as well as hormonal imbalance, can significantly alter the homeostatic fluid balance in the body.

TABLE 6-2 | **Effects of Volume Change on Fluid Levels**

Type	Key Examples	ECF Volume	ICF Volume	ECF Osmolarity	Hct and Serum [Na$^+$]
Isosmotic volume expansion	Isotonic fluid infusion (e.g., normal saline or lactated Ringer's)	↑	No change	No change	↓ Hct − [Na$^+$]
Isosmotic volume contraction	Diarrhea	↓	No change	No change	↑ Hct − [Na$^+$]
Hyperosmotic volume expansion	High NaCl intake	↑	↓	↑	↓ Hct ↑ [Na$^+$]
Hyperosmotic volume contraction	Sweating, Fever Diabetes insipidus	↓	↓	↑	− Hct ↑ [Na$^+$]
Hyposmotic volume expansion	SIADH	↑	↑	↓	− Hct ↓ [Na$^+$]
Hyposmotic volume contraction	Adrenal insufficiency	↓	↑	↓	↑ Hct ↓ [Na$^+$]

−=no change; *ECF*=extracellular fluid; *Hct*=hematocrit; *ICF*=intracellular fluid; *SIADH*=syndrome of inappropriate secretion of antidiuretic hormone From Costanzo LS. BRS Physiology, 2nd ed. Baltimore: Williams & Wilkins, 1998:139.

VIII. Electrolyte balance in the nephron (Figure 6-5)

FIGURE
6-5 Electrolyte balance in the nephron

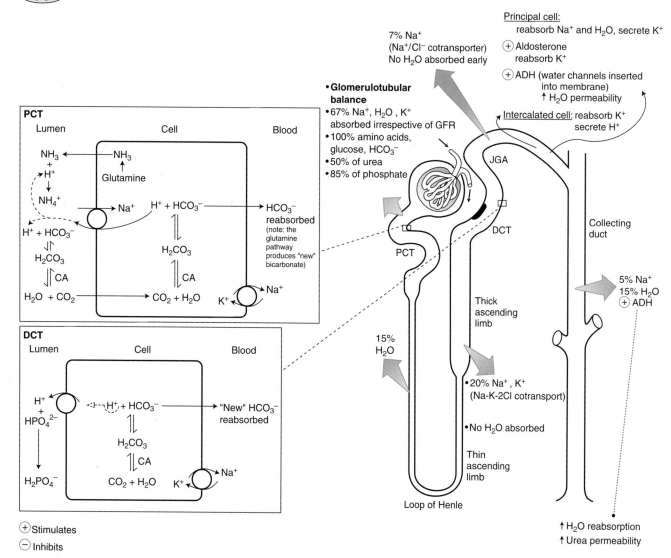

ADH=antidiuretic hormone; CA=carbonic anhydrase; Cl^-=chloride; CO_2=carbon dioxide; DCT=distal convoluted tubule; H^+=hydrogen ion; HCO_3^-=bicarbonate; H_2CO_3=carbonic acid; H_2O=water; HPO_4^{2-}, $H_2PO_4^-$=two forms of phosphate ions; JGA=juxtaglomerular apparatus; K^+=potassium; Mg^{2+}=magnesium; Na^+=sodium; NH_3=ammonia; NH_4^+=ammonium; PCT=proximal convoluted tubule.

Acidosis or alkalosis is determined by evaluating blood pH, arterial P_{CO_2}, and bicarbonate concentration. Anion gap (AG) is calculated using the following equation: $AG = Na^+ - (Cl^- + HCO_3^-)$. A normal anion gap is between 10 and 16 mEq/L. Certain acidotic conditions result in an elevated anion gap by altering the concentration of anions not considered in the above formula (lactate, β-OH butyrate, formate). A comparison of acidosis versus alkalosis is made in Table 6-3. The effects of metabolic and respiratory acid–base disturbances are outlined in Table 6-4.

Kussmaul respiration is an increase in both the rate and volume of respirations. It is classically described as occurring in diabetic ketoacidosis. Kussmaul's sign is a loss of the normal 5- to 10-mm Hg drop in blood pressure that accompanies inspiration. This is seen in pericarditis, restrictive cardiomyopathy, and after massive pulmonary embolism.

Emphysema and bronchitis often cause chronic respiratory acidosis.

Renal tubular acidosis (RTA) is characterized by a normal anion gap. Type 1 (distal) RTA is caused by a failure to excrete titratable acid and NH_4^+. Type 2 RTA is caused by renal loss of HCO_3^-. Type 4 RTA is caused by hypoaldosteronism, which leads to poor excretion of NH_4^+ and hyperkalemia.

A patient's respiratory status affects and is affected by his or her acid–base status. This is because of the reversible conversion of CO_2 to H^+ in the following way:
$$H_2O + CO_2 \rightleftharpoons H_2CO_3 \rightleftharpoons HCO_3^- + H^+.$$
The first reaction is catalyzed by the enzyme carbonic anhydrase.

TABLE 6-3 **Acidosis and Alkalosis**

Metabolic Disturbance	Presentation	Causes
Metabolic acidosis	• Fatigue • Shortness of breath • Abdominal pain • Vomiting • **Kussmaul respirations** • Hypotension • Tachycardia	• Chronic renal failure • Lactic acidosis • Uremia • **Ketoacidosis** • Intoxication (aspirin, methanol, ethylene glycol) • ***Diarrhea** • ***Renal tubular acidosis** • *Acetazolamide
Respiratory acidosis	• **Hypercapnia** • Confusion • Blunted sensation and pain • **Asterixis** • Papilledema	• Respiratory depression by drugs • Cerebral disease • Cardiopulmonary arrest response • Neuromuscular disease (e.g., myasthenia gravis) • Poor ventilation secondary to disease (e.g., asthma, pneumonia, bronchitis, emphysema)
Metabolic alkalosis	• No specific signs or symptoms • Can cause apathy, stupor, and confusion • If coupled with low calcium, can cause tetany	• Diuretics (Loop and thiazide) • Vomiting • Milk alkali syndrome • Large intake of alkaline substance • **Cushing's syndrome** • Primary aldosteronism
Respiratory alkalosis	• **Hyperventilation** • Numbness • Tingling • Paresthesia • Tetany, if severe	• Asthma • Pneumonia • Pulmonary edema • Heart disease with cyanosis • Pulmonary fibrosis • Aspirin intoxication • **Gram-negative sepsis** • Fever • Anxiety • Pregnancy • Drugs • Conditions that stimulate the medullary respiratory center (e.g. altitude)

*=Normal anion gap acidosis (acidosis items not starred have an increased anion gap)

TABLE 6-4 Effects of Metabolic and Respiratory Acid–Base Disturbances

Primary Disorder	pH	$[H^+]$	$[HCO_3^-]$	Pco_2	Respiratory Compensation	Renal Compensation
Metabolic acidosis!	↓	↑	↓ * (lost by buffering)	↓	Hyperventilation	↑ H^+ excretion (NH_3) ↑ "New" HCO_3^- reabsorption
Metabolic alkalosis	↑	↓	↑ *	↑	Hypoventilation	↑ HCO_3^- excretion
Acute respiratory acidosis	↓	↑	↑	↑ *	None	Not yet
Chronic respiratory acidosis	↓ (more normal)	↑	↑↑	↑ *	None	↑ H^+ excretion (NH_4^+) ↑ "New" HCO_3^- reabsorption
Acute respiratory alkalosis	↑	↓	↓	↓ *		Not yet
Chronic respiratory alkalosis	↑ (more normal)	↓	↓↓	↓ *		↓ H^+ excretion ↓ HCO_3^- reabsorption

*=primary disorder; ↑=increased; ↓=decreased

GLOMERULAR DISEASES

I. Nephrotic syndrome
A. **Features**
   1. **Proteinuria** of more than 3.5–4.0 g of protein/day
   2. Hypoalbuminemia
   3. Edema
   4. Hyperlipidemia
B. **Etiology**
   1. Idiopathic—75%
   2. Systemic disease—25%
C. Common types (Table 6-5)

II. Nephritic syndrome
A. **Features**
   1. **Hematuria**
   2. Hypertension
   3. Oliguria
   4. Azotemia

TABLE 6-5 **Nephrotic Glomerular Diseases**

Glomerular Disease	Etiology	Clinical Features	Notes
Minimal change disease (lipoid nephrosis)	Fusion of foot processes on the basement membrane leads to loss of negative charge and changes the protein selectivity; altered appearance of villi on epithelial cells	Electron microscopy shows **fusion of podocyte foot processes,** and lipid-laden renal cortices	**Common in young children** (usually under 5 years of age); responds well to steroids; albumin usually selectively secreted
Membranous glomerulonephritis	Idiopathic; secondarily caused by SLE, hepatitis B, syphilis, gold, penicillamine, malignancy	Basement membrane thickening; **"spike and dome"** with **subepithelial IgG and C3 deposits**	Common in young adults
Diabetic nephropathy	Microangiopathy leading to thickening of basement membrane	Basement membrane thickening	Two types: diffuse and nodular glomerulosclerosis; nodular has **Kimmelstiel-Wilson nodules;** usually leads to renal failure
Renal amyloidosis	Subendothelial or mesangial amyloid deposits; associated with multiple myeloma	Stains: periodic acid-Schiff (PAS) (−); **Congo Red (+)**	Increasing severity leads to renal failure
Lupus nephropathy	**Anti ds-DNA**	WHO classifications: • WHO I: normal • WHO II: mesangial proliferation; little clinical relevance • WHO III (focal proliferative): <1/2 of glomeruli affected • **WHO IV (diffuse proliferative):** worst prognosis; **wire-loop lesions;** (subendothelial immune complex deposition of IgM and IgG + C3) • WHO V: membranous glomerulonephritis	Degree of kidney involvement correlates to SLE prognosis; may have nephritic qualities
Focal and segmental glomerulosclerosis	Has four possible etiologies: idiopathic; superimposed on preexisting pathology; associated with loss of renal mass; secondary to other disorders (e.g., heroine abuse or HIV)	Sclerosis of some glomeruli; only capillary tuft is involved in affected glomeruli	Clinically similar to minimal change disease, but affects older population

C3=third component of complement; *ds-DNA*=double-stranded deoxyribonucleic acid; *HIV*=human immunodeficiency virus; *IgG*=immunoglobulin G; *IgM*=immunoglobulin M; *SLE*=systemic lupus erythematosus; *WHO*=World Health Organization

THE RENAL SYSTEM

B. Common types of nephritic glomerular diseases (Table 6-6)

TABLE 6-6 Nephritic Glomerular Diseases

Disease	Etiology	Special Features	Notes
Poststreptococcal glomerulonephritis	Poststreptococcal pharyngitis or impetigo; hepatitis B; high ASO titer; low C3; type III hypersensitivity	**"Lumpy bumpy"** deposits of IgG and C3; subepithelial humps on electron microscopy	Common in children; self-resolving; most common organisms are group A hemolytic streptococci; red cell casts in urine
Rapidly progressive **(crescentic)** glomerulonephritis	**ANCA positive;** poststreptococcal etiology 50%; renal failure within weeks or months	Accumulation of fibrin, macrophages, and PMNs in Bowman's capsule; wrinkling of basement membrane on electron microscopy **(crescents)**	If also involves upper respiratory system, then termed **Wegener's**
Goodpasture's syndrome	**Anti-glomerular basement membrane and alveolar basement membrane antibodies**	**Linear pattern** of IgG on fluorescence microscopy; may be associated with hemoptysis and pulmonary hemorrhage	Usually **males in their mid-20s**
Alport's syndrome	Hereditary structural defect in collagen IV leads to leaky basement membrane	Glomerular basement membrane splitting on electron microscopy	Appears before age 20; associated with deafness and ocular problems

ANCA=antineutrophil cytoplasmic antibody; *ASO*=antistreptolysin O; *C3*=third component of complement; *IgG*=immunoglobulin G; *PMN*=polymorphonuclear leukocyte

III. Nonnephritic, nonnephrotic glomerular diseases (Table 6-7)

TABLE 6-7 Nonnephritic, Nonnephrotic Glomerular Diseases

Disease	Etiology	Clinical Features	Notes
IgA nephropathy (Berger's disease)	IgA deposits in mesangium; hematuria; usually follows infection	Mesangial cell proliferation on electron microscopy	Minimal clinical significance; common
Membranoproliferative glomerulonephritis	Type 2 has IgG autoantibody; C3 is reduced in both types	Basement membrane thickens and appears as two layers; **"train-track"** appearance on electron microscopy	Two types: type 1 and type 2 (dense deposit disease); may lead to either nephrotic or nephritic syndromes

C3=third component of complement; *IgA*=immunoglobulin A; *IgG*=immunoglobulin G

IV. Glomerular deposits in disease (Figure 6-6)

FIGURE 6-6 Glomerular deposits in disease

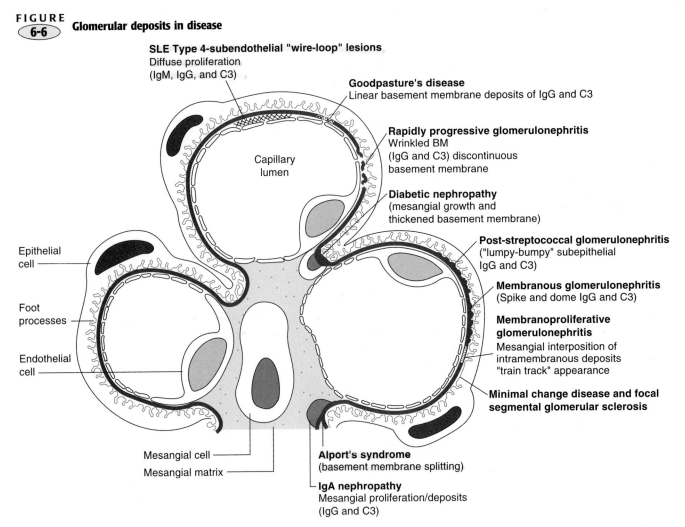

BM=basement membrane; C3=third component of complement; Ig=immunoglobulin; SLE=systemic lupus erythematosus.

URINARY TRACT INFECTIONS (UTIs)

I. Cystitis

A. Characteristic clinical features
  1. **Dysuria**
  2. **Frequency**
  3. **Urgency**
  4. Suprapubic pain

B. Etiology and pathogenesis
  1. Bacteria gain access to the urinary tract via the urethra.
  2. Cystitis most frequently involves normal colonic flora.
      a. *Escherichia coli* is the most common cause (approximately 80%).
      b. *Proteus, Klebsiella,* and *Enterobacter* have also been implicated.
      c. *Staphylococcus saprophyticus* causes 10%–15% of infections in young women.
  3. **Women** have a higher incidence of infection because they have shorter urethras.
  4. Other risk factors include sexual activity, pregnancy, urinary obstruction, neurogenic bladder, and vesicoureteral reflux.

C. Diagnostic findings
  1. Characteristic clinical features are present.
  2. **Pyuria** (more than 8 leukocytes/high-power field)
  3. Bacterial culture yields **greater than 10^5 organisms/mL.**
D. Treatment
  1. Cystitis is treated with antibiotics.
  2. Recurrent cystitis may require prophylactic antibiotics.

II. Acute pyelonephritis

A. **Characteristic clinical features**
  1. **Flank pain** or **costovertebral angle** (CVA) **tenderness**
  2. **Dysuria**
  3. **Fever**
  4. Chills
  5. Nausea and vomiting
  6. Diarrhea
B. Etiology and pathogenesis
  1. Bacteria **ascend** from an infected urinary bladder to the kidney via **vesicoureteral** reflux.
  2. Infection may also spread **hematogenously** to the kidney (may not necessarily be preceded by acute cystitis).
  3. Causative organism is usually *E. coli.*
C. **Diagnostic findings**
  1. Characteristic clinical features are present.
  2. Bacteriuria, pyuria, and **white blood cell casts** are seen on urine microscopy.
  3. Urine and blood cultures are performed to determine infection.
D. Treatment
  1. Treatment is with **antibiotics,** often **intravenously.**
  2. Recurrent infection can lead to chronic pyelonephritis. This condition has several complications:
    a. **Scarring and deformity of the renal pelvis and calyces**
    b. Interstitial fibrosis and tubular atrophy
    c. Ischemia of the tubules leads to microscopic **"thyroidization"** of the kidney.

MAJOR CAUSES OF ACUTE RENAL FAILURE (Figure 6-7)

FIGURE
6-7   **Etiology of acute renal failure**

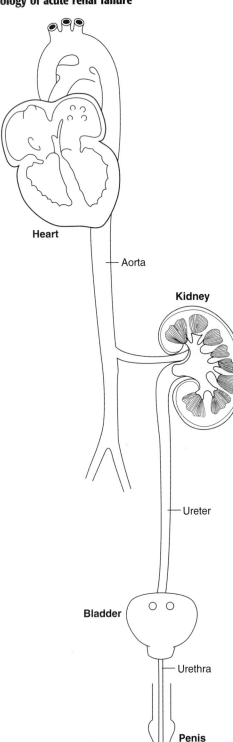

Heart

— Aorta

Kidney

— Ureter

Bladder

— Urethra

Penis

Prerenal causes

- Hypovolemia
- Low cardiac output
- Increased systemic vascular resistance
- Drugs: Cyclooxygenase inhibitors (COX ⊖)
- Angiotensin-converting enzyme inhibitors (ACE ⊖)

Renal (intrinsic) causes

- Renovesicular obstruction
- Glomerulonephritis
- Hemolytic uremic syndrome (HUS)
- Thrombotic thrombocytic purpura (TTP)
- Disseminated intravascular coagulation (DIC)
- Systemic lupus erythematosus (SLE)
- Scleroderma
- Acute tubular necrosis (ATN)
- Interstitial nephritis

Postrenal causes

- Ureteric obstruction (bilateral)
- Prostatic hyperplasia
- Bladder-neck obstruction
- Stricture
- Phimosis

THE RENAL SYSTEM

I. Prerenal failure is defined as oliguria and an increase in BUN and creatinine with inherently normal renal function.

   A. Hypovolemic states
     1. Hemorrhage
     2. Burns
     3. Dehydration
     4. Vomiting
     5. Diarrhea
     6. Diuretics
     7. Pancreatitis

   B. Low cardiac output states
     1. Arrhythmias
     2. Pulmonary embolus
     3. Myocardial or valvular disease
     4. Cardiac tamponade
     5. Pulmonary hypertension

   C. **Renal vasoconstrictive states** resulting in ischemia may be caused by the following:
     1. Cirrhosis with ascites
     2. Vasoconstrictive drugs: epinephrine, norepinephrine, cyclosporine, amphotericin B

   D. Intrinsic decrease of renal perfusion
     1. Cyclooxygenase (COX) inhibitors
     2. ACE inhibitors

II. Acute intrinsic renal failure is inherent malfunction of the renal tissue. It may be glomerular, tubular, or interstitial. For a comparison of prerenal versus intrinsic renal failure, see Table 6-8.

QUICK HIT

COX is inhibited by aspirin and other nonsteroidal anti-inflammatory drugs (NSAIDs), but not by acetaminophen.

TABLE 6-8 Prerenal Versus Intrinsic Renal Failure

	Prerenal Renal Failure	Intrinsic Renal Failure
Fractional excretion of Na⁺	<1	>1
Urine sodium concentration	<10 mg/dL	>20 mg/dL
Urine creatinine to plasma creatinine	>40	>20
Urine casts	Hyaline	Muddy brown and granular
Plasma BUN to creatinine ratio	>20	<10–15

BUN=blood urea nitrogen; Na⁺=sodium

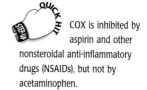

QUICK HIT

Acute renal failure and acute tubular necrosis are often used synonymously. However, acute renal failure can occur without acute tubular necrosis.

   A. Acute tubular necrosis (ATN)
     1. Drugs that may lead to ATN are exogenous toxins (contrast, cyclosporine, aminoglycosides, ethylene glycol, acetaminophen, heavy metals) or endogenous toxins (myoglobin, uric acid, oxalate).
     2. Ischemia can result in ATN via causes related to prerenal failure.

   B. Obstruction of renal vasculature from atherosclerosis, vasculitis, or other factors may also cause acute intrinsic renal failure.

   C. Diseases that affect the glomeruli or microvasculature include the following:
     1. Disseminated intravascular coagulopathy (DIC)
     2. Glomerulonephritis
     3. Hemolytic uremic syndrome (HUS)
     4. Thrombotic thrombocytopenic purpura (TTP)

QUICK HIT

Fractional excretion of Na⁺ is calculated using the formula:

$$FENa^+ = \frac{\dfrac{urine\ [Na^+]}{serum\ [Na^+]}}{\dfrac{urine\ [creatinine]}{serum\ [creatinine]}}(100)$$

QUICK HIT

Sheehan's syndrome (pituitary necrosis) is also caused by postpartum hemorrhage and leads to loss of gonadotropins, thyroid-stimulating hormone (TSH), and ACTH, which clinically manifests itself as fatigue, weight loss, and amenorrhea.

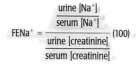

THE RENAL SYSTEM

HUS and TTP cause a "flea-bitten" kidney.

The most **common** cause of acute renal failure (ARF) is **therapeutic drugs.**

Renal transplant rejection rates can be decreased by administration of cyclosporine and muromonab-CD3 (OKT(C).

Finasteride, a 5-α-reductase inhibitor, is used to treat benign prostatic hyperplasia (BPH). Cold medicines and α-agonists exacerbate BPH.

     5. Pregnancy
     6. Scleroderma
     7. Systemic lupus erythematosus (SLE)
  D. **Interstitial nephritis** can have many causes.
     1. β-Lactams
     2. Sulfonamides
     3. Trimethoprim (TMP)
     4. Rifampin
     5. COX inhibitors
     6. Diuretics
     7. Captopril
     8. Infection
     9. Idiopathic
  E. Acute renal transplant rejection is a cause of ATN.

III. Postrenal failure is bilateral obstruction of the ureters or obstruction of the urethra. It accounts for less than 5% of acute renal failure (ARF) and has a variety of causes.
  A. Urolithiasis (see section on stone formation)
  B. Prostatic hyperplasia
  C. Tumor obstructing the bladder or the ureters bilaterally
  D. Neurogenic bladder

Chronic Renal Failure (CRF) and Uremia (Figure 6-8)

FIGURE 6-8 Manifestations of chronic renal failure and uremia

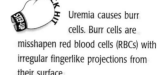

Uremia causes burr cells. Burr cells are misshapen red blood cells (RBCs) with irregular fingerlike projections from their surface.

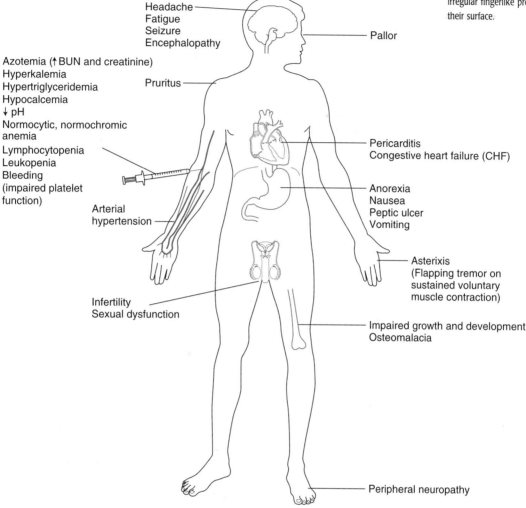

Headache
Fatigue
Seizure
Encephalopathy

Pallor

Azotemia (↑BUN and creatinine)
Hyperkalemia
Hypertriglyceridemia
Hypocalcemia
↓ pH
Normocytic, normochromic anemia
Lymphocytopenia
Leukopenia
Bleeding (impaired platelet function)

Pruritus

Pericarditis
Congestive heart failure (CHF)

Arterial hypertension

Anorexia
Nausea
Peptic ulcer
Vomiting

Asterixis
(Flapping tremor on sustained voluntary muscle contraction)

Infertility
Sexual dysfunction

Impaired growth and development
Osteomalacia

Peripheral neuropathy

BUN=blood urea nitrogen.

I. Major causes of CRF
A. **Hypertension**
B. **Diabetes mellitus**

II. Profound loss of renal function leads to uremia.
A. GFR is reduced to 50%–65% of normal.
B. Byproducts of amino acid and protein metabolism (especially urea) cause a variety of signs and symptoms.
   1. **Endocrine and electrolyte findings**
      a. Hyperkalemia
      b. Hypertriglyceridemia
      c. Hyperuricemia
      d. Hypocalcemia and osteomalacia as a result of decreased 1,25 dihydroxy cholecalciferol levels
      e. Impaired growth and development
      f. Infertility and sexual dysfunction
      g. Metabolic acidosis

2. **Gastrointestinal findings**
   a. Anorexia
   b. Nausea
   c. Peptic ulcer
   d. Vomiting
3. **Renal findings:** azotemia
4. **Cardiovascular and pulmonary findings**
   a. Arterial hypertension
   b. Congestive heart failure
   c. Pericarditis
5. **Dermatologic findings**
   a. Pallor
   b. Pruritus
6. **Neuromuscular findings**
   a. Asterixis
   b. Headache and fatigue
   c. Peripheral neuropathy
7. **Hematologic findings**
   a. Increased susceptibility to infection
   b. Lymphocytopenia and leukopenia
   c. Normocytic, normochromic anemia

KIDNEY STONE FORMATION (Figure 6-9)

FIGURE 6-9 Comparison of different types of kidney stones

Calcium Stones

A. Calcium Oxalate (CO)   B. Calcium Phosphate (CP)

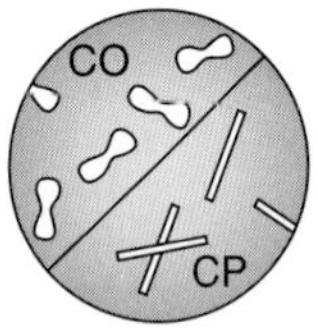

80% of stones
Men
20–30 years of age
Multiple (every 2–3 years)
Familial predisposition
Radiopaque
May be caused by primary hyperthyroidism

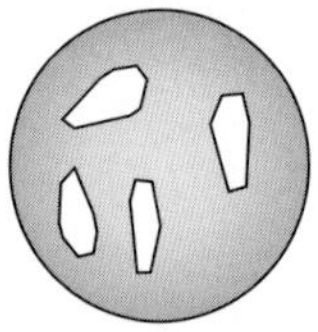

Struvite

12% of stones
Women
Risk factors:
Catheter, UTIs (especially *Proteus*)
May fill renal pelvis and calyces ("staghorn")
Radiopaque

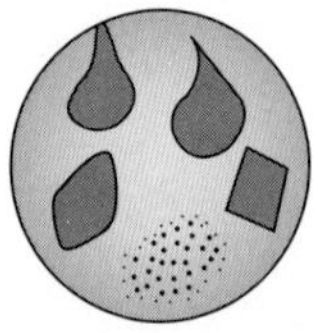

Uric acid

7% of stones
Men
Risk factors:
50% have gout
Strong negative birefringence
Radiolucent
Associated with cell lysis (e.g., chemotherapy, leukemia)

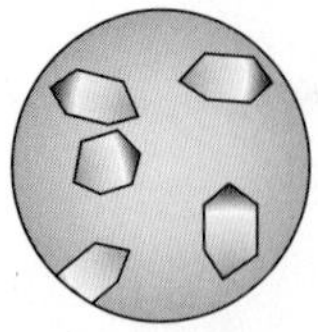

Cystine

1% of stones
Uncommon
Hereditary
Radiopaque (because of sulfur component)

Clinical manifestations of kidney stones include hematuria and flank pain. UTI=urinary tract infection.

ADULT POLYCYSTIC KIDNEY DISEASE (APKD) VERSUS NORMAL KIDNEY (Figure 6-10)

FIGURE
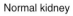 Adult polycystic kidney disease versus normal kidney

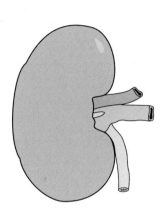 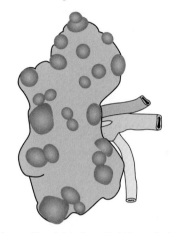

Normal kidney   Kidney with adult polycystic kidney disease

I. Etiology of APKD

A. **Autosomal dominant**

B. Occurs in midlife

II. Clinical features of APKD

A. Bilateral

B. Kidney parenchyma is partially replaced with cysts

C. **Hematuria**

D. Hypertension

E. **Large palpable kidneys**

F. Progressively worsening renal function leading to renal failure

III. APKD is associated with berry aneurysms of circle of Willis and cystic disease in other organs, especially the liver.

RENAL CANCERS (Table 6-9)

TABLE 6-9	Renal Cancers		
Malignancy	**Etiology**	**Clinical Features**	**Notes**
Renal cell carcinoma	**Smoking;** alteration of chromosome 3 (as seen in **von Hippel Lindau disease**)	Afflicts men 45–65 years of age; hematuria; mass; pain; fever; **secondary polycythemia;** paraneoplastic syndrome; usually extends from renal poles; with **clear cells**	Most common renal malignancy; may be associated with increased erythropoietin (EPO)
Wilms' tumor (nephroblastoma)	Chromosome 11 abnormality; **WAGR**	**Palpable flank mass** in children 2–5 years old; hematuria	Most common renal malignancy of childhood (see below)
Transitional cell carcinoma	Cyclophosphamide treatment; **smoking;** aniline dye exposure; **phenacetin** abuse	Hematuria	Most common tumor of the collecting system

WAGR=Wilms' tumor, aniridia, genitourinary abnormalities, and mental retardation

I. **The classic triad of hematuria, flank pain, and a flank mass is seen only in 10%–20% of renal cancer patients. Most are sporadic; however, smoking accounts for 20%–30% of cases.**

II. **Nephroblastoma (Wilms' tumor)**
   A. **Most common malignant renal tumor in children**
   B. Malignant tissue is derived from embryonic nephrogenic tissue.
   C. Peak incidence is between 2 and 4 years of age.
   D. The **two-hit theory** of oncogenesis, which explains the etiology of Wilms', requires a mutation of both copies of the Wilms' tumor-1 (WT-1) tumor suppressor gene on chromosome 11p.
   E. **Characteristic clinical features**
      1. Hematuria
      2. Hypertension
      3. Large abdominal mass
      4. Intestinal obstruction
   F. Part of **WAGR syndrome** (Wilms' tumor, Aniridia, Genital anomalies, Mental Retardation)

THERAPEUTIC AGENTS

I. Effects of diuretics on the nephron (Figure 6-11)

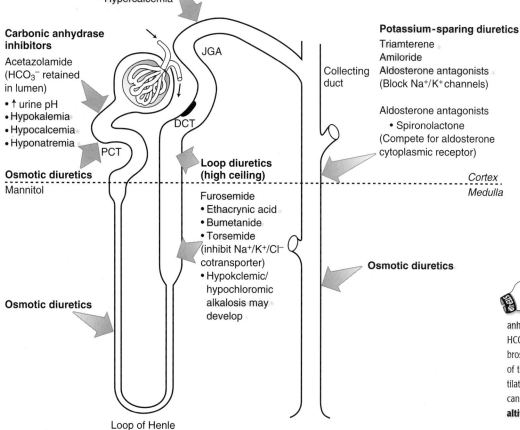

FIGURE 6-11 Effects of diuretics on the nephron

Thiazides
Hydrochlorothiazide
Chlorothiazide
(Inhibit NaCl cotransporter)
• Hypokalemia
• Hypercalcemia

Carbonic anhydrase inhibitors
Acetazolamide
(HCO_3^- retained in lumen)
• ↑ urine pH
• Hypokalemia
• Hypocalcemia
• Hyponatremia

JGA

DCT

PCT

Collecting duct

Potassium-sparing diuretics
Triamterene
Amiloride
Aldosterone antagonists
(Block Na^+/K^+ channels)

Aldosterone antagonists
• Spironolactone
(Compete for aldosterone cytoplasmic receptor)

Cortex
Medulla

Osmotic diuretics
Mannitol

Loop diuretics (high ceiling)
Furosemide
• Ethacrynic acid
• Bumetanide
• Torsemide
(inhibit $Na^+/K^+/Cl^-$ cotransporter)
• Hypoklemic/ hypochloromic alkalosis may develop

Osmotic diuretics

Osmotic diuretics

Loop of Henle

Cl^-=chloride; DCT=distal convoluted tubule; HCO_3^-=bicarbonate; JGA=juxtaglomerular apparatus; K^+=potassium; Na^+=sodium; PCT=proximal convoluted tubule.

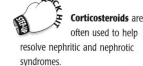 **Corticosteroids** are often used to help resolve nephritic and nephrotic syndromes.

 Besides causing metabolic acidosis, carbonic anhydrase inhibitors also block HCO_3^- secretion into the cerebrospinal fluid (CSF). The acidification of the CSF and subsequent hyperventilation means that these diuretics can be used to prevent and treat **altitude sickness.**

 Loop diuretics, which have direct **pulmonary vasodilatory** properties, are particularly useful in the treatment of pulmonary edema.

 Mannitol and other osmotic diuretics also 'pull' fluid into the bloodstream, thus decreasing pressure in glaucoma and **increased intracranial pressure.**

 Thiazide diuretics are sulfa derivatives and should be used with caution in patients with sulfa drug allergies.

A. The **diuretics** in Figure 6-11 may be grouped into five main categories, each with a different mechanism of action (Table 6-10). The side effects of each type of diuretic are also different, which means that certain diuretics are better-suited for certain patients.

B. **Antidiuretic hormone (ADH)** causes an increase in the expression of **water channels** in the collecting tubule, which results in an increase in the reabsorption of water. Urine output drops, and concentration increases.

1. In the syndrome of inappropriate secretion of ADH (SIADH), **lithium** or **demeclocycline,** which block the effects of ADH, can be administered to prevent excessive water retention.

2. In central diabetes insipidus, **desmopressin,** an ADH analog, or ADH can be given to prevent the excessive loss of dilute urine. These drugs are not useful in the nephrogenic (also known as the peripheral) form of diabetes insipidus, in which the kidneys do not respond to ADH.

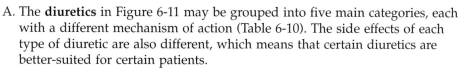

THE RENAL SYSTEM

TABLE 6-10 **Diuretics**

Diuretic Class	Mechanism of Action	Electrolytes Lost in Urine	Properties
Carbonic anhydrase inhibitors	Inhibit carbonic anhydrase in **PCT,** which prevents HCO_3^- reabsorption	Na^+, HCO_3^-, K^+	Results in **metabolic acidosis** Causes decreased secretion of HCO_3^- in aqueous humor Also used in treatment of **glaucoma**
Loop diuretics	Prevent cotransport of Na^+, K^+, and Cl^- in **thick ascending limb**	Na^+, Cl^-, Ca^{2+}, K^+	Has rapid onset and short duration of action, which is ideal for relieving acute edema Produces side effects such as **hypokalemic metabolic alkalosis** and ototoxicity
Osmotic diuretics	Prevent isosmotic reabsorption of filtrate in **PCT, loop of Henle,** and **collecting tubule** Readily filtered and not reabsorbed	Na^+ and all other filtered solutes	Results in increased urine volume Also used in maintenance of urine flow in rhabdomyolysis
Potassium-sparing diuretics	Bind to intracellular aldosterone steroid receptors in **collecting tubules** Blocks induction of Na^+ channels and Na^+/ATPase synthesis	Na^+, Cl^-	Results in decreased secretion of K^+ and H^+, which can lead to **hyperkalemic metabolic acidosis** Often given in combination with a thiazide Can cause **gynecomastia**
Thiazides	Inhibit transport of Na^+ and Cl^- into cells of **DCT**	Na^+, Cl^-, K^+	Causes decreased Ca^{2+} excretion, can lead to K^+ wasting with chronic therapy Results in **increased glucose and lipid levels** in some patients

ATPase=adenosine triphosphatase; Ca^{2+}=calcium; Cl^-=chloride; *DCT*=distal convoluted tubule; K^+=potassium; Na^+=sodium; *PCT*=proximal convoluted tubule

II. **Gout** is a condition in which **uric acid** crystals in joints trigger intermittent inflammatory reactions. The etiologic process can be blocked at different stages (Table 6-11).

Uricosuric agents are both secreted and reabsorbed in the kidney by **weak acid transporters,** which are also used by many other compounds, including aspirin, penicillin, and uric acid. At low doses, uricosurics and **aspirin** can inhibit uric acid excretion and precipitate a gouty attack.

TABLE 6-11 | **Drugs Used to Treat Gout**

Basic Mechanism	Drug	Notes
Inhibition of uric acid production	Allopurinol	Converted to oxypurinol by the enzyme **xanthine oxidase,** which also produces uric acid; allopurinol and oxypurinol inhibit xanthine oxidase Side effects: diarrhea and occasional peripheral neuritis Use: **chronic** therapy
Increased secretion of uric acid (uricosuric)	Probenecid	Competes with uric acid for **reabsorption in the kidney** Caution: should not be used in patients with sulfa allergies Use: **chronic** therapy
	Sulfinpyrazone	Competes with uric acid for **reabsorption in the kidney** Caution: should not be used in patients with sulfa allergies Use: **chronic** therapy
Anti-inflammatory	Colchicine	Interrupts **microtubule formation,** thus interfering with normal mitosis and inhibiting WBC migration and phagocytosis Side effect (common): diarrhea Use: **acute** therapy
	NSAIDs (e.g., indomethacin)	Decrease **prostaglandin** production, thereby interrupting the inflammatory process Side effects (indomethacin): bone marrow suppression and renal damage Use: **acute** therapy

NSAID=nonsteroidal anti-inflammatory drug; *WBC*=white blood cell

A. Inhibition of the production of uric acid from the breakdown of DNA **purines**

B. Increased excretion of uric acid in the urine

C. Blunting the body's **inflammatory response** to the gout crystals (The body's reaction to gout crystals actually causes the pain and damage associated with gout.)

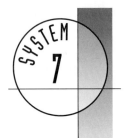

The Endocrine System

DEVELOPMENT

I. Hypothalamus
   A. A division of the **diencephalon**
   B. Forms from the embryologic forebrain (see System 2 "The Nervous System")

II. Pituitary gland consists of two lobes
   A. Anterior lobe: forms from **Rathke's pouch,** an ectodermal diverticulum of the primitive mouth that invaginates upward
   B. Posterior lobe: forms from an invagination of the **hypothalamus**

III. Thyroid gland
   A. Forms from the endoderm of the floor of the pharynx.
   B. Begins as a diverticulum that migrates caudally
   C. Thyroid follicular cells are derived from endoderm.
   D. The calcitonin-producing **parafollicular cells (C-cells)** originate from the fourth pharyngeal pouch.

IV. Parathyroid glands
   A. **Inferior parathyroid glands** develop from the **third pharyngeal pouch.**
   B. **Superior parathyroid glands** develop from the **fourth pharyngeal pouch.**
   C. The parathyroid glands migrate caudally and come to lie on the dorsal surface of the thyroid gland.

V. Adrenal glands
   A. **Gross description**
      1. Paired adult adrenal glands weigh 4 g each.
      2. They are located immediately anterosuperior to the superior renal poles.
      3. They are enclosed in renal fascia.
   B. **Adrenal cortex**
      1. Forms from the mesoderm
      2. Includes three major parts
         a. **Zona glomerulosa** and **zona fasciculata** are present at birth.
         b. **Zona reticularis** is not completely formed until 3 years of age.
   C. Medulla of adrenal gland: **Chromaffin cells** form from neural crest cells that invade the adrenal glands during development.

VI. Pancreas
   A. Forms from a ventral and dorsal bud of endoderm from the foregut
      1. The ventral bud forms the uncinate process and part of the pancreatic head.
      2. The dorsal bud forms part of the head, body, and tail.
   B. Exocrine pancreas: Acinar cells and ducts form from endoderm surrounded by mesoderm.
   C. Endocrine pancreas: Mesodermal cells aggregate to form **pancreatic islet cells.**

VII. Gonads (see System 8 "The Reproductive System")

CONGENITAL MALFORMATIONS (Table 7-1)

There is a wide spectrum of developmental abnormalities involving the endocrine system. Some of these malformations are anatomic, whereas others are biochemical.

TABLE 7-1 Congenital Malformations	
Malformation	**Description**
Craniopharyngioma	Cystic tumor of the pituitary that forms from the remnants of **Rathke's pouch**
Thyroglossal duct cysts	A remnant of the descending migratory path of the thyroid that persists into adult life Most are asymptomatic, but an infection may cause swelling and produce a progressively enlarging moveable mass
Absence of parathyroid glands	Occurs in **DiGeorge syndrome** (thymic aplasia) (see System 10 "The Hematopoietic and Lymphoreticular System") Inability to produce parathyroid hormone leads to hypoparathyroidism
Congenital adrenal hyperplasia	See Figure 7-8
Annular pancreas	Ventral and dorsal pancreatic buds form a ring around the duodenum May cause **duodenal obstruction**
Accessory pancreatic tissue	Normal pancreatic tissue found within the wall of the stomach Most common type of choristoma (normal tissue found misplaced within another organ)

QUICK HIT

Thyroglossal duct cysts are **midline** cysts of the neck. Branchial cleft cysts lie laterally anywhere along the anterior border of the sternocleidomastoid muscle.

HORMONES (Table 7-2)

Hormones are biologically active chemicals formed in an organ and carried through the blood to act on adjacent cells of the same organ or on a different body part.

TABLE 7-2 Hormones				
Hormone	**Secreted by**	**End-Organ Effects of Hormones**	**Stimulated by**	**Inhibited by**
GnRH	Hypothalamus	LH/FSH secretion	Puberty	Progesterone; testosterone
FSH	Anterior pituitary gland	Growth of follicles and estrogen secretion (acts on granulosa cells); maturation of sperm (acts on Sertoli's cells)	Pulsatile release of GnRH	Constant GnRH release; Inhibin
LH	Anterior pituitary gland (basophils)	Ovulation; formation of corpus luteum; estrogen/progesterone synthesis (acts on theca lutein cells); synthesis/secretion of testosterone (acts on Leydig's cells)	Pulsatile release of GnRH	Constant GnRH release; progesterone; testosterone

(continued)

(text continued on page 162)

Finasteride, a 5α-reductase inhibitor, is used in the treatment of benign prostatic hypertrophy. Flutamide, a competitive androgen receptor blocker, is used to treat prostatic carcinoma.

The hormone human chorionic gonadotropin (hCG) is increased in normal pregnancy, hydatidiform moles, choriocarcinomas, gestational tumors, ectopic pregnancy, and pseudocyesis.

The anti-inflammatory effect of cortisol is mediated by its induction of **lipocortin**, which inhibits phospholipase A_2 and prostaglandin synthesis. Cortisol also inhibits the production of interleukin 2 (IL-2).

TABLE 7-2 Hormones (Continued)

Hormone	Secreted by	End-Organ Effects of Hormones	Stimulated by	Inhibited by
Estrogen	Ovary (granulosa cells)	Proliferative phase of menstrual cycle; development of female reproductive organs	FSH	Estrogen
Progesterone	Ovary (granulosa lutein cells)	Breast development; secretory activity during luteal phase	LH	Progesterone
Testosterone	Testes (Leydig's cells)	Spermatogenesis; conversion of testosterone to dihydrotestosterone via 5α-reductase stimulates development of secondary male sex characteristics	LH	Testosterone
hCG	Placenta (syncytiotrophoblast)	Increased estrogen/ progesterone synthesis		
ACTH	Anterior pituitary	Synthesis and secretion of adrenal cortical hormones	CRH; stress	Cortisol
Cortisol (glucocorticoids)	Adrenal cortex (zona fasciculata)	Anti-inflammatory effects (via inhibition of phospholipase A_2); immunosuppressive effects; stimulation of gluconeogenesis; increased blood sugar	ACTH	Cortisol
Aldosterone	Adrenal cortex (zona glomerulosa)	Increased renal sodium reabsorption and potassium secretion; increased in blood volume	Decrease in blood volume; angiotensin II; hyperkalemia; hyponatremia	Hypernatremia; hypokalemia; fluid overload
TSH	Anterior pituitary	Synthesis and secretion of thyroid hormone (T_4, T_3)	TRH	T_4, T_3
T_4, T_3	Thyroid	Growth; maturation of CNS; increased basal metabolic rate, cardiac output, and nutrient utilization	TSH; estrogen	Somatostatin; dopamine
Somatostatin (somatotropin-inhibiting hormone)	Hypothalamus	Inhibited secretion of growth hormone	Growth hormone; somatomedins (IGF)	
GH (somatotropin)	Anterior pituitary (acidophils)	Decreased glucose uptake; increased protein synthesis, growth, organ size, and lean body mass	GHRH; exercise; sleep; puberty; hypoglycemia; estrogen; stress; endogenous opiates	Somatomedins (IGF); somatostatin; obesity; pregnancy; hyperglycemia

(continued)

TABLE 7-2 Hormones (Continued)

Hormone	Secreted by	End-Organ Effects of Hormones	Stimulated by	Inhibited by
Prolactin	Anterior pituitary (acidophils)	Stimulation of milk production and secretion; breast development; inhibition of ovulation	Prolactin-stimulating factor; TRH	Prolactin-inhibiting factor (dopamine)
Oxytocin	Hypothalamus via posterior pituitary	Milk ejection from breast (milk letdown); uterine contraction	Suckling; dilation of the cervix	Alcohol; stress
PTH	Parathyroid gland (chief cells)	Increased serum calcium; increased renal calcium absorption; inhibition of phosphate reabsorption; activates vitamin D to increase intestinal calcium absorption	Decreased serum calcium; mild decreased serum magnesium	Severe decrease in serum magnesium
Vitamin D (1,25 dihydroxycholecalciferol)	Kidney (active form produced by activity of 1α-12-hydroxylase); sun-exposed skin	Increased intestinal calcium and phosphorus absorption; increased bone calcium resorption; increased kidney phosphate and calcium reabsorption	Decreased serum calcium; increased PTH; decreased serum phosphate	
ADH (vasopressin)	Hypothalamus via posterior pituitary	Increased water permeability in distal tubules and collecting duct to regulate osmolarity (V_2 receptor); constriction of vascular smooth muscle (V_1 receptor)	Volume contraction; nicotine; opiates; increased serum osmolarity	Ethanol; ANF; decreased serum osmolarity
Glucagon	Pancreatic islet cells (α cells)	Increased blood glucose; increased glycogenolysis and gluconeogenesis in the liver; increased lipolysis and ketone production	Decreased blood glucose; increased amino acids, ACh	Increased blood glucose; insulin; somatostatin
Insulin	Pancreatic islet cells (β cells)	Decreased blood glucose caused by increased uptake into muscle and fat; decreased glycogenolysis and gluconeogenesis; increased protein synthesis; increased fat deposition; inhibition of lipolysis	Increased blood glucose, amino acids; glucagon; ACh	Decreased blood glucose; somatostatin

ACh=acetylcholine; ACTH=adrenocorticotropic hormone; ADH=antidiuretic hormone; ANF=atrial natriuretic factor; CNS=central nervous system; CRH=corticotropin-releasing hormone; FSH=follicle stimulating hormone; GH=growth hormone; GHRH=growth hormone-releasing factor; GnRH=gonadotropin-releasing hormone; hCG=human chorionic gonadotropin; IGF=insulin-like growth factor; LH=luteinizing hormone; PTH=parathyroid hormone; T_3=triiodothyronine; T_4=thyroxine; TRH=thyrotropin-releasing hormone; TSH=thyroid-stimulating hormone

QUICK HIT Somatostatin is also secreted in the brain, gastrointestinal (GI) tract, and δ cells of the pancreas. It functions to systemically decrease secretion of insulin, glucagon, and gastrin.

QUICK HIT Glucose enters cells through facilitated transporters designated GLUT-1 through GLUT-5. GLUT-4 is abundant in skeletal muscle and adipocytes, whereas GLUT-1 is found on erythrocytes.

THE ENDOCRINE SYSTEM

Hormone function can be localized or systemic. Hormones can alter the activity or structure of the target organ(s) depending on the specificity of the hormone's effects. Hormones play an essential role in homeostasis, reproductive function, and metabolism, but are vital in nearly every other body system as well.

I. Hormones of the hypothalamo-pituitary axis (Figure 7-1)

FIGURE 7-1 Hypothalamo-pituitary axis

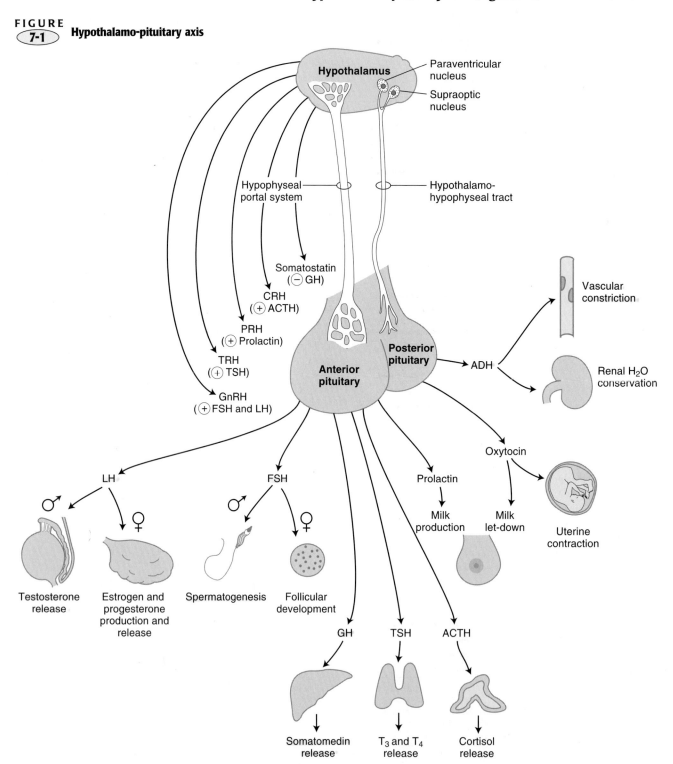

ACTH=adrenocorticotropic hormone; ADH=antidiuretic hormone; CRH=corticotropin-releasing hormone; GH=growth hormone; GnRH=gonadotropin-releasing hormone; FSH=follicle-stimulating hormone; LH=luteinizing hormone; PRH=prolactin-releasing hormone; T_3=triiodothyronine; T_4=thyroxine; TRH=thyrotropin-releasing hormone; TSH=thyroid-stimulating hormone.

THE ENDOCRINE SYSTEM

II. Hormones of the adrenal gland (Figure 7-2)

FIGURE 7-2 Hormones of the adrenal gland

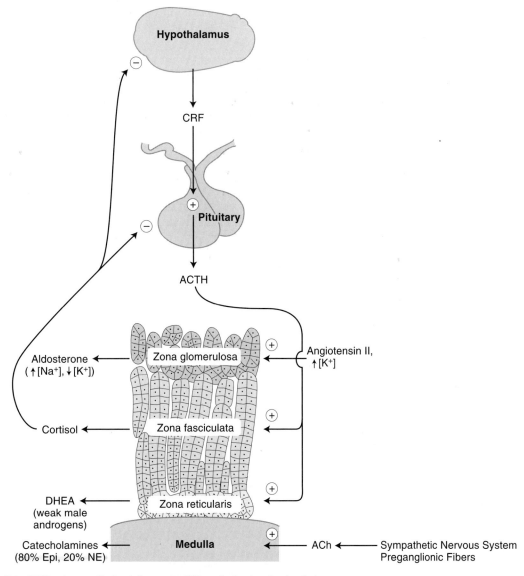

ACh=acetylcholine; ACTH=adrenocorticotropic hormone; CRF=corticotropin-releasing factor; DHEA=dehydroepiandrosterone; Epi=epinephrine; K^+=potassium; Na^+=sodium; NE=norepinephrine.

III. Hormone second-messenger systems

Second-messenger systems are the process by which extracellular signals are translated into cellular responses. Biologically active chemicals, such as hormones, bind to receptor sites on the cell membrane, resulting in phosphorylation of intracellular proteins or changes in ion channel conductivity and subsequent cellular modulation (Table 7-3) (Figure 7-3).

QUICK HIT

Luteinizing hormone (LH), follicle-stimulating hormone (FSH), and thyrotropin (TSH) are hormones consisting of two subunits: α and β. The α subunits in these hormones are identical, whereas the β subunit is unique for each hormone.

TABLE 7-3 Hormone Second Messenger Systems

cAMP	cGMP	IP₃	Steroid	Tyrosine Kinase
β₁ Agonists	ANP	α₁ Agonists	Aldosterone	Insulin
β₂ Agonists	EDRF	GnRH	Estrogen	IGF-1
LH		TRH	Glucocorticoids	Prolactin
FSH		GHRH	Testosterone	GH
TSH		Angiotensin II	Progesterone	
ADH (V₂)		ADH (V₁)	Thyroid	
hCG		Oxytocin	Vitamin D	
CRH				
PTH				
Calcitonin				
Glucagon				

(see also abbreviation key to Table 7-2) *cGMP*=cyclic guanine monophosphate; *IGF*=insulin-like growth factor; *IP₃*=inositol-1,4,5-triphosphate

FIGURE 7-3 Hormone second-messenger systems

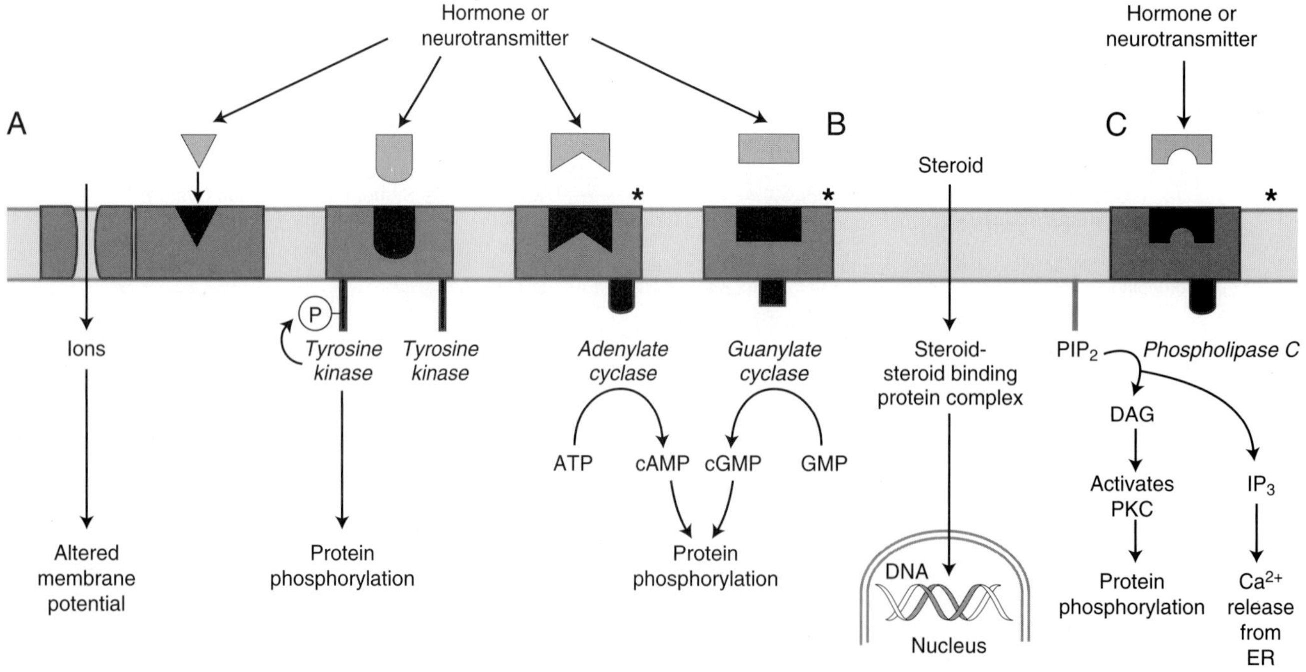

ATP=adenosine triphosphate; *Ca²⁺*=calcium; *cAMP*=cyclic adenosine monophosphate; *cGMP*=cyclic guanosine monophosphate; *DAG*=diacylglycerol; *DNA*=deoxyribonucleic acid; *ER*=endoplasmic reticulum; *GDP*=guanosine diphosphate; *GMP*=glucose monophosphate; *GTP*=guanosine triphosphate; *IP₃*=inositol-1,4,5-triphosphate; *P*=phosphate; *P [enclosed in circle]*=phosphorylated; *PIP₂*=phosphatidylinositol biphosphate; *PKC*=protein kinase C.

FIGURE
7-3 Hormone second-messenger systems *(continued)*

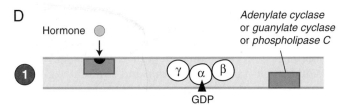

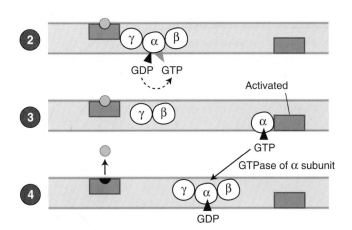

D

*Adenylate cyclase
or guanylate cyclase
or phospholipase C*

A. Peptide mechanism. Peptide binds to hormone receptor site and influences various second messenger systems. These hormones are typically short-acting and do not involve gene regulation, in contrast to steroid hormones, which have a slower onset of action.

B. Steroid mechanism. Lipid-soluble steroid penetrates cell membrane and binds to steroid binding protein. This complex enters the nucleus and influences DNA synthesis.

C. Phospholipase C mechanism.

D. G protein mechanism.

1. Messenger system before hormone binding.

2. After hormone binding, GTP replaces GDP on G protein.

3. GTP, attached to α subunit, dissociates from the β-γ complex and converts ATP to cAMP.

4. Hormone is released from binding site and complex returns to inactive state when GTPase cleaves GTP to GDP.

★ Mechanism utilizing a G protein, as shown in D

CALCIUM HOMEOSTASIS (Figure 7-4)

FIGURE
7-4 Calcium homeostasis

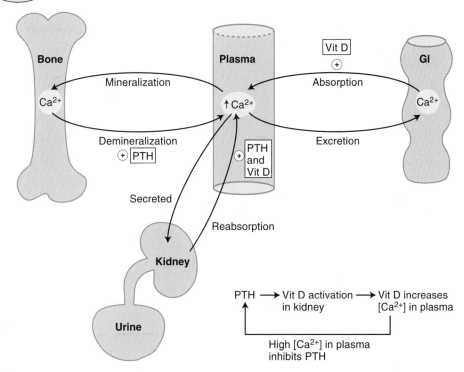

Ca^{2+}=calcium; *GI*=gastrointestinal tract; *PTH*=parathyroid hormone; *Vit D*=vitamin D.

INSULIN AND GLUCAGON

Insulin is a polypeptide hormone that serves to regulate several physiologic processes. Its primary role, in conjunction with the polypeptide hormone glucagon, is to **maintain blood glucose levels.** When blood glucose levels rise after a meal, insulin is released from the β **cells** of the pancreatic islets of Langerhans. Insulin interacts with surface receptors on muscle and adipose tissue and stimulates glucose absorption and triacylglycerol synthesis. In the liver, insulin inhibits gluconeogenesis and glycogen breakdown.

Insulin is formed from two polypeptides linked by disulfide bridges (Figure 7-5). The insulin receptor is **tyrosine kinase** linked; binding of insulin to the α subunit causes phosphorylation of the tyrosine kinase connected to the β subunit. This stimulates recruitment of glucose transporters (GLUTs) to the cell membrane (GLUT 4 in muscle) and increases the uptake of glucose (Figure 7-6).

FIGURE
7-5   **Formation of insulin**

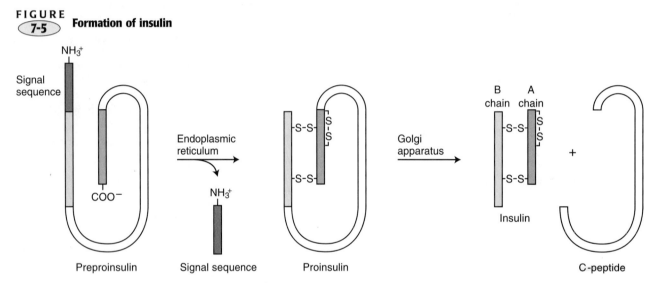

C=carbon; H=hydrogen; N=nitrogen; O=oxygen; S=sulfur (Adapted from Champe PC, Harvey RA. Lippincott's Illustrated Reviews: Biochemistry, 2nd ed. Philadelphia: Lippincott-Raven Publishers, 1994:270. Used by permission of Lippincott Williams & Wilkins.)

THE ENDOCRINE SYSTEM

FIGURE
7-6 **Insulin recruitment of glucose transporters**

2 Activated receptor promotes recruitment of glucose transporters from intracellular pool to cell membrane.

1 Insulin binds to its receptor in the cell membrane.

3 Glucose transporters increase insulin-mediated uptake of glucose into cell.

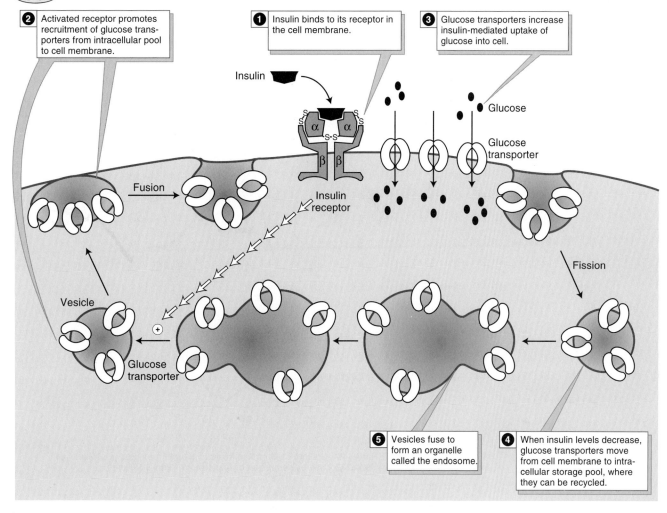

Insulin

Glucose

Glucose transporter

Insulin receptor

Fusion

Fission

Vesicle

Glucose transporter

5 Vesicles fuse to form an organelle called the endosome.

4 When insulin levels decrease, glucose transporters move from cell membrane to intracellular storage pool, where they can be recycled.

(Adapted from Champe PC, Harvey RA. Lippincott's Illustrated Reviews: Biochemistry, 2nd ed. Philadelphia: Lippincott-Raven Publishers, 1994:274. Used by permission of Lippincott Williams & Wilkins.)

Glucagon counteracts the actions of insulin. It is a single polypeptide secreted by the α **cells** of the islets of Langerhans. Glucagon is secreted in response to low blood glucose, increased amino acids in the blood, and epinephrine, and leads to a rise in blood glucose concentration via **gluconeogenesis** and **glycogenolysis.** Glucagon is also responsible for the formation of ketone bodies and increased uptake of amino acids by the liver.

THE ENDOCRINE SYSTEM

● **Blood Levels of Insulin and Glucagon After a High Carbohydrate Meal** (Figure 7-7)

FIGURE 7-7 Blood levels of glucose, insulin, and glucagon after a high-carbohydrate meal

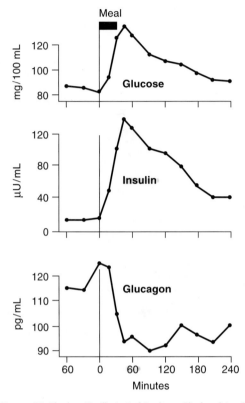

(Adapted from Champe PC, Harvey RA. Lippincott's Illustrated Reviews: Biochemistry, 2nd ed. Philadelphia: Lippincott-Raven Publishers, 1994:272. Used by permission of Lippincott Williams & Wilkins.)

BLOOD GLUCOSE LEVELS

I. Hypoglycemia
  A. **Causes**
    1. Excess insulin administration (in a diabetic patient)
    2. Sulfonylurea administration
    3. Alcohol ingestion
    4. Insulinoma
    5. Factitious hyperinsulinism
  B. **Symptoms**
    1. Sweating
    2. Palpitations
    3. Anxiety
    4. Tremor
  C. Whipple's triad (required for diagnosis)
    1. Low blood glucose
    2. Hypoglycemic symptoms
    3. Improvement of symptoms with glucose administration
  D. In diabetic patients, these symptoms may not be present, and blood glucose may be allowed to drop to dangerous levels, and coma or death may result.
  E. Therapy
    1. Glucose or intravenous (IV) dextrose should be given after measuring blood glucose levels.

    2. Glucagon should be administered.

    3. Epinephrine is sometimes appropriate therapy.

II. Hyperglycemia

  A. Causes

    1. Diabetes mellitus

    2. Chronic pancreatitis

    3. Acromegaly

    4. Cushing's syndrome

    5. Adverse drug reactions

      a. Furosemide

      b. Glucocorticoids

      c. Growth hormone

      d. Oral contraceptives

      e. Thiazides

  B. Acute symptoms

    1. Ketoacidosis or hyperosmolar nonketotic coma

    2. Polyuria

    3. Polydipsia

    4. Polyphagia

    5. Weight loss

    6. Encephalopathy

      a. Tremulousness

      b. Convulsions

      c. Coma

The chronic symptoms of hyperglycemia mimic the chronic complications of diabetes (Table 7-4).

DIABETES MELLITUS

Diabetes mellitus (or simply, diabetes) refers to a group of disorders that are characterized by hyperglycemia and affect 1%–2% of the U.S. population. Although the pathogenesis of these disorders is varied, individuals with diabetes lack the ability to produce sufficient insulin to meet their metabolic needs. Furthermore, all diabetic patients are vulnerable to complications such as nephropathy, neuropathy, and retinopathy. Monitoring and control of blood sugar, insulin replacement, and proper diet can significantly reduce the morbidity and mortality of this disease.

I. Diagnosis of diabetes mellitus (see Table 7-4)

TABLE 7-4 **Diagnosis of Diabetes Mellitus**

	Normal	Impaired Glucose Tolerance	Diabetes Mellitus
Fasting blood glucose level	<115 mg/dL	<140 mg/dL	126 mg/dL
		or	or
Blood glucose level after oral glucose tolerance test (OGTT)	<140 mg/dL	140–199 mg/dL	200 mg/dL

II. Type 1 versus type 2 diabetes mellitus is compared in Table 7-5.

TABLE 7-5 **Type 1 Versus Type 2 Diabetes Mellitus**

	Type 1 Diabetes (IDDM) 15%	Type 2 Diabetes (NIDDM) 85%
Cause	Possible **autoimmunity** to β cells triggered by viral cause	Increased **insulin resistance,** decreased receptors, or decreased conversion of proinsulin to insulin
Chromosomal association	6 (HLA DQ)	Unknown
Family history	Weak predictor	Strong predictor
Age of onset	Under 25 years of age	Over 40 years of age
Body habitus	Normal to thin	Obese
Plasma insulin	Low	Normal to high
Plasma glucagon	High but suppressible	High and resistant to suppression
Pancreas morphology	Atrophy and fibrosis; β cell depletion	Atrophy and amyloid deposits; variable β cell population
Acute complication (see Table 7-6)	Ketoacidosis	Hyperosmolar coma
Common symptoms	**Polydipsia, polyuria, polyphagia (symptoms of hyperglycemia)**	Variable: from asymptomatic to polydipsia, polyuria, polyphagia
Response to insulin therapy	Responsive	Variable
Response to sulfonylurea therapy	Unresponsive	Responsive

IDDM=insulin-dependent diabetes mellitus; *NIDDM*=non–insulin-dependent diabetes mellitus

III. Diabetic ketoacidosis (DKA) and nonketotic hyperosmolar (NKH) states (Table 7-6)

TABLE 7-6 **Diabetic Ketoacidosis (DKA) and Nonketotic Hyperosmolar (NKH) State**

	DKA	NKH
Pathology	Increased serum **ketone bodies** (>2 mmol/L); anion gap metabolic acidosis (pH < 7.2); **hyperglycemia** (glucose > 300 mg/dL because of increased production and decreased uptake)	**Hyperglycemia** (>600 mg/dL); **hyperosmolarity** (>320 mg/dL); pH > 7.3
Patient	Type 1 (IDDM)	An older type 2 (NIDDM)
Precipitating event	50% **infection** (look for fever); 25% insufficient insulin	**Decreased ability to sense thirst or obtain enough water;** infection; vascular event (CVA, MI)
Fluid loss	5–7 L	9 L
Clinical presentation	Nausea and vomiting; **Kussmaul respiration;** osmotic diuresis; shock; coma	Usually **coma** if serum osmolarity > 350 mg/dL

(continued)

THE ENDOCRINE SYSTEM

TABLE 7-6 Diabetic Ketoacidosis (DKA) and Nonketotic Hyperosmolar (NKH) State (Continued)

	DKA	NKH
Mortality	10%	17%
Treatment	Insulin; saline; K$^+$ replacement	Saline (essential); insulin
Complications	**Cerebral edema;** hyperchloremic (non-gap) metabolic acidosis	Dehydration is more severe (older patients have lower body water stores)

CVA=cerebrovascular accident; *IDDM*=insulin-dependent diabetes mellitus; *MI*=myocardial infarction; *NIDDM*=non–insulin-dependent diabetes mellitus

 Diabetic ketoacidosis (DKA) and nonketotic hyperosmolar state (NKH) are not mutually exclusive. Patients may present with features of both.

 Kussmaul respirations are rapid and deep.

IV. Chronic symptoms of diabetes (Table 7-7)

TABLE 7-7 Chronic Symptoms of Diabetes Mellitus

Anatomic Location	Clinical Features
Red blood cells	Glycosylation (**HbA1c**); measure of long-term control of diabetes (reflects past 3 months)
Blood vessels	**Atherosclerosis;** coronary artery disease; gangrene; peripheral vascular disease
Eyes	**Retinopathy;** hemorrhage; hard exudates; cotton-wool spots; cataracts; glaucoma
Gastrointestinal tract	Constipation, gastroparesis
Kidneys	Nephropathy; **nodular sclerosis; Kimmelstiel-Wilson nodules;** chronic renal failure; azotemia
Penis	Impotence as a result of autonomic neuropathy
Feet	**Stocking-glove peripheral neuropathy;** ulcers

V. Treatment of diabetes mellitus

The goal of treatment of both type 1 and type 2 diabetes mellitus is steady control of blood glucose levels. However, because the pathogenesis underlying these two disease processes is different, the therapy is also different.

Type 1 diabetes mellitus, which can be viewed simply as a total deficiency of insulin, may be treated with careful administration of exogenous **insulin.** This agent, the only treatment option for type 1 diabetes mellitus for many years, remains so today. However, advances have been made in both the type of insulin and method of delivery. To maintain steady glucose levels, different preparations of human insulin have been designed, each with a characteristic rate of onset and duration of action (Table 7-8). Insulin, a peptide hormone, cannot be given orally. It is typically administered subcutaneously and, in emergencies, intravenously.

Some combination of these types of insulin usually can be found that provides adequate glucose control during both the fed and fasting states. Treatment of type 1 diabetes mellitus is essentially a balancing act; too much insulin causes hypoglycemia, and too little leads to hyperglycemia, which over time leads to the long-term complications of diabetes mellitus. Type 2 diabetes mellitus, which is more complex than type 1 disease, is characterized primarily by insulin resistance. In some cases, a strict regimen of diet and exercise completely reverses the course of the disease. However, drugs are required to control blood sugar levels in many cases. The most commonly used drugs in type 2 diabetes mellitus include metformin

TABLE 7-8	Commonly Used Insulin Preparations		
Insulin Preparation	**Onset of Activity**	**Time of Peak Activity**	**Duration of Action**
Regular insulin	30 min	2–4 hr	6–8 hr
NPH insulin	1–2 hr	6–12 hr	18–24 hr
Lente insulin	1–3 hr	6–12 hr	18–24 hr

and the insulin sensitizers. **Metformin,** which is considered by many to be the first-line drug of choice in type 2 diabetes mellitus, acts primarily by decreasing hepatic glucose production. Advantages include the very low risk of hypoglycemia as well as the weight loss and improvement in lipid profiles in many patients. The one feared adverse reaction is lactic acidosis, a rare but serious complication.

Pioglitazone and **rosiglitazone** are the two most common insulin sensitizers. Their mechanism of action is poorly understood. Like metformin, these agents can be used alone or as part of a multidrug regimen for diabetic blood sugar control. Both drugs have a low risk of hypoglycemia. However, they have been known to exacerbate congestive heart failure.

Sulfonylureas were once the mainstay of treatment for type 2 diabetes, but they are used infrequently today. These drugs, which include agents such as glipizide and glyburide, act by increasing release of insulin from the pancreas. To a lesser extent, these agents also decrease glucagon levels and increase insulin binding at target sites in the periphery. The primary side effect of these drugs is hypoglycemia.

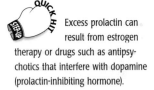 Excess prolactin can result from estrogen therapy or drugs such as antipsychotics that interfere with dopamine (prolactin-inhibiting hormone).

PITUITARY DISORDERS (Table 7-9)

The pituitary gland sits in the sella turcica. The anterior portion is regulated by the hypothalamus. The posterior portion contains extensions of hypothalamic neurons.

TABLE 7-9	Pituitary Disorders			
Disorder	**Etiology**	**Clinical Features**	**Laboratory Diagnosis**	**Treatment**
Prolactinoma	Lactotrophic (chromophobic) anterior pituitary tumor; **most common** pituitary tumor	Decreased libido; amenorrhea; gynecomastia; galactorrhea; virilization	Minimal or no increase in serum prolactin after TRH given	Bromocriptine or surgery
Acromegaly (adults)/gigantism (children)	Somatotrophic (acidophilic) anterior pituitary adenoma	Prominent forehead, jaw; **large hands, feet; enlargement of viscera;** hyperglycemia; renal failure; hypertension; mental disturbances	Excess growth hormones and somatomedins (IGF-1)	Transsphenoidal surgery, bromocriptine, radiation, or octeotide
Cushing's disease	Hypersecretion of ACTH from basophilic adenoma of pituitary	(see Table 7-11)	Suppression of ACTH secretion during high-dose dexamethasone test	Surgery or pituitary irradiation
Simmonds' disease	Pituitary tumors, ischemia, trauma; DIC; sickle cell anemia	Marked wasting; **panhypopituitarism;** headache; vomiting	Decreased levels of FSH, LH, ACTH, TSH	Hormone replacement

(continued)

TABLE 7-9 **Pituitary Disorders (Continued)**

Disorder	Etiology	Clinical Features	Laboratory Diagnosis	Treatment
SIADH	Pituitary hypersecretion; ectopic production of ADH (**small cell lung cancer**)	Decreased urinary output; fatigue; mental disturbances	Hyponatremia; high urine osmolality	Fluid restriction
Diabetes insipidus	**Neurogenic** (central): ADH insufficiency **Nephrogenic:** lack of end-organ (kidney) response	Dehydration; thirst; polyuria; recent trauma to the head or anoxia	See Table 7-9; hypernatremia	Neurogenic: desmopressin (DDAVP) acts as ADH Nephrogenic: fluid restriction and thiazide response diuretics (works by a paradoxical effect)

(see also Table 7-2 abbreviation key) *DDAVP*=1-deamino-8-D-arginine vasopressin; *DIC*=disseminated intravascular coagulation; *SIADH*=syndrome of inappropriate secretion of antidiuretic hormone

DIABETES INSIPIDUS (Table 7-10)

Diabetes insipidus is a disease characterized by excessive, low osmolality urine output. There are two forms: central and nephrogenic.

TABLE 7-10 **Diabetes Insipidus**

	Urine Osmolality Greater Than 280 mOsm/kg With Dehydration	Response to ADH After Dehydration
Normal	+	−
Central diabetes insipidus	−	+
Partial diabetes insipidus	+	+
Nephrogenic diabetes insipidus	−	−
Primary polydipsia	+	+

ADH=antidiuretic hormone

 Sheehan's syndrome is a form of Simmonds' disease caused by postpartum pituitary necrosis resulting from blood loss and ischemia during childbirth.

 Surprisingly, diabetes insipidus can be treated with hydrochlorothiazide (a diuretic).

Primary polydipsia, a psychological condition of drinking excess water, causes a decrease in plasma osmolality and therefore can be differentiated from diabetes insipidus, which causes an increase in plasma osmolality. Patients who present with primary polydipsia are generally young or middle-aged women with a history of neurosis.

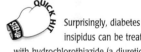

21-Hydroxylase deficiency is the **most common** adrenal enzyme deficiency.

THE ADRENAL GLANDS

I. Congenital adrenal hyperplasia (Figure 7-8)

FIGURE
7-8
Congenital adrenal hyperplasia (CAH)

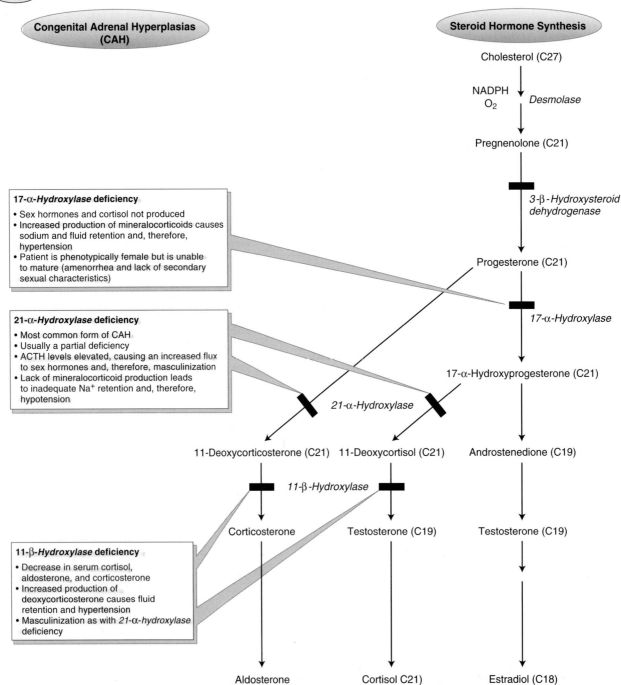

Congenital Adrenal Hyperplasias (CAH)

Steroid Hormone Synthesis

Cholesterol (C27)

NADPH
O_2 — *Desmolase*

Pregnenolone (C21)

3-β-Hydroxysteroid dehydrogenase

Progesterone (C21)

17-α-Hydroxylase

17-α-Hydroxyprogesterone (C21)

11-Deoxycorticosterone (C21)   11-Deoxycortisol (C21)   Androstenedione (C19)

21-α-Hydroxylase

11-β-Hydroxylase

Corticosterone   Testosterone (C19)   Testosterone (C19)

Aldosterone   Cortisol C21)   Estradiol (C18)

17-α-Hydroxylase deficiency
- Sex hormones and cortisol not produced
- Increased production of mineralocorticoids causes sodium and fluid retention and, therefore, hypertension
- Patient is phenotypically female but is unable to mature (amenorrhea and lack of secondary sexual characteristics)

21-α-Hydroxylase deficiency
- Most common form of CAH
- Usually a partial deficiency
- ACTH levels elevated, causing an increased flux to sex hormones and, therefore, masculinization
- Lack of mineralocorticoid production leads to inadequate Na$^+$ retention and, therefore, hypotension

11-β-Hydroxylase deficiency
- Decrease in serum cortisol, aldosterone, and corticosterone
- Increased production of deoxycorticosterone causes fluid retention and hypertension
- Masculinization as with *21-α-hydroxylase* deficiency

ACTH=adrenocorticotropin; *Na$^+$*=sodium; *NADPH*=nicotinamide adenine dinucleotide phosphate (reduced form); *O_2*=oxygen. (Adapted from Champe PC, Harvey RA. Lippincott's Illustrated Reviews: Biochemistry, 2nd ed. Philadelphia: Lippincott-Raven Publishers, 1994:224. Used by permission of Lippincott Williams & Wilkins.)

THE ENDOCRINE SYSTEM

The adrenal glands are anatomically divided into a medulla and a cortex. The cortex is itself divided into three anatomic layers. The four anatomic layers of the adrenal glands are responsible for a variety of metabolic functions in the body.

II. Adrenal cortex pathology (Table 7-11)

TABLE 7-11	**Adrenal Cortex Pathology**	
Disease	**Etiology**	**Clinical Features**
Cushing's syndrome	Excess cortisol as a result of **iatrogenic corticosteroid therapy (most common cause),** adrenal adenoma (more common than carcinoma); ectopic ACTH from neoplasm (especially **small cell lung carcinoma**)	Peripheral muscle wasting and weakness; **central obesity** with "moon facies" and "buffalo hump"; easy bruising with abdominal striae; bone demineralization, osteoporosis, psychosis, acne; hirsutism; hyperglycemia; hypertension
Cushing's disease	Excess cortisol as a result of **pituitary hypersecretion of ACTH;** bilateral hyperplasia of adrenal cortex; **second most common** cause of Cushing's syndrome	Identical to Cushing's syndrome
Conn's syndrome (primary hyperaldosteronism)	Adrenal cortex **adenoma** (more common than hyperplasia, which is more common than carcinoma); sodium retention; **low plasma renin**	**Hypertension;** hypokalemic alkalosis
Secondary hyperaldosteronism	Renal tumors; renal ischemia; edematous conditions (cirrhosis, nephrotic syndromes, CHF); **increased plasma renin**	**Hypertension;** hypokalemic alkalosis
Addison's disease	Most commonly **idiopathic** cortisol deficiency; possibly autoimmune; may be caused by tumor, infections (i.e., tuberculosis)	**Hypotension;** low serum sodium; **hyperpigmentation;** increased serum potassium
Waterhouse-Friderichsen syndrome	***Neisseria meningitides*** infection (meningitis) leads to DIC; hemorrhagic adrenal **necrosis** and collapse	Acute hypotension and salt wasting; **shock;** more common in children; death within hours if not treated

ACTH=adrenocorticotropic hormone; *CHF*=congestive heart failure; *DIC*=disseminated intravascular coagulation

III. Adrenal medulla pathology (Table 7-12)

TABLE 7-12	**Adrenal Medulla Tumors**	
Tumor	**Pathology**	**Clinical Manifestation**
Neuroblastoma	**Malignant;** excess catecholamine secretion; **N-*myc*** (oncogene) amplification	**Children;** degree of N-*myc* amplification related to prognosis
Pheochromocytoma	**Benign** (10% malignant); tumor of chromaffin cells; seen in MEN IIa and IIb	**Adults;** hypertension (usually paroxysmal); palpitations, sweating, and headache; urinary vanillylmandelic acid (**VMA**)

MEN=multiple endocrine neoplasia

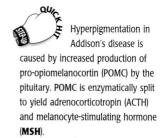
Hyperpigmentation in Addison's disease is caused by increased production of pro-opiomelanocortin (POMC) by the pituitary. POMC is enzymatically split to yield adrenocorticotropin (ACTH) and melanocyte-stimulating hormone (**MSH**).

Extraadrenal chromaffin cell tumors are called paragangliomas (e.g., tumors originating in the organ of Zuckerkandl).

The pheochromocytoma rule of tens: 10% malignant, 10% multiple, 10% bilateral, 10% familial, 10% extraadrenal, 10% children.

THE ENDOCRINE SYSTEM

THYROID

I. Formation of thyroid hormone (Figure 7-9)

FIGURE
7-9 **Formation of thyroid hormone**

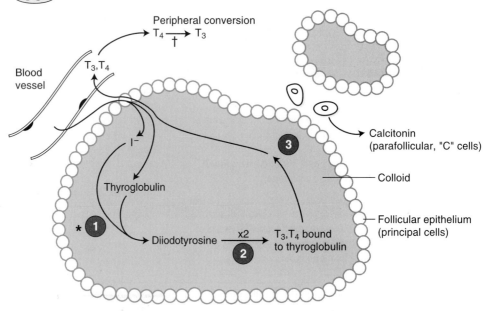

① Oxidation of I⁻ by peroxidase followed by iodination of thyroglobulin

② Condensation

③ Proteolytic release of hormone from follicle

✱ Inhibited by propylthiouracil and methimazole

† Inhibited by propylthiouracil

I^-=iodide; T_3=triiodothyronine; T_4=thyroxine.

II. Myxedema

A. Can be described as hypothyroidism of the **adult**

B. Causes
1. **Hashimoto's thyroiditis** (see below)
2. Idiopathic causes
3. Iodine deficiency
   a. A problem in geographic areas with poor nutrition
   b. Deficiency in pregnant women can lead to cretinism in the child (see below).
4. High doses of iodine, paradoxically, lead to a decrease in thyroid hormone production.
5. **Over-irradiation** of the thyroid using iodine 131 for treatment of hyperthyroidism

C. Clinical features of the hypothyroid state
1. Cold intolerance
2. Weight gain
3. Constipation
4. Lowering of voice
5. Menorrhagia
6. Slowed mental and physical function
7. Dry skin with coarse and brittle hair
8. Reflexes showing slow return phase

D. Treatment is usually with levothyroxine (T_4)

III. Cretinism

A. Can be described as **hypothyroidism** of the **fetus or child**
B. Causes
 1. **Iodine-deficient diet** in the mother, or during the early life of the child
 2. Thyroid-related enzyme deficiency
 3. Thyroid developmental defect
 4. Failure of thyroid descent during development
 5. Transfer of antithyroid antibodies from mother with autoimmune disease to fetus
C. Clinical features
 1. Impaired physical growth
 2. **Mental retardation**
 3. Enlarged tongue
 4. Enlarged, distended abdomen

IV. Hashimoto's thyroiditis

A. An **autoimmune** disorder causing **hypothyroidism** and a **painless goiter**
 1. Dense infiltrate of lymphocytes into the thyroid gland
 2. Antithyroglobulin and anti-thyroid peroxidase (formerly antimicrosomal) antibodies
 3. **5:1 female predominance**
 4. Incidence increases with age.
 5. Associated with human leukocyte antigen DR5 **(HLA-DR5)** and **HLA-B5**
B. Is the **most common form of hypothyroidism in those with adequate iodine** intake.
C. Clinical features
 1. Slowly progressing course with stages of euthyroid state, hyperthyroid state, and hypothyroid state.
 2. May lead to a scarred and shrunken gland in hypothyroid state.
 3. Microscopically, thyroid resembles lymph node.
D. Associated with other autoimmune disorders
 1. Diabetes mellitus
 2. Pernicious anemia
 3. Sjögren's syndrome

V. Subacute (De Quervain's) thyroiditis

A. Transient hyperthyroidism with **painful** goiter
 1. Focal destruction of thyroid
 2. Granulomatous inflammation
 3. 3:1 female predominance
 4. Associated with HLA-B35
B. Causes—possibly as a result of recent viral infection with coxsackie virus, echovirus, adenovirus, measles, or mumps
C. Clinical features
 1. Acute febrile state
 2. Rapid painful enlargement of the thyroid
 3. Transient hyperthyroidism owing to gland destruction
D. Self-limited disease

VI. Graves' disease

A. **Autoimmune** disorder causing **hyperthyroidism** and a **goiter**
 1. Thyroid-stimulating immunoglobulin (**TSI**) is an immunoglobulin G (IgG) antibody to the thyroid-stimulating hormone (TSH) receptor.
 2. Binding of TSI to the TSH receptor stimulates thyroid hormone production and hyperplasia of the thyroid gland.
 3. Associated with **HLA-DR3 and B8**
 4. **4:1 female** predominance

Thyroxine (T₄) is converted to triiodothyronine (T₃) in the periphery, with T₃ being 3–5 times more potent than T₄. T₄ has a half-life of 5 to 7 days, whereas T₃ has a half-life of 1 day.

Because of its long half-life, T₄ is ideal as a hormone replacement in patients with hypothyroidism. Even with once-a-day dosing, steady serum levels of T₄ and T₃ can be achieved.

Because of the devastating effects that **hypothyroidism** can have on children (cretinism), thyroid hormone levels are routinely evaluated at birth in the United States (along with **galactosemia** and **phenylketonuria**).

B. Clinical features of Graves' disease
  1. Hyperthyroidism and goiter caused by autoimmune immunoglobulins
     a. Increased total thyroxine (T_4)
     b. Increased triiodothyronine (T_3)
     c. Decreased TSH level
     d. Increased resin radioactive T_3 uptake
     e. Increased radioactive iodine
  2. **Exophthalmos**
  3. Warm, moist, and flushed skin
  4. Thin, fine hair
  5. Cardiovascular system
     a. Increased heart rate and cardiac output
     b. **Palpitations** and **fibrillations**
  6. Muscle atrophy
     a. Weakening of skeletal muscles occurs.
     b. Vital capacity of lungs decreases owing to weakened respiratory muscles.
  7. **Weight loss** occurs despite an increased appetite.
  8. Diarrhea is common.
  9. Menstrual flow may decrease or stop.
C. Treatment
  1. Antithyroid drugs (i.e., propylthiouracil or methimazole)
  2. A **β-blocker** to reduce the cardiac effects
  3. Radioactive iodine (^{131}I)
  4. Surgery

VII. Thyroid neoplasms (Table 7-13)

TABLE 7-13 Thyroid Carcinomas	
Tumor	**Description**
Papillary tumor	• **Most common** thyroid cancer • **Best prognosis** of the thyroid cancers • **3:1 female predominance** • Usually occurs in third to fifth decade of life • "Ground glass" nuclei of neoplastic cells, also called "Orphan Annie eyes" • **Psammoma bodies** may be present • Forms papillary projections covered with cuboidal epithelium within glandular spaces
Follicular tumor	• Worse prognosis than papillary • **3:1 female predominance** • Uniform cuboidal cells lining follicles • Lacks the distinctive nuclear features of papillary carcinoma
Medullary tumor	• Parafollicular cell neoplasm • **Secretes calcitonin** • Associated with MEN IIa and MEN IIb (MEN III)
Anaplastic thyroid carcinoma	• Anaplastic, undifferentiated neoplasm • More common in older patients • Rapidly fatal
MEN=multiple endocrine neoplasia	

THE ENDOCRINE SYSTEM

PARATHYROID PATHOLOGY (Table 7-14)

TABLE 7-14 Parathyroid Disorders		
Condition	**Etiology**	**Clinical Features**
Primary hyperparathyroidism	**Adenoma** (most common); hyperplasia more common than carcinoma; seen in MEN I and IIa; excess PTH; **hypercalcemia**	**Osteitis fibrosa cystica** (cystic "brown tumors" of bone); **renal calculi** and nephrocalcinosis; duodenal ulcers
Secondary hyperparathyroidism	**Hypocalcemia** caused by **chronic renal failure** (loss of vitamin D activation); parathyroid hyperplasia; excess PTH; high alkaline phosphatase; ectopic PTH (squamous cell lung carcinoma)	Cystic bone lesions; **metastatic calcification** of organs
Hypoparathyroidism	Most commonly secondary to **thyroidectomy;** seen inDiGeorge's syndrome; **hypocalcemia**	Tetany; positive **Chvostek's** and **Trousseau's** signs
Pseudohypoparathyroidism	Autosomal recessive; deficient organ response to PTH	**Short stature;** underdeveloped fourth and fifth digits
MEN=multiple endocrine neoplasia; *PTH*=parathyroid hormone		

Pancreatitis leads to fat necrosis because of release of pancreatic enzymes. The excess lipid binds calcium in a process called saponification and produces hypocalcemia.

MULTIPLE ENDOCRINE NEOPLASIA (MEN) SYNDROMES (Table 7-15)

The multiple endocrine neoplasia (MEN) syndromes are autosomal dominant conditions in which more than one endocrine organ is affected by either hyperplasia or neoplasia.

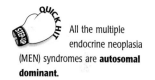

All the multiple endocrine neoplasia (MEN) syndromes are **autosomal dominant.**

TABLE 7-15 Multiple Endocrine Neoplasia (MEN) Syndromes		
Type I (Wermer's syndrome)	**Type IIa (Sipple's syndrome)**	**Type IIb (or type III)**
Hyperplasia or tumors of the thyroid, adrenal cortex, parathyroid, pancreas, or pituitary	Pheochromocytoma, medullary carcinoma of the thyroid, hyperparathyroidism	Pheochromocytoma, medullary carcinoma of the thyroid, multiple mucocutaneous neuromas (particularly of the GI tract)
GI=gastrointestinal		

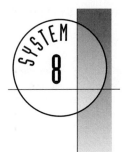

The Reproductive System

DETERMINATION OF SEX

Before the seventh week of gestation, the fetal gonads have not differentiated into either the male or female genotype. The presence or absence of the Y chromosome and the sex-determining region of the Y chromosome (SRY) determines gonadal differentiation. Gender determination, which occurs after the seventh week, depends on the type of gonads present.

FEMALE REPRODUCTIVE SYSTEM DEVELOPMENT

I. Ovaries and other female reproductive structures
   A. Primordial follicles contain **primary oocytes (XX genotype)** and follicular (granulosa) cells that form the ovaries.
   B. As the upper abdomen grows, the ovaries "descend" toward the perineum.
   C. The gubernaculum assists in this descent and then becomes the ovarian ligament and the round ligament of the uterus.
   D. The paramesonephric ducts develop into the uterine tubes and eventually into the uterus.

II. Vagina and uterus (Figure 8-1)

FIGURE
8-1 **Development of the female genital tract**

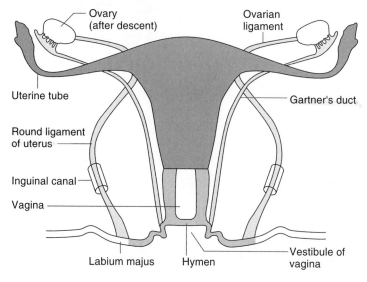

A. Reproductive system of the newborn female

Structures arising from:
- ▦ Paramesonephric duct
- ▦ Urogenital sinus
- ▢ Mesonephric duct

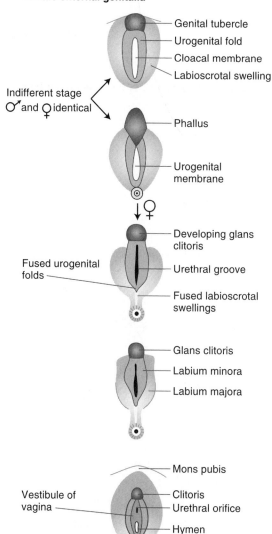

B. Stages of development of the female external genitalia

(Adapted from Moore KL, Persaud TVN. The Developing Human: Clinically Oriented Embryology, 6th ed. Philadelphia: WB Saunders, 1998.)

III. Breasts

A. Only the main lactiferous ducts develop during fetal life.

B. Glands enlarge during puberty owing to increased levels of estrogens, progestins, prolactin, and growth hormone.

MALE REPRODUCTIVE SYSTEM DEVELOPMENT

I. Testes and other male reproductive organs

A. Primary sex cords contain primordial germ cells of **XY genotype.** The Y chromosome codes for the testes-determining factor (**TDF**), which allows for male gonadal differentiation.

B. Müllerian-inhibiting factor (**MIF**) is secreted by **Sertoli's cells.** MIF causes regression of the Müllerian (paramesonephric) ducts and their associated female genital structures.

C. The mesonephric ducts, under the influence of testosterone, become the ductus deferens, the seminal vesicles, and the ejaculatory ducts in the adult male.

II. The prostate gland forms from the urogenital sinus (Figure 8-2).

FIGURE 8-2 Development of the male genital tract

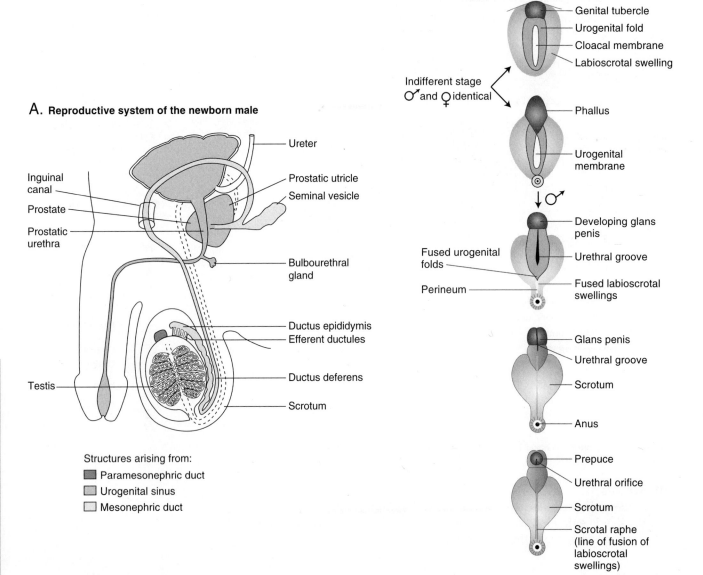

A. Reproductive system of the newborn male

- Ureter
- Prostatic utricle
- Seminal vesicle
- Inguinal canal
- Prostate
- Prostatic urethra
- Bulbourethral gland
- Ductus epididymis
- Efferent ductules
- Ductus deferens
- Testis
- Scrotum

Structures arising from:
- Paramesonephric duct
- Urogenital sinus
- Mesonephric duct

B. Stages of development of the male external genitalia

- Genital tubercle
- Urogenital fold
- Cloacal membrane
- Labioscrotal swelling

Indifferent stage ♂ and ♀ identical

- Phallus
- Urogenital membrane

♂

- Developing glans penis
- Urethral groove
- Fused urogenital folds
- Perineum
- Fused labioscrotal swellings

- Glans penis
- Urethral groove
- Scrotum
- Anus

- Prepuce
- Urethral orifice
- Scrotum
- Scrotal raphe (line of fusion of labioscrotal swellings)

(Adapted from Moore KL, Persaud TVN. The Developing Human: Clinically Oriented Embryology, 6th ed. Philadelphia: WB Saunders, 1998.)

THE REPRODUCTIVE SYSTEM

THE REPRODUCTIVE SYSTEM ● 183

III. External genitalia

A. Testosterone is responsible for masculinization of genitalia.

B. The **genital tubercle** enlarges to become the glans penis.

C. The **urogenital fold** becomes the shaft of the penis.

D. The **labioscrotal swellings** fuse in the midline and become the scrotum.

Spermatogenesis versus oogenesis (Figure 8-3)

FIGURE
8-3 **Spermatogenesis versus oogenesis**

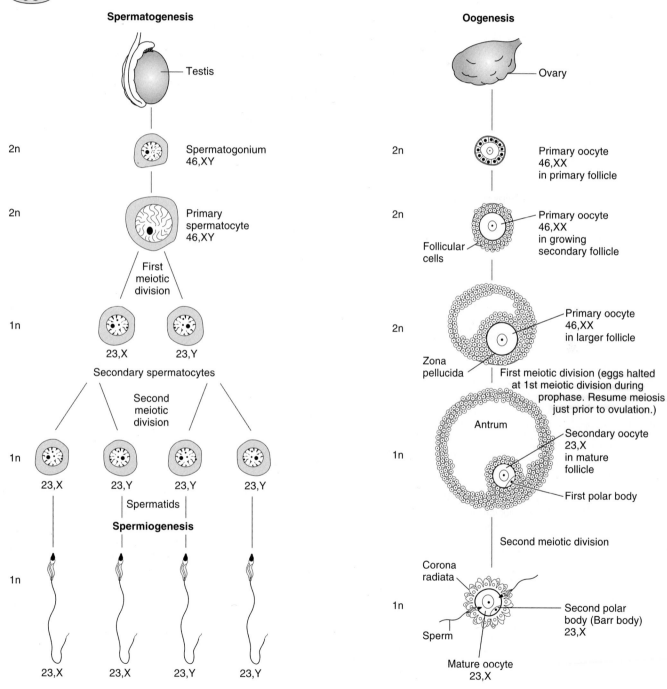

(Adapted from Moore KL, Persaud TVN. The Developing Human: Clinically Oriented Embryology, 6th ed. Philadelphia: WB Saunders, 1998.)

Important anatomic features of the perineum (Figure 8-4)

FIGURE
8-4   **Important anatomic features of the perineum**

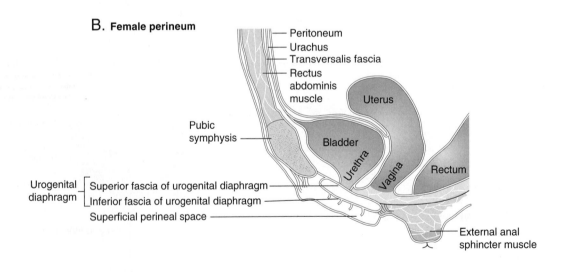

A. **Male perineum**

Pubic symphysis

Bladder

Prostate gland

Membranous layer of superficial fascia of abdomen (Scarpa's)

Superior fascia of urogenital diaphragm
Muscles within deep perineal space
Inferior fascia of urogenital diaphragm
— Urogenital diaphragm

Membranous layer of superficial fascia of penis (Buck's)

Corpus cavernosum
Urethra
Corpus spongiosum
Bulbospongiosus muscle
Membranous layer of superficial fascia of urogenital region (Colles')
— Contents of superficial perineal space near midsagittal plane

B. **Female perineum**

Peritoneum
Urachus
Transversalis fascia
Rectus abdominis muscle

Uterus

Pubic symphysis

Bladder

Urethra

Vagina

Rectum

Urogenital diaphragm
— Superior fascia of urogenital diaphragm
Inferior fascia of urogenital diaphragm
Superficial perineal space

External anal sphincter muscle

CONGENITAL MALFORMATIONS (Table 8-1)

Congenital malformations are most often caused by exposure to teratogens during the third to eighth weeks of pregnancy, which is the period of organogenesis.

TABLE 8-1 **Congenital Malformations**	
Malformation	**Clinical Features**
Hypospadias	• Urethra opens on the **ventral** side of the penis • Spongy urethra does not form properly or the **urogenital folds** do not fuse • Paucity of hormone receptors or too little hormone produced from the testes may play a role • More common than epispadias
Epispadias	• Urethra opens on the **dorsum** of the penis
Undescended testis (cryptorchidism)	• Most are of unknown cause • May be unilateral or bilateral • Most testes descend before 1 year of life • If testes remain undescended, **sterility or testicular cancer** can result
Congenital inguinal hernia (indirect hernia)	• A communication is formed between the **tunica vaginalis** (adjacent to the testis) and the peritoneal cavity • A loop of intestine may herniate into the opening and become entrapped, resulting in obstruction
True hermaphroditism	• **Both testicular** and **ovarian tissue** is present • External genitalia are ambiguous • Usually 46,XX
Female pseudohermaphroditism	• XX genotype with **virilization** of the external genitalia is present • The cause is **excess androgen exposure** • This malformation is most often caused by congenital adrenal hyperplasia, a **21-hydroxylase deficiency** (autosomal recessive disease with low cortisol and high ACTH)
Male pseudohermaphroditism	• XY genotype with varying ambiguities of the external genitalia • The cause is a **lack of MIF and testosterone**
Androgen insensitivity syndrome (testicular feminization)	• **XY** genotype with female phenotype • Caused by a **defective androgen receptor** • Vagina ends blindly (no uterus) • Normal female pubertal development occurs but pubic hair is scant and there are no menses
Double uterus completely	• The cause is failure of the **paramesonephric ducts** to fuse • The condition may appear in two forms: uterus divided internally by a thin septum; or a division of only the superior part of the uterus (bicornuate uterus)
Kallmann's syndrome	• A deficiency of GnRH results in decreased FSH and LH • No secondary sexual characteristics are present • Associated with hypoplasia of the olfactory bulbs **(anosmia)**

FSH=follicle-stimulating hormone; *GnRH*=gonadotropin-releasing hormone; *LH*=luteinizing hormone; *MIF*=Müllerian inhibiting factor

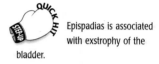

Epispadias is associated with exstrophy of the bladder.

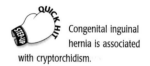

Congenital inguinal hernia is associated with cryptorchidism.

THE REPRODUCTIVE SYSTEM

GENETIC ABNORMALITIES

The incidence of genetic abnormalities as a result of aberrant chromosomes significantly increases when the mother is older than 35 years of age. In these patients, additional consideration should be given to genetic testing.

● **Genetic Abnormalities Caused by Abnormal Somatic Chromosomes** (Table 8-2)

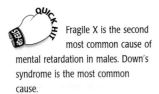

Fragile X is the second most common cause of mental retardation in males. Down's syndrome is the most common cause.

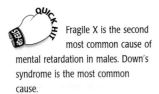

There is an increased incidence of trisomy 21 in women over 35. The incidence of the Robertsonian translocation type of Down's syndrome is familial and does not increase with the age of the mother.

TABLE 8-2	Genetic Abnormalities Caused by Abnormal Somatic Chromosomes	
Syndrome	**Genotype**	**Description**
Down's syndrome	Trisomy 21 (95%), or Robertsonian translocation of 14 and 21	• **Mental retardation** • Epicanthal folds • Large tongue • Brushfield's spots on iris • Simian crease in hands • Increased incidence of congenital heart disease, acute leukemia, and dementia of the Alzheimer type later in life • Duodenal atresia
Edward's syndrome	Trisomy 18	• Mental retardation • Micrognathia • **Rocker bottom feet** • Second digit overlaps third and fourth • Increased incidence of congenital heart disease
Patau's syndrome	Trisomy 13	• Mental retardation • Microophthalmia • Polydactyly • Cleft lip and palate
Cri-du-chat syndrome	Deletion of 5p (5p–)	• Catlike cry • Mental retardation • Microcephaly • Hypertelorism

● **Genetic Abnormalities Caused by Abnormal Sex Chromosomes** (Table 8-3)

TABLE 8-3	Genetic Abnormalities Caused by Abnormal Sex Chromosomes	
Syndrome	**Genotype**	**Description**
Turner's syndrome	45,X0	• **Monosomy** of the X chromosome • Absent Barr body • Short stature • Webbed neck • Widely spaced nipples • Wide "shieldlike" chest • Wide carrying angle of arms • Lack of sexual maturity • Amenorrhea • Coarctation of the aorta
Klinefelter's syndrome	47,XXY	• Tall with long limbs • Often presents with gynecomastia • Hyalinization of seminiferous tubules • Lack of spermatogenesis leading to sterility • One Barr body
XYY syndrome	47,XYY	• Normal-appearing male, often tall • Often associated with **aggressive behavior** • May be over-represented in the population of incarcerated males
XXX syndrome	47,XXX	• Usually asymptomatic • Rarely associated with **menstrual irregularities** and mild mental retardation • Two Barr bodies
Fragile X syndrome	46,XY	• The end of the X chromosome appears delicate • **Macroorchidism** • Common cause of **mental retardation** • Long face • Low-set, large ears
Prader-Willi syndrome	−15q12 (no paternal contribution, imprinting disorder)	• Obesity • **Hyperphagia** • **Hypogonadism** • Short stature • Mental retardation
Angelman syndrome	−15q12 (no maternal contribution, imprinting disorder)	• Ataxia • Mental retardation • **Inappropriate laughter** • Patient appears to act like a **"happy puppet"**

QUICK HIT

Puberty in males, usually occurring at age 15, is marked by increased testosterone, leading to greater hair distribution, growth of genitalia, nocturnal emissions, deepening of the voice, and increased muscle mass. Precocious puberty in males has a similar pathology to that in females, with the exception that it has a later age of onset.

THE REPRODUCTIVE SYSTEM

MENARCHE, MENSTRUATION, AND MENOPAUSE (Figure 8-5)

FIGURE 8-5 Hormone regulation from infancy to menopause

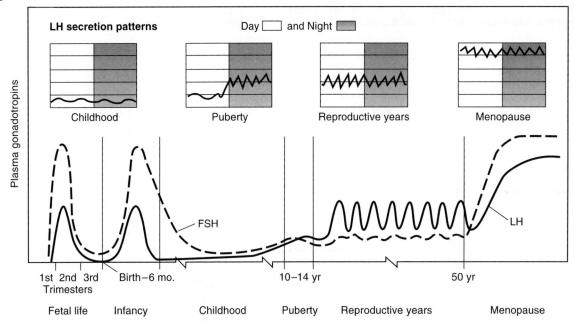

FSH=follicle-stimulating hormone; LH=luteinizing hormone. (Adapted from Harrison TR, Fauci AS. Harrison's Principles of Internal Medicine, 14th ed. New York: McGraw-Hill, 1997.)

I. Menarche

A. Is the final maturation of ovarian follicles

B. Is the first menstruation and usually occurs **between 11 and 14 years of age**

C. Follows thelarche (development of breast buds) by 2 years

D. Precocious puberty

    1. Pubertal changes before 9 years of age in boys and 8 years of age in girls

    2. True precocious puberty

        a. Early, but normal pubertal development

        b. **Usually idiopathic**

        c. May cause emotional and social adjustment problems

    3. Incomplete precocious puberty

        a. Premature development of a single pubertal characteristic

        b. Types

            (1) Premature thelarche: breast budding before 8 years of age

            (2) Premature adrenarche: growth of axillary hair

            (3) Premature pubarche: growth of pubic hair

        c. Generally self-limiting

    4. Etiology

        a. Central—increased follicle-stimulating hormone (FSH) and luteinizing hormone (LH)

        b. Peripheral—caused by increased sex steroids

Breast surgery should not be performed in girls with precocious puberty because the excision of a "lump" in premature thelarche leads to loss of entire breast.

THE REPRODUCTIVE SYSTEM

II. Menstruation and fertilization

A. Hormone formation and function (Figure 8-6)

FIGURE 8-6 Hormone function within the menstrual cycle

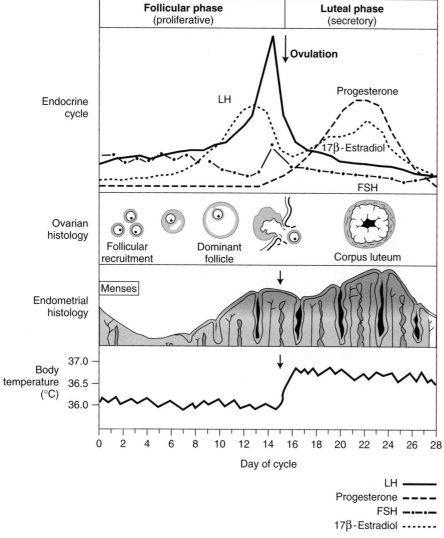

FSH=follicle-stimulating hormone; LH=luteinizing hormone.

1. Ovarian **steroids** are synthesized from **cholesterol.**
2. LH regulates the conversion of cholesterol to pregnenolone (the first step in estrogen synthesis) in the theca cells.
3. FSH regulates the final step in estrogen synthesis in the granulosa cells.
4. Estrogen
   a. Secreted by the **ovary**
   b. Induces development of secondary sex characteristics
      (1) Binds to the estrogen receptor
      (2) Activated estrogen-receptor complex interacts with nuclear chromatin
      (3) Initiates hormone-specific RNA synthesis
      (4) Results in protein synthesis
   c. Stimulates uterine growth and development
   d. Stimulates growth of endometrial spiral arteries
   e. Causes thickening of vaginal mucosa

           f. Induces development of the breast ductal system

           g. Bone growth (increased osteoblastic activity)

        5. Progesterone

           a. Secreted by the **corpus luteum** produced in response to LH

           b. Converts proliferative endometrium to secretory

           c. Induces proliferation of endometrium

           d. Inhibits uterine contractions

           e. Increases viscosity of cervical mucus

           f. Increases basal body temperature

           g. Induces development of breast glandular system

      B. Menstrual cycle (Figure 8-7)

FIGURE 8-7 The menstrual cycle

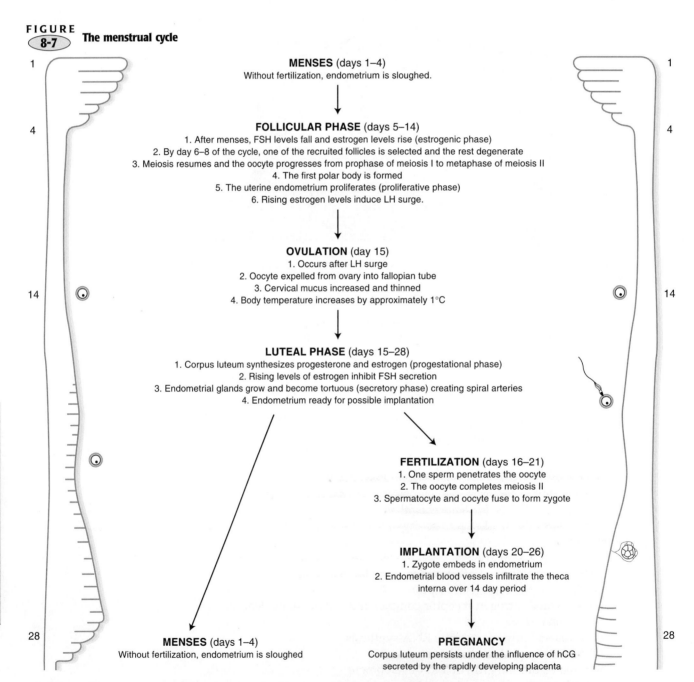

MENSES (days 1–4)
Without fertilization, endometrium is sloughed.

FOLLICULAR PHASE (days 5–14)
1. After menses, FSH levels fall and estrogen levels rise (estrogenic phase)
2. By day 6–8 of the cycle, one of the recruited follicles is selected and the rest degenerate
3. Meiosis resumes and the oocyte progresses from prophase of meiosis I to metaphase of meiosis II
4. The first polar body is formed
5. The uterine endometrium proliferates (proliferative phase)
6. Rising estrogen levels induce LH surge.

OVULATION (day 15)
1. Occurs after LH surge
2. Oocyte expelled from ovary into fallopian tube
3. Cervical mucus increased and thinned
4. Body temperature increases by approximately 1°C

LUTEAL PHASE (days 15–28)
1. Corpus luteum synthesizes progesterone and estrogen (progestational phase)
2. Rising levels of estrogen inhibit FSH secretion
3. Endometrial glands grow and become tortuous (secretory phase) creating spiral arteries
4. Endometrium ready for possible implantation

FERTILIZATION (days 16–21)
1. One sperm penetrates the oocyte
2. The oocyte completes meiosis II
3. Spermatocyte and oocyte fuse to form zygote

IMPLANTATION (days 20–26)
1. Zygote embeds in endometrium
2. Endometrial blood vessels infiltrate the theca interna over 14 day period

MENSES (days 1–4)
Without fertilization, endometrium is sloughed

PREGNANCY
Corpus luteum persists under the influence of hCG secreted by the rapidly developing placenta

FSH=follicle-stimulating hormone; *hCG*=human chorionic gonadotropin; *LH*=luteinizing hormone.

1. One cycle is defined as the time from the onset of one menses to the next, usually **28 days.**
2. Some oocytes within the ovaries undergo developmental changes during the cycle (Figure 8-8).

FIGURE
8-8 **Developmental changes in the ovary**

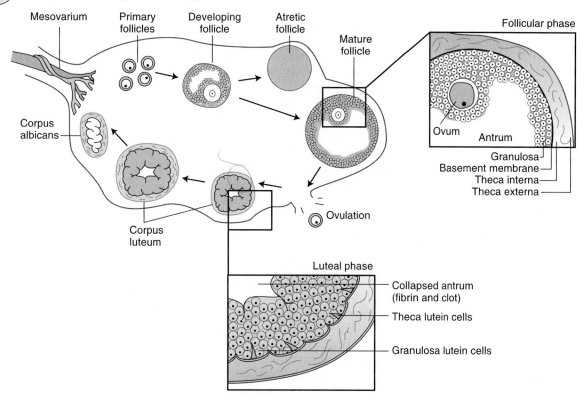

C. Disorders
   1. Dysfunctional uterine bleeding
      a. A functional menstrual disorder with excessive bleeding during, or bleeding between, menstrual periods
      b. **Most common gynecological problem** during reproductive years
      c. Caused by
         (1) Leiomyoma (fibroids)
         (2) Anovulatory cycle
         (3) Organic lesions (tumors, polyps)
         (4) Complications of pregnancy (ectopic pregnancy, cesarean section, abortion)
         (5) Endometrial hyperplasia
         (6) Corpus luteum cysts
   2. Polycystic ovary syndrome (Stein-Leventhal syndrome)
      a. Triad of **secondary amenorrhea, obesity, and hirsutism**
      b. Increased LH and testosterone
      c. Stromal fibrosis and small follicular cysts in the ovary
   3. Endometriosis
      a. Nonneoplastic endometrial tissue located outside the uterus
      b. Responds to hormonal variations of menstrual cycle
      c. Most commonly occurs in the ovary (bilateral)
      d. Presents as pain and excessive bleeding during menstruation
      e. Large blood-filled sacs (**chocolate cysts**) seen
      f. May result in infertility
      g. **Danazol,** a mild androgen, can be used as a treatment modality.

III. Menopause

A. Last physiologic menstrual cycle usually occurs in the **mid 40s or early 50s.**

B. Estrogen levels fall (owing to reduced ovarian function) and FSH levels increase.

C. Early signs
   1. Anxiety
   2. Mood swings
   3. Irritability
   4. Depression
   5. **Hot flashes:** bouts of flushing and sweating

D. Late signs
   1. Vaginal dryness
   2. Painful intercourse
   3. Urinary tract infections
   4. Atrophy of breast tissue because of lack of estrogen stimulation
   5. **Osteoporosis**
   6. **Decreased high-density lipoproteins (HDL)** leading to an increased risk of **coronary artery disease**
   7. Does not result in a decreased libido

E. Management of patients who are menopausal or postmenopausal may involve estrogen replacement therapy.
   1. Effects
      a. Decreases sleep disturbances
      b. Provides a protective effect against cardiovascular disease by increasing HDL and decreasing low-density lipoprotein (LDL)
      c. Decreases postmenopausal vaginal atrophy
      d. Decreases bone resorption and osteoporosis
      e. Decreases frequency of "hot flashes" by reestablishing hypothalamic control of norepinephrine secretion
   2. Risks and contraindications
      a. History of estrogen-dependent cancer
      b. Increased risk of breast and endometrial cancer
      c. Combined with progestin to prevent endometrial carcinoma in patients who have had a hysterectomy as women with a hysterectomy may have a higher risk of developing endometrial cancer secondary to the unopposed estrogen.

IV. Oral contraceptives

A. Agents that interfere with ovulation to prevent pregnancy

B. Combination pills contain progestin and estrogen.
   1. The estrogen component suppresses ovulation.
   2. The progestin component prevents implantation in the endometrium.

C. Other agents
   1. Progestin only
      a. Available as pills and progestin implants
      b. Higher failure rate
      c. Increased rate of menstrual irregularities
   2. Mifepristone (RU 486), a progestin antagonist
      a. Results in fetal abortion when given early in pregnancy (within 1st 6 weeks)
      b. Interferes with progesterone and decreases human chorionic gonadotropin (hCG)

D. Side effects
   1. Cardiovascular disease
      a. Women older than 35 years of age who smoke are at greatest risk from thromboembolism.

Tamoxifen, a competitive inhibitor of estrogen at the estrogen receptor, can be used to treat advanced breast cancer and certain types of endometrial cancer in postmenopausal women. It can lead to regression of estrogen-stimulated tumors in some cases.

THE REPRODUCTIVE SYSTEM

b. Progestin-predominant preparations can lead to an increase in the LDL/HDL ratio.
2. Benign liver hepatomas and hemangiomas
3. Emotional changes

PREGNANCY AND ITS ASSOCIATED COMPLICATIONS

I. Normal pregnancy

A. For clinical purposes, assume that a **woman of childbearing age is pregnant** unless proven otherwise.

B. Normal gestation is **40 weeks.**

C. Clinical signs include missed periods, swollen breasts, fatigue, nausea, and **elevated β-hCG** (serum).

D. Hormonal regulation
1. During fertilization, **β-hCG** produced by the placenta **prevents corpus luteum regression.**
2. During the first trimester, the **corpus luteum** produces estrogen and progesterone.
3. Second and third trimester
   a. Progesterone is produced by the **placenta.**
   b. Estrogen production is regulated by the interplay among fetal adrenal gland, fetal liver, and placenta.
4. The initiating event in parturition is unknown, but delivery can be induced by oxytocin.
5. Lactation
   a. Estrogen and progesterone block the effect of prolactin on the breast.
   b. Prolactin levels rise throughout pregnancy and suppress ovulation.
   c. Estrogen/progesterone levels fall after delivery.

E. Prenatal diagnostic procedures
1. **Amniocentesis** is an aspiration of fluid from the amniotic sac at 10–14 weeks after fertilization.
   a. α-Fetoprotein (**AFP**) assay for neural tube defects
   b. **Spectrophotometry** to determine hemolytic disease of the newborn (see System 10 "The Hematopoietic and Lymphoreticular System")
   c. Sex chromatin studies for X-linked disease
   d. **Cell culture** studies for chromosomal abnormalities
   e. Enzyme and DNA analysis
2. Maternal serum AFP
   a. Elevated in neural tube defects
   b. Reduced in Down's syndrome
3. Chorionic villus sampling (CVS)
   a. Can be performed at 10 weeks of pregnancy
   b. Cells are aspirated from the chorionic villi.
   c. Cells are evaluated for genetic abnormalities.
4. **Ultrasound**
   a. Can be performed at 12 weeks of pregnancy
   b. Measures fetal size, determines sex, and diagnoses fetal malformations

F. Apgar score
1. Used for physical assessment of child 1 minute and 5 minutes after birth
2. Five categories are scored 0, 1, or 2, with 2 being indicative of better performance.
   a. Color (blue = 0, trunk pink = 1, all pink = 2)
   b. Heart rate (0 = 0, <100 = 1, 100+ = 2)
   c. Reflexes (none = 0, grimace = 1, grimace and irritable = 2)
   d. Muscle tone (none = 0, some = 1, active = 2)
   e. Respiration (none = 0, irregular = 1, regular = 2)

Clomiphene interferes with the negative feedback provided by estrogen and causes an increase in gonadotropin-releasing hormone (GnRH). This leads to stimulation of ovulation and can be used to treat infertility associated with anovulatory cycles.

A pudendal nerve block can be performed to alleviate the pain of childbirth. One hand is inserted into the vagina to locate the ischial spine, which is used as a landmark, while the other hand inserts a needle, which contains anesthetic for the skin lateral to the vaginal opening.

The narrowest diameter that the fetus must transverse during birth is the pelvic outlet, from ischial spine to ischial spine (interspinous distance).

II. Abnormal placental attachment
  A. **Abruptio placentae**
    1. Placenta separates from the uterine wall before parturition
    2. Usually leads to fetal **death**
    3. May result in disseminated intravascular coagulation (**DIC**) in mother
  B. **Placenta accreta**
    1. Direct connection of uterus wall to placenta
    2. Caused by prior surgery or trauma during pregnancy
    3. Improper separation results in massive **hemorrhage.**
  C. **Placenta previa**
    1. Placenta attaches to lower uterus and blocks the cervical os.
    2. Associated with **bleeding**

III. Ectopic pregnancy
  A. Risk factors
    1. **Pelvic inflammatory disease (PID)** (e.g., chronic salpingitis)
    2. Previous surgery
    3. Endometriosis
    4. Previous ectopic pregnancy
  B. Clinical features
    1. Amenorrhea
    2. Pelvic pain and cervical tenderness
    3. Tissue mass (usually in the fallopian tubes)
    4. Abnormally elevated β-hCG levels

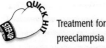

Treatment for preeclampsia includes magnesium sulfate or terbutaline. However, the treatment of choice to deliver a complete cure is delivery of the fetus if feasible.

IV. Preeclampsia
  A. Triad of **hypertension, proteinuria,** and **edema**
  B. Most common in the last trimester of first pregnancy
  C. May result in eclampsia if untreated
    1. Eclampsia has similar manifestations to preeclampsia, but also includes seizures and possibly DIC.
    2. Eclampsia can be characterized by **H**ypertension, **E**levated **L**iver enzymes, and **L**ow **P**latelets (**H-EL-LP** syndrome).

Hydatidiform moles usually precede gestational choriocarcinoma (a malignant neoplasm of trophoblastic cells).

V. Hydatidiform mole
  A. Placental villi that enlarge abnormally early in pregnancy
  B. **"Cluster of grapes"** with marked increase in β-hCG
  C. Manifests as vaginal bleeding and an increase in uterine size
  D. "Snow storm" pattern seen on ultrasound.
  E. Two types
    1. **Complete mole**
      a. Diploid XX karyotype
      b. No embryo present
      c. Completely paternal in origin
    2. **Partial mole**
      a. Triploid (XXX or XXY) karyotype
      b. Embryo present

VI. Gestational diabetes
  A. Insulin resistance occurs in normal pregnancy.
  B. Mother may be unable to meet the increased metabolic demands of pregnancy.
  C. Two or more of the following venous glucose values must be reached after a 100-g oral glucose load.
    1. Fasting > 105 mg/dL
    2. 1 hour > 190 mg/dL

3. 2 hour > 165 mg/dL
4. 3 hour > 145 mg/dL

D. High blood glucose leads to hypoglycemia in the infant, macrosomia (enlarged body), increased risk of trauma, and increased likelihood of cesarean section because of large size of fetus.

VII. Infections causing birth defects (TORCHES)

A. The **TORCHES** are **t**oxoplasmosis, **o**ther infections, **r**ubella, **c**ytomegalovirus infection, **her**pes simplex, and **s**yphilis.

B. This group of infectious organisms can cause birth defects if the mother is infected during pregnancy, especially in the first trimester.

1. Infection with herpes simplex more commonly occurs during passage through the birth canal.

C. Important agents in the "other" category are HIV and hepatitis B.

GYNECOLOGIC DIAGNOSTIC TESTS

I. Wet mount

A. Vaginal epithelial scrapings placed on a glass slide with a drop of saline

B. Microbes detected

1. *Trichomonas* appears as pear-shaped organisms with sporadic movement.

2. Bacterial vaginosis appears as vaginal epithelium with roughened edges (**clue cells**).

II. Potassium hydroxide (KOH) preparation

A. KOH is added to a microscope slide prepared with vaginal epithelial scrapings.

B. Epithelium is dissolved with KOH.

C. Microbes detected

1. *Candida*, which is resistant to KOH, remains on the slide and is identified by its **budding cells with short hyphae.**

2. KOH reacts with bacterial amines producing a "**fishy odor**" characteristic of bacterial vaginosis ("**whiff test**").

III. Papanicolaou (Pap) smear

A. Cells from the cervix are scraped and fixed onto a glass slide.

B. Microbes detected

1. Human papilloma virus (HPV) is characterized by **koilocytes** (large epithelial cells with perinuclear clearing).

2. Cytomegalovirus (CMV) appears as intranuclear inclusions with a halo around them (**owl's eye** cells).

3. Herpes simplex virus (HSV) appears as intranuclear inclusions and multinucleated giant cells.

C. Precancerous lesions detected: cervical intraepithelial neoplasia (**CIN**) 1, 2, and 3

D. Cancers detected

1. Invasive **squamous cell carcinoma** (most common)

2. Endometrial adenocarcinoma

SEXUALLY TRANSMITTED DISEASES (STDS) (Table 8-4)

Between 20% and 50% of those patients with one sexually transmitted disease (STD) will have a coexisting infection with another. The sexual partners of those diagnosed with an STD should be treated. However, the physician cannot inform the partner, except when the physician believes that the patient is unreliable and the partner will go untreated.

Chlamydia is the most common STD in the world in part because of the fact that it goes undetected when the patient is coinfected with *N. gonorrhoeae*. Treatment for gonorrhea should also be supplemented with chlamydia therapy for both the patient and their partner.

Pelvic inflammatory disease (PID) can be diagnosed via bimanual pelvic examination eliciting "**the chandelier sign**" (exquisite cervical motion tenderness).

Salpingitis, often associated with PID, can lead to infertility if left untreated.

Some nonsexually transmitted infections of the genitourinary (GU) tract include *Candida albicans*, which causes vulvovaginitis, *Staphylococcus aureus*, which can result in toxic shock syndrome, and *Escherichia coli* and *Staphylococcus saprophyticus*, which can both cause urinary tract infections (UTIs).

Toxic shock syndrome results from bacterial (*Staphylococcus aureus*) overgrowth on tampons. The enterotoxin involved acts as a supertoxin causing excess activation of T-helper cells, resulting in increased cytokine production and septic shock.

CA125 (cancer antigen 125) is elevated in greater than 80% of ovarian carcinomas.

75% of ovarian neoplasms are epithelial in origin. These tumors are usually seen in middle-aged to elderly women.

TABLE 8-4	Sexually Transmitted Diseases (STDs)
Microbe	**Disease**
Calymmatobacterium granulomatis	Granuloma inguinale; biopsy shows **Donovan bodies**
Chlamydia trachomatis	Urethritis; **acute PID;** ulcerative lesions of the genitalia (L1, L2, L3 serotypes)
Gardnerella vaginalis	Vulvovaginitis
Haemophilus ducreyi	Chancroid; ulcerative lesions of the genitalia
Herpes simplex virus-2	Genital herpes; urethritis; **painful** ulcerative lesions of the genitalia
HIV type 1 and 2	**AIDS**
Human papilloma virus especially (serotypes 6 and 11)	**Condyloma acuminatum** of vulva
Human papilloma virus (especially serotypes 16, 18, 31, 45)	Genital or anal **warts; squamous cell carcinoma** of cervix, vagina, anus, or penis; cervical intraepithelial neoplasia (CIN)
Neisseria gonorrhoeae	Urethritis; **acute PID;** pharyngitis; monoarticular **arthritis**
Treponema pallidum	Syphilis; **painless** ulcerative lesions of the genitalia Primary syphilis—hard chancres Secondary syphilis—gray wartlike lesions on the genitalia (condyloma lata) Tertiary syphilis—neurologic manifestations such as tabes dorsalis and ascending aortic aneurysm
Trichomonas vaginalis	Vulvovaginitis; male urethritis

AIDS=acquired immunodeficiency syndrome; *HIV*=human immunodeficiency virus; *PID*=pelvic inflammatory disease

FEMALE GYNECOLOGIC NEOPLASMS

Tumors of the gynecologic organs may manifest themselves as dysfunctional uterine bleeding (DUB), and as such, a heightened level of suspicion must be maintained with this presentation. Many of these neoplasms can be detected and even prevented (as is the case with cervical cancer) by routine gynecologic examinations.

I. Ovarian neoplasms of epithelial origin (Table 8-5)

TABLE 8-5	Ovarian Neoplasms of Epithelial Cell Origin	
Neoplasm	**Morphology**	**Clinical Presentation**
Serous cystadenoma	Cystic	Benign; frequently bilateral
Serous cystadenocarcinoma	Cystic	Malignant; frequently bilateral; most common (50% of ovarian neoplasms)
Mucinous cystadenoma	Mucin-filled cysts	Benign
Mucinous cystadenocarcinoma	Mucin-filled cysts	Malignant; **pseudomyxoma peritonei** (diffuse peritoneal metastasis secreting mucin)
Endometrioid adenocarcinoma	Resembles endometrium	Malignant
Brenner tumor	Resembles **transitional epithelium**	Benign; rare tumor
Clear cell cancer	Abundant **clear cytoplasm**	Usually unilateral; rare

(text continued on page 199)

II. Ovarian neoplasms of germ cell origin (Table 8-6)

TABLE 8-6	Ovarian Neoplasms of Germ Cell Origin	
Neoplasm	**Morphology**	**Clinical Features**
Dysgerminoma	Large cells with clear cytoplasm	Malignant; **equivalent of seminoma; occurs in** children
Endodermal sinus (yolk sac)	Resembles yolk sac	Malignant; produces α-fetoprotein **(AFP)**
Immature teratoma	Elements from multiple embryonic layers; poorly differentiated; resembles fetal or embryonic tissue	Malignant
Mature teratoma (dermoid cyst)	Elements from multiple embryonic layers; including: hair, bone, tooth, and nervous tissue; duplication of maternal genetics; resembles adult tissue	**Most common germ cell neoplasm** (90%); **benign** (vs. malignant in males)
Monodermal teratoma	Elements from multiple embryonic layers; one tissue type develops, most commonly thyroid tissue **(struma ovarii)**	Benign; hyperthyroidism
Choriocarcinoma	Usually seen in combination with other germ cell tumors	Malignant; produces β-human chorionic gonadotropin (**β-hCG**)
Granulosa-theca tumor	Lipid-laden cells; fibroblast proliferation; cuboidal cells in cords; eosinophilic follicles **(Call-Exner bodies)**	Benign; may secrete estrogen leading to precocious puberty or endometrial hyperplasia or carcinoma
Thecoma-fibroma	Fibroblast proliferation	Benign; rare; in combination with ascites and hydrothorax referred to as **Meigs' syndrome**
Sertoli-Leydig cell tumor	Tubules containing sertoli and leydig cells	Produces testosterone; virilization
Metastasis	Most commonly from GI, breast, or ovary; **Krukenberg tumor:** primary in stomach with signet-ring cells bilaterally	Only 5% of ovarian neoplasms

GI=gastrointestinal tract

QUICK HIT Germ cell tumors account for only 25% of ovarian neoplasms, but are the most common ovarian tumors found in women younger than 20 years of age.

III. Tumors of the uterus (cervix and body) (Table 8-7)

TABLE 8-7	Tumors of the Uterus (Cervix and Body)
Neoplasm	**Clinical Features**
Cervical intraepithelial neoplasia (CIN)	• May be classified as CIN I, CIN II, or CIN III • Neoplastic changes in the endometrium beginning at the **squamocolumnar junction** • CIN I: mild dysplasia extending less than 1/3 of the thickness of the epithelium • CIN II: cells appear more malignant with increased mitotic figures and variation in nuclear size; approximately 2/3 of the epithelium involved • CIN III: also called carcinoma in-situ (CIS); involves the full thickness of the cervical epithelium • Associated with human papilloma virus (HPV) 16, 18, 31, 33, 45 infection
Squamous cell carcinoma of the cervix	• Evolves from a progression of CIN • Increased incidence is associated with **early sexual activity** and **multiple sex partners**
Leiomyoma	• Benign tumor of the uterine body • The **most common tumor of women** (the most common malignancy in women is breast cancer) • Often multiple • Size increases with pregnancy and decreases with menopause
Leiomyosarcoma	• Uncommon • Does not arise from a preexisting dysplastic or neoplastic condition
Endometrial carcinoma	• The **most common malignancy** of the female genital tract • Associated with nulliparity • More often found in older women • Exogenous **estrogen** administration or estrogen-producing tumors may be predisposing factors • Other risk factors are diabetes, tamoxifen, hypertension, and obesity • Usually presents as vaginal bleeding

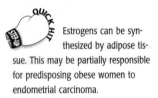

Estrogens can be synthesized by adipose tissue. This may be partially responsible for predisposing obese women to endometrial carcinoma.

IV. Tumors of the vulva and vagina (Table 8-8)

TABLE 8-8	Tumors of the Vulva and Vagina
Tumor	**Description**
Papillary hidradenoma	• **Most common** benign tumor of the vulva • Often presents as an ulcerated and bleeding nodule • Originates from apocrine sweat glands • Can easily be surgically removed
Squamous cell carcinoma of the vulva	• Similar to squamous cell carcinoma of the cervix • Highest occurrence in **older women** • Vulvar dystrophy precedes carcinoma • Associated with infection of human papillomavirus (HPV) 16, 18, 31, 33, 45
Paget's disease of the vulva	• Histologically similar to Paget's disease of the breast • Is not always associated with underlying adenocarcinoma (vs. Paget's disease of the breast)

(continued)

THE REPRODUCTIVE SYSTEM

TABLE 8-8 **Tumors of the Vulva and Vagina** *(Continued)*

Tumor	Description
Malignant melanoma	• Similar to malignant melanoma of the skin • 10% of malignant tumors of the vulva
Squamous cell carcinoma of the vagina	• The vagina is rarely a primary site of cancer formation • Usually an extension of squamous cell carcinoma of the cervix
Clear cell adenocarcinoma	• A rare malignant tumor • Occurs in the daughters of women given **diethylstilbestrol (DES)** during pregnancy
Sarcoma botryoides	• A type of rhabdomyosarcoma • Usually occurs in **girls under 5** years of age • **"Bunch of grapes"** that protrude from the vagina

BREAST PATHOLOGY (Table 8-9)

Risk factors for breast cancer include being older than 45 years of age, nulliparity, early menarche, late menopause, high-fat diet, HER-2/neu oncogene activation, first-degree relative with positive history, and a history of breast cancer in the contralateral breast.

TABLE 8-9 **Breast Pathology**

Condition	Pathology	Clinical Features
Acute mastitis	Entry of ***Staphylococcus aureus*** through nipple; abscess	Most often occurs during **nursing;** may be caused by eczema
Fibrocystic changes	Breast mass; tender during menstruation; usually **bilateral; "blue-domed"** cysts	**Most common breast disorder;** nonneoplastic; predisposition to cancer only with evidence of cellular atypia
Fibroadenoma	Painless; rubbery mass	Benign; **most common tumor in patients under 25 years of age**
Intraductal papilloma	Tumor of the lactiferous ducts	Benign; may present as serous or bloody discharge
Phyllodes tumor	Large mass; cysts; ulceration of skin	Malignant potential; may recur
Invasive ductal carcinoma	Firm mass; cells form glands; fibrous stroma	Malignant; **most common carcinoma of the breast**
Lobular carcinoma	Cancer cells fill ducts; **bloody discharge;** may be bilateral; cells line up **"Indian file"**	Malignant; may be progression of lobular carcinoma in situ
Paget's disease	Superficial lesion of nipple or areola; **Paget cells** in epidermis (large cell with marginal clearing seen)	Malignant; indicative of **underlying ductal carcinoma**
Medullary carcinoma	Soft, fleshy tumor; characterized by lymphocytic infiltrate	Malignant

 Breast cancer is the **most common cancer** of women, but the second leading cause of cancer death after lung cancer. The most common location is the **upper, outer quadrant.**

 The presence of estrogen or progesterone receptors on breast cancer reflects a good prognosis because of the ability to use hormonal (antiestrogen) therapy.

 Gynecomastia (enlargement of the breast tissue in males) can be caused by alcoholism, cimetidine, ketoconazole, spironolactone, and digitalis.

 Male breast cancer represents 1% of all breast cancer.

THE REPRODUCTIVE SYSTEM

THE PROSTATE (Figure 8-9)

FIGURE 8-9 The prostate

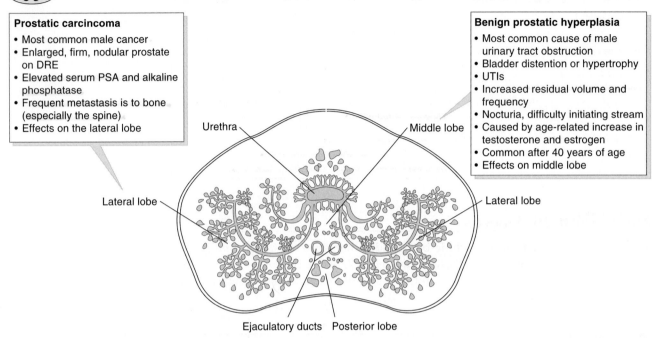

Prostatic carcincoma
- Most common male cancer
- Enlarged, firm, nodular prostate on DRE
- Elevated serum PSA and alkaline phosphatase
- Frequent metastasis is to bone (especially the spine)
- Effects on the lateral lobe

Benign prostatic hyperplasia
- Most common cause of male urinary tract obstruction
- Bladder distention or hypertrophy
- UTIs
- Increased residual volume and frequency
- Nocturia, difficulty initiating stream
- Caused by age-related increase in testosterone and estrogen
- Common after 40 years of age
- Effects on middle lobe

Urethra — Middle lobe

Lateral lobe — Lateral lobe

Ejaculatory ducts   Posterior lobe

DRE=digital rectal examination; *PSA*=prostate-specific antigen; *UTI*=urinary tract infection.

 Benign prostatic hyperplasia (BPH) is not a precancerous disorder, and it cannot be accurately diagnosed by measuring prostate-specific antigen (PSA).

 Prostate cancer is the second most common cause of cancer death in males. The leading cause is lung cancer.

 The digital rectal examination (DRE) is essential, because many of the male pelvic organs can be assessed. When the examining finger is introduced into the rectum, anal tone (S2–S4 innervation) can be evaluated. Anteriorly, from inferior to superior, lie the lower border of the prostate, the posterior aspect of the prostate, and the bladder if distended.

TESTICULAR PATHOLOGY

Anatomic disorders of the testis occur more often in young children, whereas the infectious and neoplastic diseases are more likely to occur in the young adult, sexually active population. Routine testicular examinations can often prevent and detect serious complications. When detected early, testicular neoplasms are one of the most curable cancers.

I. Testicular disorders (Table 8-10)

TABLE 8-10 Testicular Disorders

Disorder	Clinical Features
Hydrocele	• **Serous fluid** collects in the tunica vaginalis • Caused by **patency** between the peritoneal cavity and the tunica vaginalis
Hematocele	• **Blood** collects in the tunica vaginalis • Usually caused by **trauma**
Varicocele	• **Engorgement of the veins** of the spermatic cord • Most noticeable when patient is standing
Spermatocele	• Epididymal cyst containing **sperm**
Cryptorchidism	• **Failure** of one or both of the testes to **descend** • Increased incidence of **germ cell testicular cancer,** such as seminoma and embryonal carcinoma (see Table 8-11 on testicular neoplasms) • Failure of descent leads to testicular **atrophy** and **sterility**

(continued)

(text continued on page 203)

TABLE 8-10 | **Testicular Disorders (Continued)**

Disorder	Clinical Features
Testicular torsion	• **Twisting** of the spermatic cord • If untreated, will result in **testicular necrosis**
Orchitis	• Testicular infection and inflammation • May be viral or bacterial in origin • Can lead to **sterility if bilateral**
Epididymitis	• **Inflammation and infection** of the epididymis • Most often caused by **Neisseria gonorrhoeae, Chlamydia trachomatis,** Escherichia coli, Mycobacterium tuberculosis

II. Testicular neoplasms (Table 8-11)

TABLE 8-11 | **Testicular Neoplasms**

Neoplasm	Site of Origin; Morphology	Clinical Features
Seminoma	Germ cell; arranged in lobules or nests	Malignant; incidence highest in 35- to 40-year-olds; painless enlargement of testis; **most common germ cell tumor;** similar to dysgerminoma of the ovary; radiosensitive and curable
Embryonal carcinoma	Germ cell; variable morphology with papillary convolutions	Malignant; highest incidence in 20s; more aggressive than seminomas; very common in mixed tumors
Yolk sac tumor (endo-dermal sinus tumor)	Germ cell; anastomosing cords	Malignant; presents with pain or metastasis; similar to ovarian tumor; peak incidence in childhood (infants to 3 years of age); **increased AFP**
Teratoma	Two or more embryonic layers; **multiple tissue types** such as cartilage, epithelium, liver, and muscle	Malignant; occurs at any age, but more common in children; mature: heterogeneous tissue in organoid fashion; immature: incompletely differentiated
Mixed germ cell tumor	Variable; variable	Malignant; aggressive; more than one neoplastic pattern; **most common**
Leydig cell tumor (interstitial)	Testicular stroma; intracytoplasmic **Reinke crystals**	Benign; produces androgens, estrogens, or corticosteroids; often seen with **precocious puberty** or gynecomastia; similar to ovarian Sertoli-Leydig cell tumor
Sertoli cell tumor	Testicular stroma; form cordlike structures	Benign; minor endocrine abnormalities; similar to ovarian Sertoli-Leydig cell tumor
Choriocarcinoma	Trophoblastic cells; villous structures resembling placenta	Malignant; hemorrhagic; **β-hCG elevated;** peaks in early adulthood

AFP=α-fetoprotein

THE REPRODUCTIVE SYSTEM

HUMAN IMMUNODEFICIENCY VIRUS (HIV) (Figure 8-10)

FIGURE 8-10 Replication of the human immunodeficiency virus and its effect

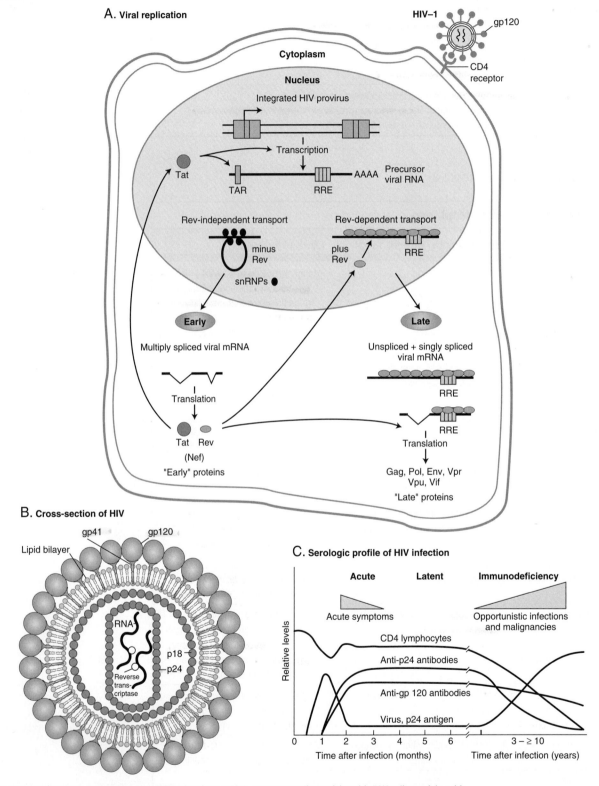

gp=glycoprotein; HIV=human immunodeficiency virus; mRNA=messenger ribonucleic acid; RNA=ribonucleic acid; snRNP=small nuclear ribonucleoprotein particle

I. Etiology

A. HIV-1 (more common) or HIV-2 **retrovirus**

B. Transmitted by

1. Sexual contact

2. **Intravenous (IV) drug** abusers sharing needles

3. Contact with bodily fluids (blood, semen, breast milk)

4. Mother to fetus (transplacentally)

C. Not transmitted through

1. Casual contact

2. Toilet seats

3. Kissing

4. Mosquitoes

D. Occupational risk to health care worker is low. A needle stick with an HIV patient's blood carries a **0.3% chance of transmission.**

II. Pathology

A. Primary infection

1. Transmitted virus infects **T-helper lymphocytes** (CD4) via the interaction of viral proteins **gp120** and **gp41** with each other and the CD4 marker (see Figure 8-10 and Table 8-12).

> **QUICK HIT**
> The gene encoding the gp120 envelope protein mutates rapidly, protecting the human immunodeficiency virus (HIV) from elimination by providing **genetic variation.**

TABLE 8-12	HIV Proteins and Function
Gene	**Product and Function**
gag	Viral core proteins p17, p24
pol	Protease, integrase, reverse transcriptase, RNAse H
env	gp 120, gp41
tat	Transcriptional transactivator (increases gene expression); essential for replication
rev	Transition from early to late gene expression; protein transport from nucleus to cytoplasm; essential for replication
nef	Transcriptional silencer; may produce latent infection
vif	Viral infectivity gene; cell to cell transmission
vpu	Viral protein U; viral particle export
vpr	Viral protein R; activates viral and cellular promoters

2. The virus also infects macrophages and monocytes (proposed portal of entry into the central nervous system [CNS]).

3. Viremia is accompanied by the **"acute retroviral syndrome"** (a flulike illness).

4. The first month is the **window period,** as p24 antigen is not yet detectable in the blood (patient is contagious).

B. Chronic infection

1. Immune response lowers viral blood counts but active replication persists.

2. **No clinical symptoms** for up to **10 years (latent period)**

3. CD4 count steadily declines.

4. Near end of latent period, constitutional symptoms develop

a. Weight loss

b. Fever

c. Night sweats

d. Adenopathy

C. Acquired immunodeficiency syndrome (AIDS)
   1. Defined as a **CD4 count of 200 cells/μL** or less coupled with the presence of certain **opportunistic** infections
   2. Infections typically seen with AIDS
      a. *Pneumocystis carinii* **pneumonia** (80%)
      b. **Kaposi's sarcoma** (HHV-8)
      c. B-cell lymphoma (brain and bone marrow)
      d. *Toxoplasma gondii* (brain tissue infection)
      e. Cytomegalovirus (CMV; leads to retinitis)
      f. *Cryptococcus neoformans* (meningeal infection)
      g. *Mycobacterium avium-intracellulare* (MAI)
      h. Tuberculosis (TB)
      i. *Candida albicans* (thrush, esophagitis)
      j. *Cryptosporidium* (chronic diarrhea)
D. Epidemiology
   1. In the United States, during the 1980s, the infection first spread among **male homosexuals.**
   2. **IV drug abusers** and **hemophiliacs** (before tests were developed to screen blood) were the next populations affected.
   3. **Heterosexual** transmission is rising in the United States and is now the leading cause of infection in Africa.
E. Laboratory diagnosis
   1. **The enzyme-linked immunosorbent assay (ELISA) test** for antibodies lends a presumptive diagnosis (screening test).
   2. This must be confirmed by the **Western blot** test, which demonstrates antibodies to gp41 or p24 (see Figure 8-10).

III. Treatment
   A. Reverse transcriptase inhibitors
      1. Zidovudine (AZT, Retrovir)
         a. This competitive inhibitor of deoxythymidine triphosphate is incorporated into viral DNA by reverse transcriptase.
         b. AZT terminates DNA synthesis; it lacks a 3' hydroxyl group.
         c. AZT is effective in reducing transmission from mother to fetus.
         d. Although AZT is toxic to bone marrow, it is not associated with fetal distress.
      2. Didanosine (ddI, Videx)
         a. This 2',3'-dideoxyadenosine analog terminates DNA synthesis; it lacks a 3' hydroxyl group.
         b. ddI can result in pancreatitis and peripheral neuropathy.
      3. Stavudine (d4T)
         a. Thymidine analog
         b. Good CNS penetration
      4. Lamivudine (3TC)
         a. Terminates synthesis of proviral DNA chain and inhibits reverse transcriptase
         b. Used in combination with AZT
   B. Protease inhibitors
      1. Protease is essential for the final step of viral proliferation and is encoded for in the HIV genome by the *pol* gene.
      2. Inhibition of the protease enzyme leads to assembly of nonfunctional viruses.
      3. Metabolism occurs by the cytochrome P-450 family of enzymes.
      4. Specific agents
         a. Saquinavir (SQV, Invirase)
         b. Ritonavir (RTV, Norvir)
         c. Indinavir (IDV, Crixivan)

THE REPRODUCTIVE SYSTEM

C. **Combination therapy** has drastically improved HIV treatment by forestalling the development of resistance to medication, and is referred to as HAART ("highly active retroviral therapy").
1. Two reverse transcriptase inhibitors and a protease inhibitor are often combined.
2. Therapy should be initiated before compromise of the immune system occurs.
3. The most common "cocktail" used is a combination of ZDV, 3TC, and IDV.
4. Ideally, therapy should be based on the virus strain isolated from the patient.

PSYCHOSOCIAL DEVELOPMENT

TIMELINE OF THE DEVELOPMENTAL STAGES OF LIFE (Figure 8-11)

FIGURE 8-11 Stages of development

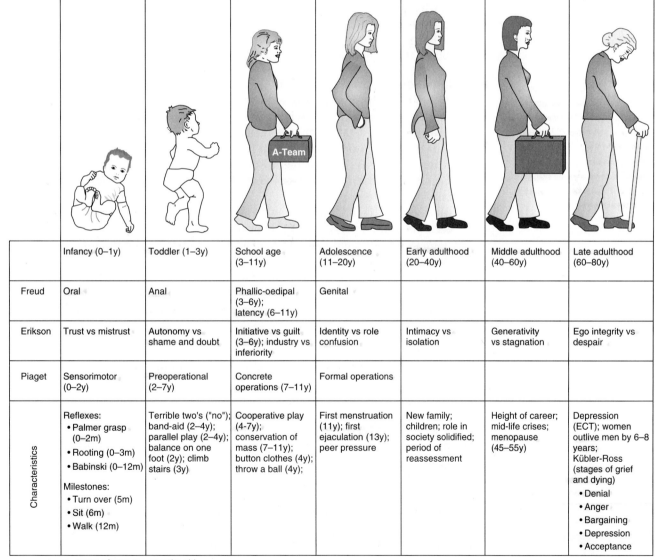

	Infancy (0–1y)	Toddler (1–3y)	School age (3–11y)	Adolescence (11–20y)	Early adulthood (20–40y)	Middle adulthood (40–60y)	Late adulthood (60–80y)
Freud	Oral	Anal	Phallic-oedipal (3–6y); latency (6–11y)	Genital			
Erikson	Trust vs mistrust	Autonomy vs shame and doubt	Initiative vs guilt (3–6y); industry vs inferiority	Identity vs role confusion	Intimacy vs isolation	Generativity vs stagnation	Ego integrity vs despair
Piaget	Sensorimotor (0–2y)	Preoperational (2–7y)	Concrete operations (7–11y)	Formal operations			
Characteristics	Reflexes: • Palmer grasp (0–2m) • Rooting (0–3m) • Babinski (0–12m) Milestones: • Turn over (5m) • Sit (6m) • Walk (12m)	Terrible two's ("no"); band-aid (2–4y); parallel play (2–4y); balance on one foot (2y); climb stairs (3y)	Cooperative play (4-7y); conservation of mass (7–11y); button clothes (4y); throw a ball (4y);	First menstruation (11y); first ejaculation (13y); peer pressure	New family; children; role in society solidified; period of reassessment	Height of career; mid-life crises; menopause (45–55y)	Depression (ECT); women outlive men by 6–8 years; Kübler-Ross (stages of grief and dying) • Denial • Anger • Bargaining • Depression • Acceptance

y = years of age; m = months old

ECT =Electro convulsive therapy; *m*=months; *y*=years.

THE FAMILY UNIT AND RELATED CONCEPTS

I. The Family Cycle
  A. Phase 1: **Marriage**
    1. Statistically, married couples are mentally and physically healthier than unmarried couples.
    2. Over half of all marriages end in divorce.
  B. Phase 2: **Child-rearing**
    1. Children raised in single-parent families have higher rates of depression, drug abuse, suicide, and criminal activity.
    2. Children from divorced families are more likely to become divorced themselves later in life.
  C. Phase 3: **Children leave home**
  D. Phase 4: **Physical decline** and final distribution of goods

The death of a child or the suicide of a spouse are the most severe psychological stressors.

II. Postpartum depression
  A. Up to 50% of all women develop a short-lived depression after giving birth (postpartum blues)
  B. Etiology
    1. Change in hormone levels
    2. Increased responsibility
    3. Fatigue
  C. Major depression seen in 5%–10% of all women after childbirth

III. Attachment of child to mother
  A. **Anaclitic depression:** sustained absence of mother between 6 and 12 months of age leads to a withdrawn and unresponsive infant
  B. **Harlow** showed that monkeys raised in **isolation** did not develop normally.
    1. Males were more affected than females.
    2. Recovery was not possible if isolation lasted longer than 6 months.
  C. **Bowlby** showed that **physical contact** between mother and child was crucial to development.
  D. **Spitz** observed that children **without proper mothering** were slow to develop and had a greater number of medical problems.
  E. **Mahler** documented development as a process in which the infant **separates** from the mother.
    1. Normal autistic phase (0–1 month): infant has little interaction
    2. Symbiotic phase (1–5 months): infant is close to mother
    3. Separation-individuation phase (5–16 months): child realizes individuality and begins to explore environment

Depression is defined as a 2-week course marked by four of the following eight criteria: (1) anhedonia, (2) increased or decreased sleep, (3) feelings of guilt, (4) decreased energy level, (5) inability to concentrate (6) changes in appetite, (7) psychomotor retardation, (8) suicidal ideation.

IV. Child abuse
  A. Includes physical abuse, sexual abuse, and emotional neglect
  B. Risk factors
    1. Substance abuse by parents
    2. Poverty
    3. Marital problems or single-parent home
  D. Physical abuse is marked by numerous fractures, bruises, subdural hematomas, or burns (at various stages of healing).
  E. Sexual abuse of children is marked by trauma to the genitalia, sexually transmitted diseases, or urinary tract infections.
  F. Abuse predisposes the child to posttraumatic stress disorder (PTSD), dissociative disorders, depression, anorexia, phobias, and personality disorders.
  G. Physician intervention is necessary and obligatory.

The **Minnesota Multiphasic Personality Inventory** (MMPI) is the most commonly used objective personality test, while the **Rorschach** test is the major projective test of personality. Intelligence is measured by the **Stanford-Binet** scale as an intelligence quotient (IQ) and is relatively stable throughout life.

V. Family therapy
  A. Involves all members of a family even though only one person might have a problem

THE REPRODUCTIVE SYSTEM

B. Identifies dysfunctional behavior and encourages communication and problem-solving
C. Based on the concept that the family system is composed of subsystems in which boundaries are established and mutual accommodation occurs

SEXUALITY

I. Gender
A. **Gender identity** is an individual's sense of being male or female, whereas **gender role** is the expression of one's gender.
B. Sexual orientation is a physical preference for one or both genders (heterosexual, homosexual, bisexual).
C. Psychological factors play a role in gender identity and sexual orientation.
   1. **Transsexual:** a person who has the sense of being in the wrong-sex body and has a strong desire to correct it
   2. **Homosexual:** a person who has a sexual preference for same-sex individuals
   3. **Transvestite:** a man who dresses in women's clothing for pleasure, usually heterosexual

II. Sexual dysfunction
A. Premature ejaculation (early climax without reaching plateau phase) is the **most common** male sexual disorder.
B. The most common sexual dysfunction in women is **sexual arousal disorder** in which lubrication cannot be maintained throughout the sexual act.
C. Impotence
   1. Failure to achieve erection or ejaculation
   2. Usually has an organic component but may be psychogenic (e.g., caused by stress or anxiety)
      a. Often related to alcohol abuse
      b. May also result from medical problems such as diabetes or illicit drug use
      c. Psychogenic cause can be confirmed by observing erections during REM sleep.
C. Vaginismus
   1. Spasm in the outer third of the vagina
   2. Difficulty during intercourse or pelvic examination
   3. Often results from rape, incest, or abuse
D. Paraphilias (Table 8-13)

QUICK HIT The four stages of normal sexual response in both the male and female are excitement, plateau, orgasm, and resolution.

TABLE 8-13	**Paraphilias**
Category	**Description (how sexual pleasure is derived)**
Exhibitionism	Exposing one's genitalia
Fetishism	Inanimate objects (e.g., women's high-heeled shoes or undergarments)
Frotteurism	Furtively rubbing genitalia against a woman (e.g., pushing up against a woman in a crowded subway)
Necrophilia	Corpses
Pedophilia	Children
Masochism	Receiving physical or psychological pain and humiliation
Sadism	Inducing physical or psychological pain and humiliation in others
Transvestic fetishism	Wearing women's clothing (such men are still attracted to women)
Voyeurism	Furtively watching individuals engage in intercourse or seductive activities
Zoophilia	Animals

 QUICK HIT Pedophilia is the **most common** paraphilia and needs to be reported to the authorities on discovery by the physician if the patient acts on this desire.

THE REPRODUCTIVE SYSTEM

1. Involves unusual objects of sexual desire
2. Are found almost exclusively in men

RAPE

I. **An act of sexual aggression in which the penis penetrates the outer vulva.**

II. **Rapists tend to be male and tend to rape women of own race.**
   A. Roughly, half of the assailants are black and half are white.
   B. Use of weapons and alcohol is common.
   C. Rapists are usually young (under 25 years of age).
   D. Rapes are underreported (usually only 15% of total).
      1. Victims are generally 15–30 years of age.
      2. Rape usually occurs inside the woman's home by an individual whom she knows.
   E. Rape usually results in rape trauma syndrome, which involves emotional lability for more than 1 year.
      1. Group therapy and support are important treatment modalities.
      2. PTSD may occur even after treatment.
         a. PTSD occurs in a subgroup of individuals exposed to trauma.
         b. Usually develops in adolescents or young adults

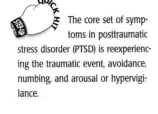

The core set of symptoms in posttraumatic stress disorder (PTSD) is reexperiencing the traumatic event, avoidance, numbing, and arousal or hypervigilance.

SUICIDE

I. **Second-leading cause of death in persons 15–24 years of age and eighth leading cause of death in the United States**

II. **Women attempt suicide 4 times more often** than men, but **men are 3 times more successful** owing to the lethality of method used.

III. **Gay and lesbian youths have a threefold increased risk of suicide because of increased societal pressures and stigmata.**

IV. **Marriage reduces the risk of suicide.**

V. **Professional women may be at an increased risk for suicide.**

VI. **Suicide risk should be assessed during the mental status examination.**
   A. Patients with a **plan** are at higher risk.
   B. Indications for hospitalization include impulsiveness, lack of social support, and a plan.

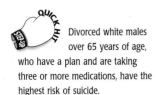

Divorced white males over 65 years of age, who have a plan and are taking three or more medications, have the highest risk of suicide.

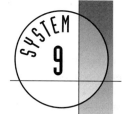

The Musculoskeletal System

DEVELOPMENT

I. Bone formation
A. **Endochondral bone**
   1. Forms over a cartilage frame
   2. Becomes the **long bones** of the skeleton (e.g., **femur**)
B. **Membranous bone**
   1. Forms without a cartilage frame
   2. Becomes the **flat bones** of the skeleton, (e.g., bones of the cranium)

II. Skeletal muscle
A. Derives from **somites**
B. Each somite produces its own **myotome**
C. Each somite produces its own **dermatome**

III. Pharyngeal arches
A. **Arch 1**
   1. Innervated by the mandibular branch of the trigeminal nerve (cranial nerve V [**CN V**])
   2. Gives rise to the following muscles
      a. Muscles of mastication (temporalis, masseter, lateral pterygoid, medial pterygoid)
      b. Two tensor muscles (tensor veli palatini, tensor tympani)
      c. Two other muscles (mylohyoid, anterior belly of the digastric)
B. **Arch 2**
   1. Innervated by the facial nerve (**CN VII**)
   2. Gives rise to the following muscles
      a. Muscles of facial expression (orbicularis oculi, obiculare oris, buccinator)
      b. Three other muscles (stylohyoid, stapedius, and the posterior belly of the digastric)
C. **Arch 3**
   1. Innervated by the glossopharyngeal nerve (**CN IX**)
   2. Gives rise to the stylopharyngeus muscle
D. **Arch 4**
   1. Innervated by the vagus nerve (pharyngeal and superior laryngeal branches of **CN X**)
   2. Gives rise to the following muscles
      a. Cricothyroid muscle
      b. All the muscles of the soft palate and pharynx except the stylopharyngeus muscle (arch 3) and tensor veli palatini (arch 1)
E. **Arch 6**
   1. Innervated by the vagus nerve (recurrent laryngeal branch of **CN X**)
   2. Gives rise to the intrinsic muscles of the larynx except the cricothyroid

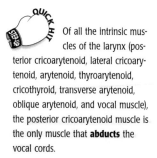 Of all the intrinsic muscles of the larynx (posterior cricoarytenoid, lateral cricoarytenoid, arytenoid, thyroarytenoid, cricothyroid, transverse arytenoid, oblique arytenoid, and vocal muscle), the posterior cricoarytenoid muscle is the only muscle that **abducts** the vocal cords.

THE MUSCULOSKELETAL SYSTEM

All the intrinsic muscles of the pharynx, except the cricothyroid, are innervated by the recurrent laryngeal branches of the vagus nerve. Therefore, bilateral injury to the recurrent laryngeal nerves leaves the cricothyroid unopposed, and the vocal cords become tense and adducted.

IV. Skin (Figure 9-1)

FIGURE 9-1 Skin histology

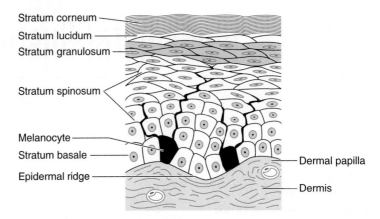

Stratum corneum
Stratum lucidum
Stratum granulosum
Stratum spinosum
Melanocyte
Stratum basale
Epidermal ridge
Dermal papilla
Dermis

Stratum basale is actively mitotic, and gives rise to the other four types.

A. Stratum basale is actively mitotic, and gives rise to the other four layers.
B. Epidermis forms from **ectoderm** and dermis forms from mesoderm.
C. Melanocytes contain melanin pigment and are derived from **neural crest**.
D. Renews every 2–3 weeks
E. Function
　1. Barrier to infection
　2. Thermoregulation
　3. Protection from desiccation
F. Two types of skin
　1. Thick skin (e.g., palms and soles of feet)
　　a. Stratum basale (deepest layer)
　　b. Stratum spinosum
　　c. Stratum lucidum
　　d. Stratum granulosum
　　e. Stratum corneum (most superficial layer)
　2. Thin skin (e.g., face, genitalia, and back of hands): stratum lucidum is absent in thin skin (although it has all the other layers).

Among the most common bacteria found on the skin are *Staphylococcus epidermidis* and various species of *Corynebacterium* and *Propionibacterium*.

BONE FUNCTION AND METABOLISM (Figure 9-2)

FIGURE 9-2 Bone histology

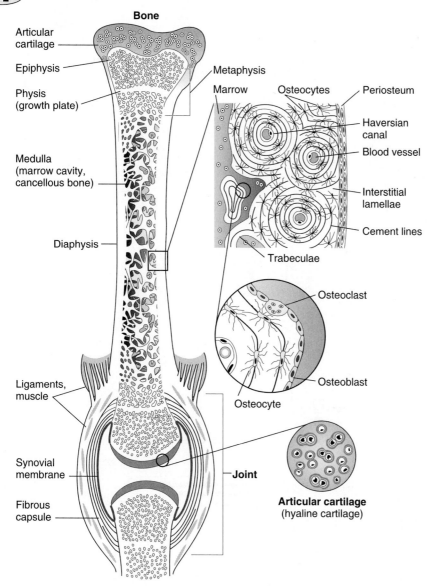

(Adapted from Damjanov IM: Histopathology: A Color Atlas and Textbook. Baltimore: Williams & Wilkins, 1996:422.)

I. Osteoblasts

A. Synthesize collagen to form osteoid (Figure 9-3)

B. Calcium and phosphate are deposited on the cartilaginous matrix to form mineralized bone.

C. Blood supply goes to osteoblasts via vessels within the **haversian canals.**

D. When osteoblasts become surrounded by bone matrix they become osteocytes.

FIGURE
9-3 Collagen synthesis

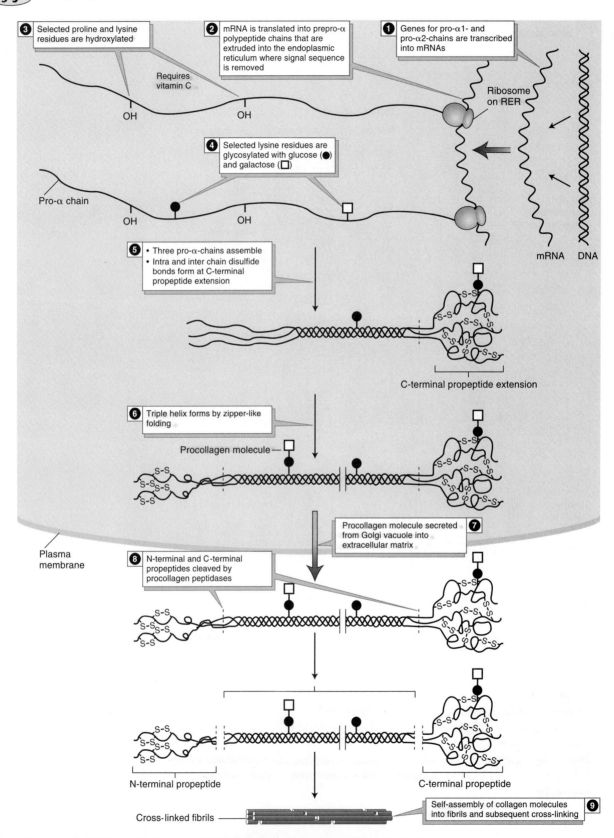

(Adapted from Champe PC, Harvey RA: Lippincott's Illustrated Reviews: Biochemistry, 2nd ed. Philadelphia: Lippincott-Raven, 1994:41. Used by permission of Lippincott Williams & Wilkins.) *DNA*=deoxyribonucleic acid; *mRNA*=messenger ribonucleic acid; *RER*=rough endoplasmic reticulum.

II. Osteocytes
A. Are influenced by parathyroid hormone (**PTH**) to stimulate osteoclastic bone resorption
B. Resorption allows Ca^{2+} to be transferred rapidly into the blood.
C. Are not directly involved in bone resorption

III. Osteoclasts
A. Multinucleated cells formed from **monocytes**
B. Contain acid phosphatase
C. Resorb bone under influence of **PTH**

IV. Hormonal control (also see Chapter 7 "The Endocrine System")
A. **Parathyroid hormone**
   1. Stimulates osteoclastic activity causing osteolysis and release of Ca^{2+} from bone
   2. Promotes the reabsorption of Ca^{2+} in the kidney
   3. Inhibits phosphate (PO_4^{3-}) reabsorption in the kidney
   4. Converts vitamin D to its active form, 1,25-dihydroxycholecalciferol
   5. Raises blood calcium and lowers blood phosphate
B. **Calcitonin**
   1. Inhibits osteoclasts, which inhibits bone resorption
   2. Lowers blood calcium
C. **Vitamin D**
   1. Assists PTH in the resorption of bone
   2. Increases Ca^{2+} absorption from the intestine
   3. Increases Ca^{2+} reabsorption from the kidney
   4. Increases PO_4^{3-} reabsorption from the kidney
   5. Raises blood calcium and phosphate
   6. Has net effect of bone growth

Exogenous estrogen administration (hormone replacement therapy) slows the rate of bone loss that occurs after menopause, by stimulating osteoblasts via estrogen receptors.

BONE, CARTILAGE, AND JOINT DISEASE

In the healthy adult, bone mass peaks between 20 and 25 years of age. Peak bone mass is typically higher in males and blacks. Bone diseases can adversely affect the mass and strength of the skeleton, predisposing the patient to fractures.

● Diseases That Affect Bone Formation (Table 9-1)

TABLE 9-1	Diseases That Affect Bone Formation	
Disease	**Etiology**	**Clinical Features**
Osteitis fibrosa cystica (von Recklinghausen's disease of bone)	Caused by increased levels of **PTH;** primary or secondary hyperparathyroidism	Cystic spaces in the bone that are lined with osteoclasts; often colored brown owing to hemorrhage, hence the name **"brown tumor of bone"**
Achondroplasia (dwarfism)	Caused by failure of long bones to elongate because of narrow epiphyseal plates and sealing of these plates with the metaphysis; **autosomal dominant** disease; **most common cause of dwarfism**	Short limbs; normal-sized head and trunk
Osteogenesis imperfecta	Group of gene mutations that cause **defective collagen synthesis;** most common type of mutation is autosomal dominant	Multiple fractures occur with only minor trauma; often called "brittle bone disease"; **blue sclera;** deformities of teeth and skin
Osteopetrosis ("marble bone disease")	**Increased density of bone** as a result of failure of reabsorption by osteoclasts; the most severe form is autosomal recessive	Multiple **fractures** despite increased density; narrowing of marrow spaces causes anemia; narrowing of other cavities causes blindness, deafness, and cranial nerve compression
Paget's disease of bone	Increased osteoblastic and osteoclastic activity by an unknown cause; occurs most commonly in the elderly; may involve one or more bones	**Skeletal deformities;** complications include bone pain owing to **fracture,** multiple **AV shunts** in bone causing high output cardiac failure, hearing loss as a result of thickening of bony structures in ear; may lead to osteosarcoma; three phases of disease: • Osteolytic phase—resorption owing to osteoclasts • Mixed phase—osteoclastic and osteoblastic activity leads to a **mosaic pattern** in the bone • Late phase—increase in bone density as a result of osteoblastic activity

AV=arteriovenous; *PTH*=parathyroid hormone

METABOLIC AND INFECTIOUS BONE DISEASE (Table 9-2)

I. Bisphosphonates

The bisphosphonates, which include **alendronate, pamidronate,** and **etidronate,** inhibit osteoclast-mediated bone resorption. The bisphosphonates are most commonly used to prevent or treat postmenopausal osteoporosis but can also be used for Paget's disease and steroid-induced osteoporosis.

The most common cause of avascular necrosis is steroid-induced vascular compression, most commonly occurring in the femoral head.

Caisson disease, which leads to necrosis via thrombosis and embolism, is caused by gas emboli resulting from decompression syndrome (e.g., rapid ascension from deep levels while scuba diving).

Patients with sickle cell disease may contract osteomyelitis as a result of *Salmonella,* whereas intravenous drug users may be infected with *Pseudomonas.* However, *Staphylococcus aureus* continues to be the most common cause of osteomyelitis in both these groups of patients.

TABLE 9-2 Metabolic and Infectious Bone Disease		
Disease	**Etiology**	**Clinical Features**
Osteoporosis	Decreased formation or increased resorption of bone as a result of physical inactivity, increased parathyroid levels, postmenopausal state, increased cortisol level, decreased calcium levels	**Decrease in bone mass** leads to fractures (especially of the weight-bearing bones of the spine); radiolucent bone seen on radiograph; DEXA scan positive
Scurvy	Lack of vitamin C intake; defective **proline and lysine hydroxylation** in collagen synthesis (see Figure 9-3)	Impaired bone formation and lesions result; painful subperiosteal hemorrhage; osteoporosis; bleeding gums
Rickets (children) Osteomalacia (adults)	Impaired calcification of bone because of deficiency of vitamin D; if caused by renal disease, termed "renal osteodystrophy"	Children: Skeletal malformations Craniotabes (thinned and softened bones of the skull) Late fontanelle closure Decreased height Rachitic rosary (costochondral junction thickening resembling string of beads) Pigeon breast owing to a protruding sternum Adults: Fractures Radiolucency on radiography
Avascular necrosis	Death of osteocytes and fat necrosis via the following mechanisms: vascular compression, vascular interruption (fracture), thrombosis (sickle cell disease, caisson disease), vessel injury	Joint pain; osteoarthritis; sites include head of the femur (**Legg-Calvé-Perthes** disease), tibial tubercle (**Osgood-Schlatter** disease)
Pyogenic osteomyelitis	Infection of bone most often caused by **_Staphylococcus aureus;_** routes of infection include hematogenous, extension from adjacent infection, open fracture or surgery	Acute febrile illness; pain; tenderness; usually affects metaphysis of distal femur, proximal tibia, and proximal humerus; forms sequestrum and involucrum
Tuberculous osteomyelitis	Tuberculous infection spreads to bone from elsewhere in body	Seen in hips, long bones, hands, feet, and vertebrae (**Pott's disease**)

DEXA = dual-energy x-ray absorptiometry

Osteochondromas generally do not undergo malignant transformation to chondrosarcoma, except in the familial variety, which is characterized by multiple lesions.

Predisposing factors for osteosarcoma include Paget's disease of the bone, mutations of the p53 gene on chromosome 17 (Li-Fraumeni syndrome), familial retinoblastoma, radiation, and bone infarcts.

The most common bone sarcoma in children is an osteosarcoma, followed by Ewing's sarcoma.

Café au lait spots are also seen in Peutz-Jeghers syndrome, neurofibromatosis type 1 (Von Recklinghausen's disease), and McCune-Albright syndrome.

II. Tumors of bone and cartilage (Table 9-3)

Tumors of the bone and cartilage, while rare, occur most commonly in the lower extremities of young males. Metastases are more common than primary tumors of the bone. Tumors of the prostate, breast, and lung account for 80% of bone metastases.

TABLE 9-3 **Tumors of Bone and Cartilage**

Tumor	Morphology	Clinical Features
Osteochondroma	Benign bone tumor; **most common benign tumor;** originates in metaphysis of long bones	Most common in men younger than 25 years of age; usually occurs on the lower end of the femur or upper end of the tibia
Giant cell tumor	Benign bone tumor; spindle-shaped cells with multinuclear giant cells; occurs on epiphyseal end of long bones	Most common in women 20–55 years of age; has **"soap bubble"** appearance on radiograph; usually occurs on the lower end of the femur or upper end of the tibia
Osteoma	Benign bone tumor; mature bone (dense tissue)	Most common in men; affects skull or facial bones; protrudes from surface
Osteoid osteoma	Benign bone tumor; **nidus** rimmed by osteoblasts and surrounded by vascular, spindled stroma	Most common in men 20–30 years of age; occurs near the ends of the tibia and femur; painful; radiolucent **nidus** is seen on radiograph
Osteosarcoma	Malignant bone tumor; origin usually in metaphyseal long bones; destructive masses with hemorrhage and necrosis	Most common in boys in their teenage years; usually occurs in tibia or femur near the knee; local pain; tenderness; swelling; metastasizes to lung first; growth under bone results in **Codman's triangle** on radiograph
Chondrosarcoma	Malignant cartilage tumor; lobulated translucent tumors; necrosis; calcification	Most common in men in mid- to late life; central skeleton is affected; radiograph shows localized area of bone destruction
Ewing's sarcoma	Malignant cartilage tumor; similar to lymphoma; **t(11;22);** sheets of small round cells producing **Homer-Wright pseudorosettes**	Most common in boys 10–15 years of age; occurs in long bones, ribs, pelvis, scapula; early metastasis; responds to chemotherapy; painful, warm, swollen mass
Fibrous dysplasia	Benign; bone replaced haphazardly by fibrous tissue	**"Chinese figures"** configuration on radiograph Three types: • single bone involvement • several bones involved • several bones involved, along with precocious puberty and café au lait spots _Albrights syndrome_
Metastasis	Malignant; usually lytic lesions unless arising from prostate or breast	Originate from prostate, breast, kidney, lung; ectopic hormone production **(parathyroid hormone related protein [PTHrP])**

III. Arthritic joint disease (Table 9-4)

The etiology of arthritic joint diseases is not well understood. For this reason, treatment is often palliative rather than curative.

Two factors to consider in the differential diagnosis of an acutely painful joint include infection and urate deposition. These two entities may be distinguished from each other, in part, by aspiration of the joint fluid with evaluation for white blood cells, bacteria on Gram stain, or crystals.

 Osteoarthritis may affect only one joint and can affect the distal interphalangeal (DIP) joints of the hands. Rheumatoid arthritis is bilaterally symmetric and does not affect the DIP joints. Also, rheumatoid arthritis is characterized by joint stiffness in the morning that is relieved as the day goes on, whereas osteoarthritis pain gets worse as the day goes on.

TABLE 9-4 Arthritic Joint Disease

Disease	Etiology	Clinical Features
Osteoarthritis (degenerative joint disease)	Degeneration of joint cartilage followed by growth of surrounding bone; the **most common type of arthritis;** primary type has no specific risk factor; secondary type related to trauma, metabolic disorder, or inflammatory arthropathy; **knee** is the most common site	**"Joint mice"** form from pieces of torn and frayed joint cartilage and broken pieces of osteophytes; erosion of cartilage results in **eburnation** (polishing) of the underlying bone; cysts visible in bone on radiograph; Heberden's nodes are osteophytes at the DIP joint; Bouchard's nodes are osteophytes of the PIP joints
Rheumatoid arthritis	Inflammation of joints and tendons most likely because of autoimmune reaction; **rheumatoid factor**—IgM antibody to IgG is characteristic; more common in women; associated with **HLA-DR4**	Acute inflammation of the synovium with edema and cellular infiltrate; synovial hypertrophy and hyperplasia; granulation tissue **(pannus)** over articular cartilage; subcutaneous rheumatoid nodules; **swan-neck and boutonniere** deformity develop owing to inflammation, muscle atrophy, and contracture; **DIP joints are spared**
Ankylosing spondylitis	Unknown cause; high association with **HLA-B27;** negative rheumatoid factor; males are more commonly affected	Chronic low back pain and stiffness; improves with movement; calcification of spinal ligaments and fusion of the facet joints produces a **"bamboo spine";** may produce extraskeletal manifestations of **apical lung fibrosis, aortic insufficiency,** or **cauda equina syndrome**
Psoriatic arthritis	Unknown cause; may present similar to rheumatoid arthritis; HLA-B27 association; **no rheumatoid factor;** no male or female preponderance	**Asymmetric** involvement of **DIP joints,** PIP joints, feet, ankles, and knees; **"pencil in a cup"** deformity of the proximal phalanges
Reiter's syndrome	Caused by reaction to systemic illness that originated either enteropathically or urogenitally; HLA-B27 association; most common in males, usually 20–40 years of age	Classic triad of genitourinary inflammation **(urethritis),** ocular inflammation **(conjunctivitis),** and acute asymmetric **arthritis**

DIP=distal interphalangeal; *HLA*=human leukocyte antigen; *Ig*=immunoglobulin; *PIP*=proximal interphalangeal

Hypertrophic osteoarthropathy, which manifests as clubbing of the digits and periostitis, is one of the sequelae of systemic disorders such as chronic lung disease, cirrhosis, inflammatory bowel disease, and congenital cyanotic heart disease.

Lesch-Nyhan syndrome is an **X-linked** deficiency of **hypoxanthine-guanine phosphoribosyl transferase** (HGPRT) that results in elevated levels of uric acid and manifests as mental retardation, gout, and self-mutilation. It can be treated with allopurinol, which blocks xanthine oxidase, an important enzyme in the formation of uric acid.

Pseudogout, caused by **calcium pyrophosphate** crystals, resembles gout in its presentation. However, calcium pyrophosphate crystals have weak **positive birefringence** under polarized light.

IV. Infectious and metabolic joint disease (Table 9-5)

TABLE 9-5 Infectious and Metabolic Joint Disease

Disease	Etiology	Clinical Features
Gout	Inflammatory reaction in joints caused by **urate crystal** deposition; IgG opsonization of the crystals followed by phagocytosis stimulates inflammation; often precipitated by a large high protein meal or by drinking excessive amounts of alcohol	Great toe involvement is called **podagra; tophi** (nodules of fibrous tissue and crystals) occur near the joints, on the ear, and on the Achilles' tendon; renal damage may occur when crystals deposit in collecting tubules; urate crystals have **strong negative birefringence** under polarized light
Nongonococcal septic arthritis	Inflammation of joints; most commonly **Staphylococcus aureus** and *Streptococcus* species	Monoarticular arthritis, usually affecting the knee; chills and fever; **positive Gram stain** and cultures of synovial fluid
Gonococcal septic arthritis	Inflammation of joints and other systemic effects secondary to dissemination of sexually acquired gonococcal infection; **most common form of arthritis in sexually active adults**	Monoarticular arthritis, usually affects the knee; chills and fever; rash (including papules and pustules); Gram stain and synovial fluid cultures often negative
Lyme disease	Infection with *Borrelia burgdorferi*, which is transmitted by the tick, *Ixodes dammini*; arthritis occurs late in the disease	**Erythema chronicum migrans,** a characteristic expanding bull's eye rash; knees are most common site of arthritis; may cause myocardial, pericardial, and neurologic manifestations

Ig=immunoglobulin

SYSTEMIC LUPUS ERYTHEMATOSUS (SLE)

I. Prototypical connective tissue disorder, which more frequently affects **women**

II. Clinical features
A. Fever, lymphadenopathy, weight loss, and general malaise
B. **Immune complex deposition** in the vessels of almost all organs
C. Pulmonary fibrosis characterized by interstitial fibrosis or diffuse alveolitis
D. **Libman-Sacks** endocarditis
  1. **Mitral valve** affected
  2. Sterile verrucous lesions seen on both sides of the leaflets
E. Pericarditis and pleuritis
F. Glomerular disease
  1. May range from mild to diffuse proliferative change
  2. Subendothelial and mesangial immune complex deposits
  3. Endothelial proliferation **(wire-loops)** and thickened basement membranes (membranous glomerulonephritis)
G. Arthralgia and arthritis
H. Vasospasm of small vessels, especially of the fingers **(Raynaud's phenomenon)**
I. Cotton-wool spot lesions in fundus of eye
J. Skin rash
  1. Characteristic **butterfly rash** over the malar eminences of the face
  2. Rashes can also be prevalent elsewhere on the body
  3. Rashes associated with exposure to sunlight (photosensitivity)

III. Laboratory findings
A. Anti-nuclear antibodies (ANA) are seen in almost all cases.
  1. ANA is a sensitive marker, but it is not specific for SLE.

2. Presence of antibodies to **double-stranded DNA** is highly specific for SLE.
3. Antibodies to **Smith antigen** (Sm) are also specific for SLE.
B. Decreased level of complement (C3 and C4) in the serum
C. Skin biopsies show immune complex deposition.
D. **False-positive test for syphilis**
E. **Hypercoagulable** state in vivo owing to anti-phospholipid antibodies

In vitro, the hypocoagulable state is due to antibodies that react with the cardiolipin test substrate. However, this reaction does not occur in vivo as the SLE patient is prone to excessive clotting, not excessive bleeding.

OTHER CONNECTIVE TISSUE DISORDERS (Table 9-6)

Inherited disorders of the bone, skin, cartilage, and blood vessels are some of the most common genetic conditions in humans. These diseases are characterized by widespread manifestations.

Xerostomia and xerophthalmia alone are characteristic of **sicca syndrome**, which is also autoimmune in nature.

TABLE 9-6 Other Connective Tissue Disorders

Disorder	Etiology	Clinical Features
Marfan's syndrome	Abnormality of **fibrillin** (a glycoprotein in microfibrils) results in skeletal, visual, and cardiovascular defects; **autosomal dominant** inheritance	Abnormally long fingers (**arachnodactyly**), arms, and legs; hyperextensible joints; tall and thin body habitus; high palate; ocular lens dislocation (**ectopia lentis**); cardiovascular defects including mitral valve prolapse, proximal aorta aneurysm, aortic valve insufficiency, and **aortic dissection**
Ehlers-Danlos syndrome	Genetic defect in collagen and **elastin** formation	Frequent hemorrhage; **hyperextensibility of joints** and skin; fragility of tissue
Progressive systemic sclerosis (scleroderma)	Diffuse fibrosis and degeneration of almost every organ owing to autoimmune reaction; **anti-scl-70** (anti-nuclear antibody); anti-centromere antibody present in **CREST** (**c**alcinosis, **R**aynaud's phenomenon, **e**sophageal dysfunction, **s**clerodactyly, and **t**elangiectasia); occurs more frequently in women	Hypertrophy of subcutaneous collagen leads to thickened skin, fixed facial expression, clawlike hand (sclerodactyly); Raynaud's phenomenon; fibrosis of esophagus, GI tract, lungs, heart, and kidney
Sjögren's syndrome	Auto-immune reaction; **anti-SS-A (Ro)** and **anti-SS-B (La)** antibodies; anti-SS-B antibody is highly specific; occurs more often in women	Classic triad: • Dry eyes (**xerophthalmia**) • Dry mouth (**xerostomia**) • Presence of **other connective tissue or autoimmune disease** (often rheumatoid arthritis) Enlarged parotid glands owing to lymphocytic infiltration; hypergammaglobulinemia
Polymyositis	Autoimmune inflammatory disorder; occurs more frequently in women; often **associated with malignancy**	Weakness in the proximal muscles of the extremities; high level of creatine kinase in serum; termed **dermatomyositis** when skin is involved
Mixed connective tissue disease (MCTD)	Autoimmune disorder; occurs more frequently in women; renal involvement is rare (as opposed to other connective tissue diseases); anti-nuclear ribonucleic protein (**anti-nRNP**) is a highly specific ANA	Raynaud's phenomenon; arthralgia; muscle inflammation; esophageal dysmotility

ANA=antinuclear antibody; *GI*=gastrointestinal tract

(text continued on page 222)

BRACHIAL PLEXUS (Figure 9-4)

FIGURE 9-4 Brachial plexus

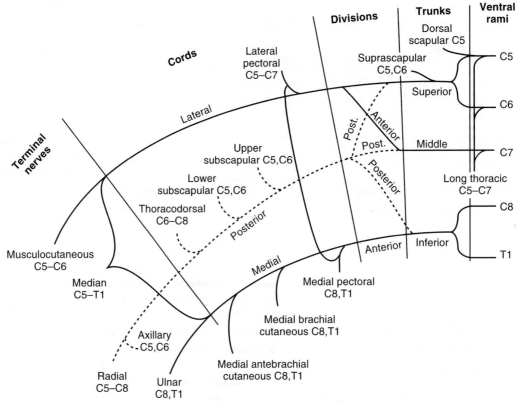

C=cervical vertebra; T=thoracic vertebra.

● Lesions of the Brachial Plexus and its Branches (Table 9-7)

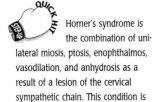

Horner's syndrome is the combination of unilateral miosis, ptosis, enophthalmos, vasodilation, and anhydrosis as a result of a lesion of the cervical sympathetic chain. This condition is often seen with a Pancoast's tumor.

Wristdrop also occurs in lead poisoning.

The radial nerve is also involved in lateral epicondylitis (tennis elbow).

The median nerve can also be damaged in fractures of the distal third of the humerus and elbow (causing total loss of thumb opposition) or slashing of the wrist.

TABLE 9-7 Lesions of the Brachial Plexus and Its Branches

Disorder	Lesion	Cause	Clinical Features
Erb-Duchenne palsy	Upper brachial plexus (C5 and C6)	**Hyperadduction** of the arm	**"Waiter's tip"** position (arm extended and adducted, forearm pronated)
Klumpke's palsy	Lower brachial plexus (C7–T1)	**Hyperabduction** of the arm	Claw hand from ulnar nerve involvement; wrist and hand dysfunction; associated with **Horner's syndrome**
Claw hand	Ulnar nerve	Occurs in children with **epiphyseal separation** of the medial epicondyle of the humerus	Weak finger adduction; medial hand numbness; dysfunction of fourth and fifth digit flexion
Radial nerve palsy	Radial nerve	**Fracture of mid-humerus**	**Wristdrop;** inability to extend wrist or fingers; loss of sensation from dorsum of hand
Carpal tunnel syndrome	Median nerve	**Repetitive wrist motion** (swelling within the flexor retinaculum compresses the median nerve)	Wrist flexion elicits pain; wrist extension relieves pain; symptoms worse at night

(continued)

Disorder	Lesion	Cause	Clinical Features
Medial winging of the scapula	Long thoracic nerve	Surgery (e.g., **mastectomy**)	Limited arm abduction and flexion; **serratus anterior paralysis;** medial scapula protrudes if patient pushes wall
Shoulder dislocation	Axillary nerve	**Anterior dislocation** (owing to forced abduction and extension)	Loss of innervation to deltoid; compromised shoulder flexion and extension; palpable depression under acromion
Surgical neck fracture of the humerus	Axillary nerve	A fall landing on the elbow	Loss of innervation to deltoid; compromised shoulder flexion and extension; palpable depression under acromion

TABLE 9-7 Lesions of the Brachial Plexus and Its Branches (Continued)

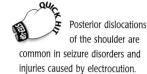

QUICK HIT
Lateral winging is caused by accessory nerve lesions leading to trapezius paralysis.

QUICK HIT
Posterior dislocations of the shoulder are common in seizure disorders and injuries caused by electrocution.

● Nerve Damage and Regeneration (Figure 9-5)

FIGURE 9-5 Nerve damage and regeneration

Nerve cell body

Nerve

Muscle fiber

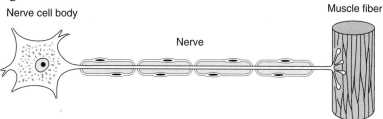

Nerve damage causes some degeneration of the distal segment. The nerve cell body undergoes chromatolysis (dispersion of Nissl substance).

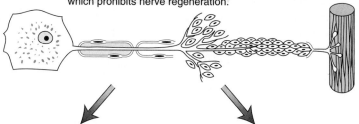

The muscle continues to atrophy for 3 weeks. In the PNS, Schwann cells proliferate and help direct the regenerating neuron. In the CNS, astrocyte proliferation forms a scar, which prohibits nerve regeneration.

If the nerve fibers don't find the degenerating segment, a neuroma is formed

Successful nerve regeneration allows the muscle fiber to return to its original size

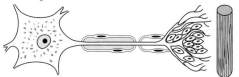

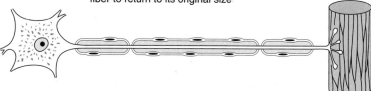

CNS=central nervous system; *PNS*=peripheral nervous system.

THE MUSCULOSKELETAL SYSTEM

LUMBOSACRAL PLEXUS (Figure 9-6)

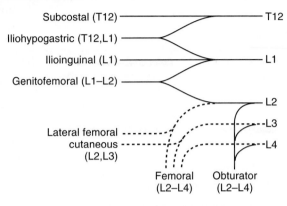

FIGURE 9-6 Lumbosacral plexus

A. The Lumbar Plexus

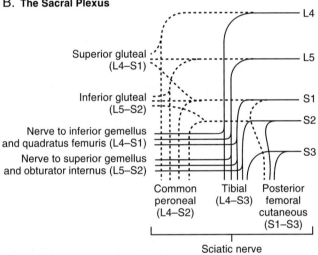

B. The Sacral Plexus

L=lumbar vertebra; *S*=sacral vertebra; *T*=thoracic vertebra.

All the nerves of the sacral plexus and the pudendal nerve (S2–S4) emerge from the pelvis through the greater sciatic foramen below the piriformis muscle except the superior gluteal nerve, which passes above the piriformis.

I. The lumbosacral plexus, which consists of the ventral rami of L1 to S4, supplies the lower extremity.

II. Motor and sensory functions of the lumbosacral plexus

Sacral plexus lesions are commonly caused by locally invading or metastasizing carcinoma from pelvic organs (e.g., bladder, prostate, ovaries). Knowledge of the motor and sensory functions of the sacral plexus can assist in determining the deficits resulting from complications of these tumors (Tables 9-8 and 9-9).

TABLE 9-8 Segmental Nerve Functions of the Lumbosacral Plexus

Spinal Nerve	Muscle Innervation	Muscle Test	Sensory Function
L1	Cremaster	Cremasteric reflex	Inguinal region
L2	Iliopsoas	Hip flexion	Upper anteromedial thigh
L3	Medial thigh Quadriceps femoris	Hip adduction Knee extension	Lower anteromedial thigh
L4	Tibialis anterior	Ankle dorsiflexion	Anteromedial leg
L5	Extensor hallucis longus	Great toe extension	Anterolateral leg, medial dorsal foot, plantar region of great toe
S1	Gastrocnemius-soleus Posterior thigh Gluteus maximus	Ankle plantarflexion Hip extension, knee flexion Power hip extension, external rotation	Heel region, plantar foot, lateral dorsal foot
S2	Gastrocnemius-soleus Foot intrinsics	Ankle plantarflexion Abduction and adduction of toes	Posterior upper thigh and leg
S3–S4	External anal sphincter Bulbospongiosus	External anal sphincter tone Bulbospongiosus reflex	Circumanal and perineal region

TABLE 9-9 Peripheral Nerve Functions of the Sacral Plexus

Nerve	Muscle Innervation	Muscle Test	Sensory Function
Genitofemoral	Cremaster	Cremasteric reflex	Skin below middle of inguinal ligament
Lateral femoral cutaneous	None	None	Skin of lateral thigh
Femoral	Anterior thigh (quadriceps)	Knee extension	Skin of anteromedial thigh and leg
Obturator	Medial thigh	Hip adduction	Hip joint and medial skin of knee
Superior gluteal	Gluteus medius-minimus	Hip abduction and internal rotation	None
Inferior gluteal	Gluteus maximus	Power hip extension and external rotation	None
Posterior femoral cutaneous	None	None	Skin of posterior thigh and upper leg
Superficial peroneal	Lateral leg	Foot eversion	Skin of anterolateral leg and dorsum of foot
Deep peroneal	Anterior leg	Ankle dorsiflexion, foot inversion, metatarsophalangeal joint extension	Skin of dorsum of web space between great and second toes
Tibial	Posterior thigh Gastrocnemius-soleus Deep posterior leg Planar muscles	Hip extensions, knee flexion, foot inversion, toe flexion	Skin of posterior leg and plantar foot

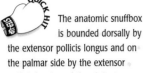

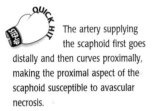

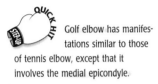

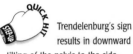

III. Other traumatic injuries (Table 9-10)

Musculoskeletal dysfunction can be caused by derangement of bone, nerve, musculature, or any combination of these elements. Insult to the body can result in problems that are acute (e.g., a torn anterior cruciate ligament) or chronic (e.g., tennis elbow).

TABLE 9-10	Other Traumatic Injuries
Injury	**Description**
Anterior cruciate ligament (ACL) tear	Positive **anterior drawer sign** (lower leg pulled forward with knee flexed); often manifests as **"terrible triad"** (i.e., torn medial collateral ligament, medial meniscus damage, and torn ACL)
Clavicle fracture	**Middle one third** of clavicle; upward displacement of proximal fragment; downward displacement of distal fragment; severe pain
Compartment syndrome	Fascial sheets separate the limbs into anterior and posterior compartments; hemorrhage into these compartments, owing to crush injury or fracture, results in **compression of neurovascular structures** and further complications; surgical emergency
Inversion sprain of ankle	Most common ankle injury; results from forced inversion; stretches or tears lateral ligaments (especially the **anterior talofibular**)
Scaphoid fracture	Tenderness in the anatomic snuffbox; may lead to **avascular necrosis** if left untreated; easily missed on radiographs
Scoliosis	Complex lateral deviation and torsion of the spine; may be idiopathic or congenital or may result from a short leg, hip displacement, or polio
Shoulder separation	Downward displacement of the clavicle as a result of laxity of the acromioclavicular and coracoclavicular ligaments
Subacromial bursitis	Inflammation of the subacromial bursa; **most common bursitis** in the body
Tennis elbow	Sprain of radial collateral ligament (lateral epicondyle); pain on wrist extension and forearm supination
Waddling gait	Limp owing to superior gluteal nerve injury affecting gluteus medius and minimus; inability to abduct thigh; results in **Trendelenburg's sign**

PAIN MANAGEMENT

I. Musculoskeletal conditions, such as fractures and soft tissue injuries, can result in significant disability, pain, and inflammation. Medical management of this pain and discomfort involves the use of nonnarcotic and narcotic preparations.

II. Acetaminophen

Acetaminophen, commonly known as Tylenol, is a nonnarcotic analgesic with antipyretic and analgesic properties. It has little anti-inflammatory action. After acetaminophen is absorbed by the gastrointestinal (GI) tract, it is metabolized in the liver. In therapeutic doses, acetaminophen has minimal significant adverse effects. However, in large doses, depletion of liver **glutathione** levels may occur, resulting in hepatic necrosis as a result of the excess *N*-acetyl-benzoquinoneimine. Treatment for acetaminophen overdose is aerosolized *N*-acetylcysteine.

III. Nonsteroidal anti-inflammatory drugs (NSAIDs)

NSAIDs are similar to acetaminophen in that they have **antipyretic** and **analgesic** properties. In addition, these agents have **anti-inflammatory** effects. NSAIDs act by inhibiting cyclooxygenase (COX) enzymes (Figure 9-7).

THE MUSCULOSKELETAL SYSTEM

FIGURE
9-7 **Mechanism of action of NSAIDs**

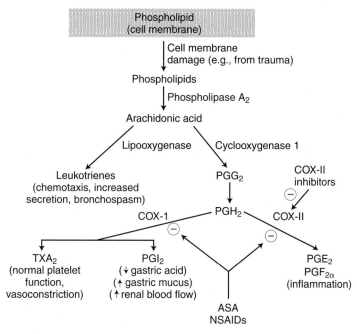

ASA=acetylsalicylic acid; COX=cyclooxygenase; NSAIDs=nonsteroidal anti-inflammatory drugs; PG=prostaglndin; TX=thromboxane.

A. Aspirin, the most common NSAID, blocks prostaglandin synthesis in the hypothalamus and in peripheral tissue. Unlike other NSAIDs, its inhibitory effect on COX enzymes is irreversible.

B. One of the major adverse effects of aspirin and NSAIDs (e.g., ibuprofen, indomethacin, naproxen, diclofenac, ketorolac) is increased risk **of GI bleeding.** By blocking prostaglandin synthesis, NSAIDs may result in GI ulcers and hemorrhage. Prostacyclin (PGI$_2$) inhibits gastric acid secretion, whereas the prostaglandins PGE$_2$ and PGF$_{2\alpha}$ help synthesize protective mucus in the stomach and small intestine. **COX-2 inhibitors,** including **celecoxib** and **rofecoxib,** may be indicated in patients who have a history of GI conditions; these NSAIDs are more specific for the inflammatory mediators (see Figure 9-7).

IV. Opioids

Opioids are useful for severe pain that is uncontrolled by NSAIDs. Opioids exert their effects by interacting with protein receptors in the central nervous system (CNS) and by inhibiting G proteins and adenylyl cyclase in the peripheral nervous system. Each family of opioid receptors—μ, κ, σ, and δ—has its own set of properties and binding potency, which correlates with the amount of analgesia provided. The μ receptors primarily mediate analgesia.

The strong agonists of the various receptor families are morphine, meperidine, methadone, fentanyl, and heroin. Moderate agonists include codeine and propoxyphene. Some of these agents can produce extreme states of euphoria and become drugs of abuse because of their binding affinity and their intrinsic effects on the CNS. Methadone, which induces less euphoria and has a longer duration of action, is often used to provide controlled withdrawal from addiction to agents such as morphine and heroin.

Opioid overdose can lead to respiratory depression, depression of the cough reflex, pinpoint pupils, constipation, bronchoconstriction, diaphoresis, and urinary retention. Naloxone and naltrexone reverse the adverse effects of opioids. A rapid-acting drug, naloxone displaces the receptor-bound opioid agents. Its effects are short-lived (approximately 2 hours). However, naltrexone works for up to 48 hours.

(text continued on page 228)

 It is believed that prostaglandin E$_2$ (PGE$_2$) sensitizes the nerve endings to the action of bradykinin, histamine, and other chemical mediators.

 Because of the irreversible effect of aspirin on thromboxane production in platelets, it can be used as an anticoagulant. A daily low dose of aspirin has been shown to have a cardioprotective effect in men.

 Opioids can also be used as effective medications to combat diarrhea and cough.

 The miosis seen in opioid overdose is a result of stimulation of the Edinger-Westphal nucleus of the oculomotor nerve, which leads to enhanced parasympathetic stimulation of the eye.

THE MUSCULOSKELETAL SYSTEM

MUSCLE FUNCTION AND DYSFUNCTION (Figure 9-8)

FIGURE
9-8 Myocyte contraction

A. The cross-bridge cycle of skeletal muscle

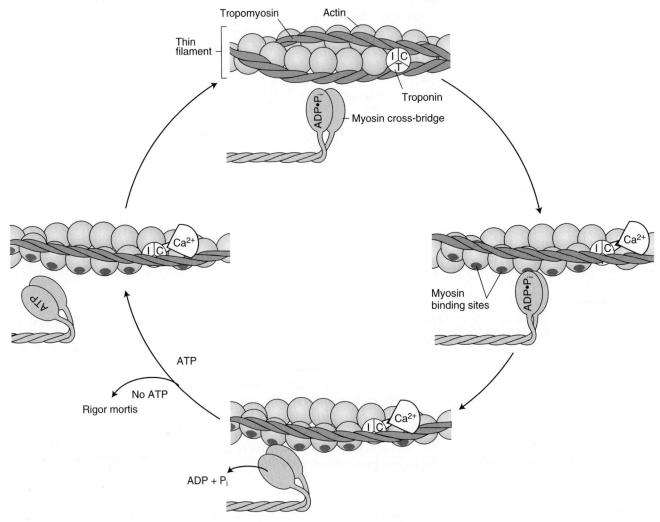

ADP=adenosine diphosphate; *ATP*=adenosine triphosphate; *Ca*=calcium; *P*=phosphate; *T*=troponin.

FIGURE 9-8 Myocyte contraction *(continued)*

B. Gross, histologic, microscopic anatomy of skeletal muscle

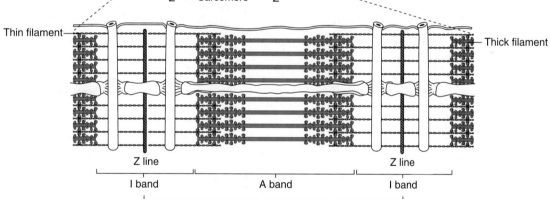

Muscle

Muscle fasciculus

Muscle fiber

Z line

H band

I band

A band

Myofibril

Z — Sarcomere — Z

Thin filament

Thick filament

Z line

I band

A band

I band

Z line

Sarcomere

I. Comparison of muscle fibers (Table 9-11)

TABLE 9-11	Comparison of Muscle Fibers		
Category	**Smooth Muscle Fiber**	**Cardiac Muscle Fiber**	**Skeletal Muscle Fiber**
Nuclei	Centrally located single nucleus	Centrally located single nucleus	Peripherally located multiple nuclei
Banding	No distinct bands	Distinct bands	Distinct bands
Z line (convergence actin filaments)	None; dense bodies present	Present	Present
Transverse (T) tubules (membrane invaginations)	None	At Z line; diads	At A–I junction; triads
Junctional communication	Gap junctions	Intercalated disks	None
Neuromuscular junction	None	None	Present
Regeneration	High	None	Some
Calcium source	Sarcoplasmic reticulum; extracellular	Sarcoplasmic reticulum; extracellular	Sarcoplasmic reticulum
Mechanism of calcium release	IP_3	Calcium-induced	Depolarization of T tubule
Calcium binding protein	Calmodulin	Troponin	Troponin

IP_3 = inositol-1,4,5-triphosphate

A. **Smooth muscle** plays a significant role in the maintenance of the lumens of the respiratory and gastrointestinal tracts, and blood vessels. **Cardiac muscle** contracts the heart and propels blood through the vasculature.

B. Skeletal muscle fiber types (Table 9-12)

TABLE 9-12	Types of Skeletal Muscle Fiber	
Category	**Type 1**	**Type 2**
Action	Sustained force; weight-bearing muscles	Sudden movement; directed action
Lipid stores	Abundant	Few
Glycogen stores	Few	Abundant
Energy utilization	Aerobic; many mitochondria	Anaerobic; few mitochondria; easily fatigued
Twitch	Slow	Fast
Color	Red (owing to blood supply)	White

Skeletal muscle maintains posture and produces movement. Muscle can be divided into **two subtypes** with differing physiologic roles.

II. Muscle tumors (Table 9-13)

Pathology of muscles can take many forms. Metabolic dyscrasias, which can be induced or inherited, are far more common than neoplasms.

The embryonal type of rhabdomyosarcoma is related to sarcoma botryoides resulting in a "bunch of grapes" appearance (see System 8 "Reproductive System").

TABLE 9-13	Muscle Tumors		
Category	**Leiomyoma**	**Leiomyosarcoma**	**Rhabdomyosarcoma**
Morphology	Benign; elongated nuclei; whorled bundles of smooth muscle cells; no larger than 2 cm	Malignant; "cigar-shaped" nuclei; dense bodies	Malignant; embryonal, alveolar, and pleomorphic types; rhabdomyoblast is diagnostic cell
Location	Smooth muscle; **uterus**	Smooth muscle; skin; deep soft tissues	Skeletal muscle; head and neck; GU tract; retroperitoneum
Immunohisto-chemistry	Antibodies to actin and desmin	Antibodies to vimentin, actin, and desmin	Antibodies to vimentin, actin, desmin, and myoglobin
Prognosis	Indolent course; easily cured	Variable; prognosis worse with increased size	Aggressive; treat with surgery, radiation, chemotherapy
Notes	Afflicts women more often than men; **most common tumor in women**	Uncommon	**Most common soft tissue sarcoma of childhood** and adolescence

GU=genitourinary tract

III. Other neuromuscular disorders (Table 9-14)

TABLE 9-14	Other Neuromuscular Disorders		
Disorder	**Etiology**	**Clinical Features**	**Notes**
Lactic acidosis	Shock; sepsis; methanol poisoning; metformin toxicity; liver failure; diabetic ketoacidosis	Increased serum lactate; **metabolic acidosis;** increased anion gap	May lead to coma or death
Myasthenia gravis	Acetylcholine receptor **autoantibodies at the neuromuscular junction;** linked to HLA-DR3; associated with thymus disorders	Muscle weakness with use; ptosis; manifests itself in facial, ocular, and limb muscles; proximal muscles affected first	Four times more common in women; anti-cholinesterase (e.g., edrophonium) improves condition
Duchenne's muscular dystrophy	**X-linked recessive;** deficiency in **dystrophin** leading to lack of actin stabilization	Progressive; proximal muscle weakens; **pseudohyper-trophy** of muscles (e.g., calf); positive Gower's maneuver; leads to death via respiratory or cardiac failure	Increased creatine kinase and lactate dehydrogenase
Mitochondrial myopathy	Transmitted via mitochondrial DNA (mtDNA); non-Mendelian inheritance	**Ragged red fibers** seen on muscle biopsy; proximal muscle weakness	**Maternal** mode of transmission

DNA=deoxyribonucleic acid; *HLA*=human leukocyte antigen

 Increased anion gap metabolic acidosis may also be caused by salicylate poisoning, alcohol intoxication, acute renal failure, diabetic ketoacidosis, and aspirin ingestion. Normal anion gap metabolic acidosis is caused by diarrhea and renal tubular acidosis.

Becker's muscular dystrophy is similar to Duchenne's, but is much less severe.

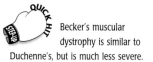

IV. Neuromuscular blocking agents

Neuromuscular blocking agents, which are most often encountered in the operating room, are used to produce the flaccid paralysis that is essential for many procedures such as abdominal operations or joint replacements. These drugs affect the muscles of the body in a typical order. The small, fast-twitch muscles of the face and eyes are first to be paralyzed, followed by the muscles of the hand, limbs, and trunk. The intercostal muscles and the diaphragm are the last to be affected. As the effects of neuromuscular blockers wear off, the muscles regain function in the reverse order.

Neuromuscular blocking agents can be categorized several ways. The most useful system divides them into central-acting and neuromuscular end-plate (NMEP) blockers. The NMEP blockers can be further divided into depolarizing and nondepolarizing agents.

Centrally acting neuromuscular blocking drugs include diazepam and baclofen. **Diazepam**, a benzodiazepine, acts at γ-aminobutyric acid (GABA) receptors in the CNS. **Baclofen**, another GABA mimetic, also acts in the CNS to decrease muscle tone. Peripherally acting drugs include curare, succinylcholine, and dantrolene. Curare and its derivatives act as nondepolarizing or competitive neuromuscular blockers.

Curare acts as a nicotinic antagonist at the motor end-plate to produce muscle relaxation. At low doses, this agent binds to and blocks the nicotinic receptor, a competitive blockade that can be overcome by increasing the concentration of acetylcholine. At higher doses, curare and the curarelike agents actually block ion channels at the NMEP (noncompetitive block).

Succinylcholine, the only depolarizing neuromuscular blocking agent, acts by binding to and activating the nicotinic receptor of the NMEP. In phase 1 block, a wave of fasciculations rapidly pass over the patient as the drug is administered. The drug then remains attached to the nicotinic receptor and is not broken down by acetylcholinesterase. In phase 2 block, the membrane of the NMEP repolarizes, the muscle relax, and the succinylcholine continues to block the nicotinic receptor. Plasma cholinesterase quickly breaks down the drug, and its duration of action is only a few minutes. The rapid onset and short duration of action of succinylcholine make it ideal for use during rapid sequence endotracheal intubation and electroconvulsive therapy.

V. Muscle glycogen storage disorders (Figure 9-9)

Dantrolene, which acts by inhibiting the release of calcium from the sarcoplasmic reticulum, is used in the treatment of malignant hyperthermia.

When succinylcholine is used in combination with halothane, it can cause **malignant hyperthermia** in certain predisposed individuals. Treatment of this condition, which is characterized by severe, prolonged muscle contractions, involves the use of dantrolene and cooling blankets.

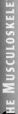

THE MUSCULOSKELETAL SYSTEM

(text continued on page 233)

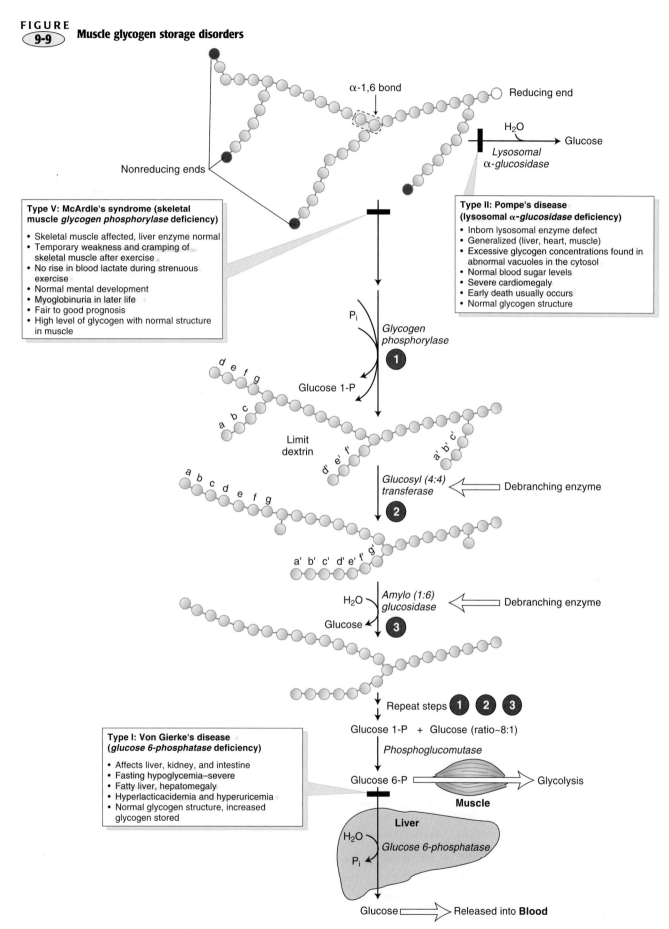

FIGURE 9-9 Muscle glycogen storage disorders

α-1,6 bond

Reducing end

H₂O → Glucose

Lysosomal α-glucosidase

Nonreducing ends

Type V: McArdle's syndrome (skeletal muscle *glycogen phosphorylase* deficiency)

- Skeletal muscle affected, liver enzyme normal
- Temporary weakness and cramping of skeletal muscle after exercise
- No rise in blood lactate during strenuous exercise
- Normal mental development
- Myoglobinuria in later life
- Fair to good prognosis
- High level of glycogen with normal structure in muscle

Type II: Pompe's disease (lysosomal *α-glucosidase* deficiency)

- Inborn lysosomal enzyme defect
- Generalized (liver, heart, muscle)
- Excessive glycogen concentrations found in abnormal vacuoles in the cytosol
- Normal blood sugar levels
- Severe cardiomegaly
- Early death usually occurs
- Normal glycogen structure

Pᵢ

Glycogen phosphorylase **1**

Glucose 1-P

Limit dextrin

Glucosyl (4:4) transferase **2** ← Debranching enzyme

H₂O

Amylo (1:6) glucosidase **3** ← Debranching enzyme

Glucose

Repeat steps **1** **2** **3**

Glucose 1-P + Glucose (ratio~8:1)

Type I: Von Gierke's disease (*glucose 6-phosphatase* deficiency)

- Affects liver, kidney, and intestine
- Fasting hypoglycemia–severe
- Fatty liver, hepatomegaly
- Hyperlacticacidemia and hyperuricemia
- Normal glycogen structure, increased glycogen stored

Phosphoglucomutase

Glucose 6-P → Glycolysis

Muscle

Liver

H₂O

Glucose 6-phosphatase

Pᵢ

Glucose → Released into **Blood**

(Adapted from Champe PC, Harvey RA: Lippincott's Illustrated Reviews: Biochemistry, 2nd ed. Philadelphia: Lippincott-Raven, 1994:140. Used by permission of Lippincott Williams & Wilkins.)

THE MUSCULOSKELETAL SYSTEM

THE INGUINAL CANAL (Figure 9-10)

FIGURE
9-10 **The inguinal canal**

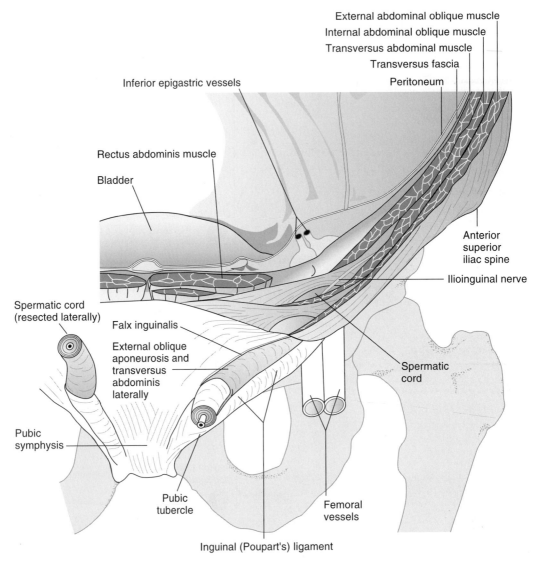

I. The inguinal canal (Table 9-15)

The inguinal canal contains the ilioinguinal nerve (sensory to the anterior aspect of labia or scrotum), spermatic cord in males (ductus deferens, testicular artery, pampiniform plexus), and the round ligament of the uterus in females.

TABLE 9-15	The Inguinal Canal
Border	**Anatomic Composition**
Superior	**Falx inguinalis:** internal abdominal oblique (IAO) and transversus abdominis muscles
Inferior	Inguinal ligament
Anterior	External abdominal oblique (EAO) aponeurosis; IAO and transversus abdominis muscles laterally
Posterior	Transversalis fascia; falx inguinalis medially

II. Hernias (Table 9-16)

Hernias may cause small bowel obstruction. However, small bowel obstructions are most commonly caused by adhesions.

TABLE 9-16	Hernias		
Hernia	**Pathology**	**Clinical Features**	**Diagnosis**
Direct inguinal hernia	Parietal peritoneum passes directly through abdominal wall (**Hesselbach's** triangle)	More common in older males	Medial to inferior epigastric artery; located above pubic tubercle
Indirect inguinal hernia	Parietal peritoneum passes through internal inguinal ring and follows the inguinal canal	**Most common** type; occurs in young adult males more frequently than in females	Lateral to inferior epigastric artery; located above and medial to pubic tubercle
Femoral hernia	Parietal peritoneum passes through the femoral canal	More common in females	Located below and lateral to pubic tubercle

Hernia complications include small bowel entrapment (incarceration) and bowel ischemia (strangulation).

Hesselbach's triangle is formed from the border of the rectus abdominis medially, inferior epigastric artery laterally, and the inguinal ligament inferiorly.

SKIN DISORDERS (Table 9-17)

Skin disorders are often characterized by pruritus, inflammation, and irritability. Skin lesions that are suggestive of malignancy demonstrate asymmetry, irregular borders, variations in color, and increasing size.

TABLE 9-17	Skin Disorders
Disorder	**Description**
Keloid scarring	• **Excessive scarring** that occurs after minor trauma • Results in raised, firm lesions on the skin • Occurs more frequently in African-Americans • Genetic predisposition is a factor
Xanthomas	• Accumulation of foam-filled histiocytes within the dermis • Often associated with **hyperlipidemia** or lymphoproliferative disorders • Often found on the Achilles tendon, the extensor tendons of the fingers, and the eyelids
Seborrheic keratosis	• Common **benign neoplasm** in the elderly • Raised papules and plaques that appear to be "pasted on"
Albinism	• **Lack of melanin pigment** production • Ocular type limited to eyes; X-linked • Oculocutaneous type involves the skin, eyes, and hair; autosomal recessive; lack of tyrosinase enzyme, which converts tyrosine to DOPA
Hemangiomas	• Large-vessel malformation composed of masses of blood-filled channels • **Port-wine stain** birthmarks are the most common manifestation • Cavernous hemangiomas are a subset with large cavernous vascular spaces that can occur in von Hippel-Lindau disease

DOPA = 3,4-dihydroxyphenylalanine

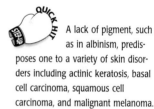

A lack of pigment, such as in albinism, predisposes one to a variety of skin disorders including actinic keratosis, basal cell carcinoma, squamous cell carcinoma, and malignant melanoma.

● Skin Cancers and Premalignant Conditions (Table 9-18)

TABLE 9-18 **Skin Cancers and Premalignant Conditions**

Disorder	Description
Acanthosis nigricans	• A thickening and **hyperpigmentation** of the axilla, neck, and groin region • Benign type—several causes (e.g., diabetes mellitus) • Malignant type—is an important marker of an underlying visceral **adenocarcinoma**
Actinic keratosis	• A series of dysplastic changes that occur before the onset of **squamous cell carcinoma** • A buildup of keratin caused by excessive exposure to sunlight leads to a **"warty"** appearance
Squamous cell carcinoma	• Malignant tumor of the skin caused by excessive exposure to sunlight • Rarely metastasizes • Characterized by ulcerated, scaling nodules • Appears microscopically as islands of neoplastic cells with **whorls of keratin** ("pearls")
Basal cell carcinoma	• **Most common** skin tumor • Appears grossly as a pearl-like papule on sun-exposed areas • Appears histologically as a dark cluster with **palisading peripheral cells** • Almost never metastasizes

Malignant melanoma	• Aggressive tumor that arises from melanocytes
	• Associated with excess exposure to sunlight
	• Two growth patterns:
	  • **Benign radial manner** (growth within skin layer)
	  • **Aggressive vertical manner** (growth through deeper layers)
	• Associated with the S-100 tumor marker

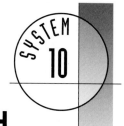

The Hematopoietic and Lymphoreticular System

HEMATOPOIESIS TIMETABLE

I. **Week 3:** Embryonic visceral mesoderm gives rise to angioblasts.

II. **1st trimester:** Yolk sac produces red blood cells (RBCs).

III. **2nd trimester:** Liver and spleen produce RBCs.

IV. **3rd trimester:** Central and peripheral skeleton produces RBCs.

V. **Adulthood:** Axial skeleton (vertebral bodies, sternum, ribs, pelvis) produces RBCs.

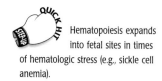

Hematopoiesis expands into fetal sites in times of hematologic stress (e.g., sickle cell anemia).

THE CELLS (Table 10-1)

The hematopoietic-lymphoreticular system is composed of a multitude of cells. Most of these cells can be found circulating in the bloodstream, although a few are found within peripheral tissues.

TABLE 10-1	The Cells of the Hematopoietic-Lymphoreticular System						
Cell	**Relative Amounts**	**Life Span**	**Morphology**		**Functions**	**Secretion**	**Notes**
Neutrophils (PMNs)	40%–75% of WBCs	Less than 7 days	Multilobed nucleus, azurophilic granules (lysosomes), **myeloperoxidase**	Neutrophil	Phagocytic, acute inflammatory response	Lysosomal contents released on cell death	Lysosomes contain lysozyme, which is **bactericidal**
Basophils	<1% of WBCs	Years	Bilobate, basophilic	Basophil	Allergies	Heparin, histamine, SRS-A	**Bind IgE** antibody to their membrane
Eosinophils	0.5%–5% of WBCs	Less than 2 weeks in connective tissues	Bilobed, azurophilic granules	Eosinophil	Phagocytic for Ag-Ab complexes, **antiparasitic,** inactivated histamine and SRS-A	Histaminase arylsulfatase	Large numbers found in lamina propria of GI tract
Mast cells	Found in connective tissue	9–18 months	Basophil-like, round nucleus	Mast cell	Bind IgE; mediate **type I hypersensitivity** reaction	ECF, histamine, leukotrienes, heparin	**Cromolyn sodium** prevents degranulation by stabilizing membrane
Macrophages	Found **only in tissues,** not in the blood	Extended life in tissues	Ameboid bacteria, RBCs, and damaged cells	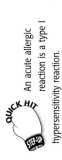 Macrophage	Phagocytize	IL-1, **IL-2**, TNFα	Activated by LPS and INF-γ

QUICK HIT

Neutrophils are hypersegmented (6–7 segments) in megaloblastic anemia.

QUICK HIT

Slow-reacting substance of anaphylaxis (SRS-A) is comprised of leukotriene C₄ and leukotriene D₄, which bronchoconstrict, vasoconstrict, and increase vascular permeability.

QUICK HIT

Eosinophilia occurs in response to trematodes (also called flukes) including Schistosomes, Clonorchis sinensis, and Paragonimus westermani; or cestodes (also called tapeworms) including Taenia solium, Taenia saginata, Diphyllobothrium latum, and Echinococcus granulosus). Eosinophilia can also result from neoplasms, allergy, asthma, and connective tissue disorders.

QUICK HIT

An acute allergic reaction is a type I hypersensitivity reaction.

Cell	Count	Lifespan	Morphology		Function	Secretions	Notes
Monocytes	3%–9% of WBCs	Less than 3 days in the blood	Large kidney-shaped nucleus	Monocyte	Differentiate into macrophages and osteoclasts	IL-1, IL-6	Chemotactically **attracted to sites of inflammation**
T lymphocytes	15%–18% of WBCs, 75% of lymphocytes	Years	Basophilic, large nucleus, scan cytoplasm	Large T-lymphocyte	**Cell-mediated immune response**	IL-2, IL-3, IL-4, IL-5, IL-6, INF-γ, TNF-α, TNF-β	Several types (see Figure 10-5)
B lymphocytes	5%–% of WBCs, 25% of lymphocytes	Months	Basophilic, large nucleus, scant cytoplasm	Plasma cell	**Humoral immune response**	INF-α	Differentiate into plasma cells and long-lived memory cells
Erythrocytes	5×10^6/mL in men, 4.55×10^6/mL in females	120 days	**Anucleate, biconcave disc**	Erythrocyte	Gas exchange	See Figure 10-3	Anaerobic metabolism exclusively
Platelets	250,000 to 400,000/mL	68 days	Irregularly shaped, membrane bound	Platelets	Prevention of bleeding by **clot formation**	Histamine, PDGF, serotonin, TXA_2	Disorders of number or function can result in bleeding

Ag-Ab= antigen-antibody; *ECF*=eosinophilic chemotactic factor; *GI*=gastrointestinal; *Ig*=immunoglobulin; *IL*=interleukin; *INF*=interferon; *LPS*=lipopolysaccharide; *RBC*=red blood cell; *SRS-A*=slow-reacting substance of anaphylaxis; *TNF*=tumor necrosis factor; TXA_2=thromboxane A_2; *WBC*=white blood cell

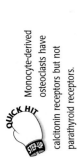

QUICK HIT
STEP-UP

Monocyte-derived osteoclasts have calcitonin receptors but not parathyroid receptors.

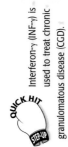

QUICK HIT
STEP-UP

Interferon-γ (INF-γ) is used to treat chronic granulomatous disease (CGD).

THE ORGANS OF THE LYMPHORETICULAR SYSTEM

I. Thymus

A. Derived from the **third pharyngeal pouch**

B. The cortex contains thymocytes (immature T lymphocytes).

C. The medulla contains mature T lymphocytes and **Hassall's corpuscles** (whorl-like bodies that contain keratin). As T lymphocytes mature, they express T-cell receptors and CD receptors. T lymphocytes that recognize "self" undergo apoptosis, whereas those that recognize "non-self" undergo clonal expansion.

II. Lymph nodes (Figure 10-1)

A. Derived from mesenchymal cells

B. Outer cortex contains B lymphocytes.

C. Inner cortex (also called the paracortex) contains T lymphocytes and is thymic dependent.

D. Medulla contains B lymphocytes, plasma cells, and macrophages.

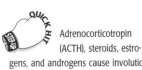

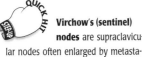

Adrenocorticotropin (ACTH), steroids, estrogens, and androgens cause involution of the thymus.

Virchow's (sentinel) nodes are supraclavicular nodes often enlarged by metastasis from gastric carcinoma.

FIGURE 10-1 The lymph node

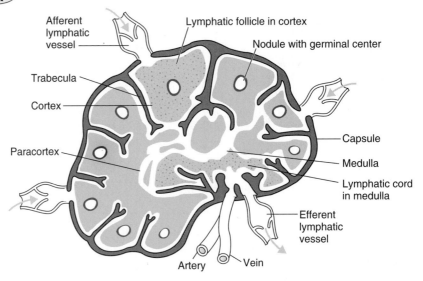

III. Lymph

A. Fluid that returns lipids, proteins, and water-soluble substances to the circulation via the lymphatic vessels

B. The left side of the head, the left thorax, the left upper limb, and everything below the diaphragm drain into the thoracic duct. This duct terminates at the junction of the left subclavian and left internal jugular veins.

C. The **right upper quadrant of body** (right side of head, right upper limb, and right thorax) empties into the **great vessels of the right side.**

IV. Spleen (Figure 10-2)

FIGURE
10-2 The spleen

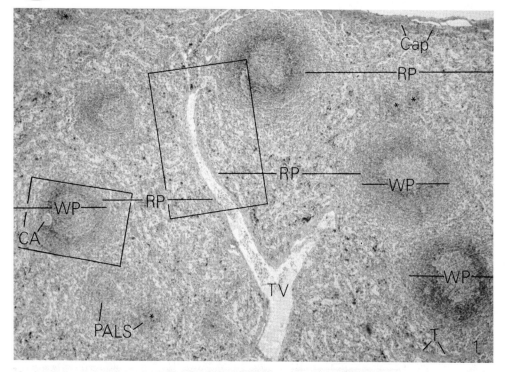

(From Ross MH, Romrell LJ, Kaye GI: *Histology: A Text and Atlas,* 3rd edition. Baltimore: Williams & Wilkins, 1995. p. 365. Used by permission of Lippincott Williams & Wilkins.) *CA*=; *Cap*=; *PALS*=periarteriolar lymphatic sheaths; *T*=trabeculae; *TV*=trabecular vein; *WP*=white pulp.

A. Derived from mesenchyme beginning in the 5th week

B. White pulp: B lymphocytes surround the central artery, and T lymphocytes are arranged into periarteriolar lymphatic sheaths (PALS).

C. Marginal zone: where blood meets spleen parenchyma; antigen-presenting cells (APCs) and macrophages are present

D. Red pulp: contains splenic (Billroth) cords separated by sinusoids; also has plasma cells, macrophages, lymphocytes, and RBCs

V. Liver

A. Endoderm of foregut (hepatic diverticulum) grows into surrounding mesoderm (septum transversum).

B. Hepatic cords from diverticulum, arranged around umbilical and vitelline veins, form hepatic sinusoids.

C. Produces **fetal hemoglobin (HbF) during second trimester**

D. Produces **clotting factors** of coagulation cascade

E. Can function to sequester and break down RBCs if spleen is removed

VI. Gut-associated lymphatic tissue

A. Found in tonsils, Peyer's patches of the jejunum, appendix, and cecum

B. M cells: present antigens to lymphocytes and secrete IgA

RED BLOOD CELL PHYSIOLOGY (Figure 10-3)

FIGURE
10-3 Red blood cell physiology

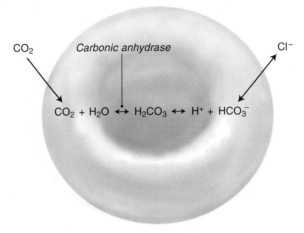

Cl^-=chloride; CO_2=carbon dioxide; H^+=hydrogen ion; HCO_3^-=bicarbonate; H_2O=water; H_2CO_3=carbonic acid.

● Hemoglobin-Oxygen Dissociation Curve (Figure 10-4)

Red blood cells deliver oxygen to tissues and carry carbon dioxide (CO_2) to the lungs. In the tissues, CO_2 diffuses into the RBC, combines with water via **carbonic anhydrase** (CA), and produces carbonic acid. This dissociates into hydrogen ions and bicarbonate. The **bicarbonate leaves** the RBC in exchange for chloride **(chloride shift).** In the lungs, this process is reversed. Thus, **bicarbonate in the plasma** is the **major route** for CO_2 transport to the lungs.

Deoxyhemoglobin exists in the **tense state,** which resists oxygen binding. Binding of the first oxygen molecule requires considerable energy and precipitates a conformational change from the tense state to the relaxed state. Binding of further oxygen molecules requires less energy (**positive cooperativity**). Certain factors affect hemoglobin affinity for oxygen (see Figure 10-4). However, carbon monoxide does not affect hemoglobin affinity for oxygen, and therefore does not shift the hemoglobin-oxygen dissociation curve. Instead, because of its 200-fold greater affinity for the oxygen binding sites on hemoglobin, carbon monoxide causes hypoxia.

> **QUICK HIT**
> Carbon monoxide poisoning causes hypoxic injury to the basal ganglia and results in a cherry-red color of the skin and viscera. The treatment is 100% oxygen.

FIGURE
10-4 Hemoglobin-oxygen dissociation curve

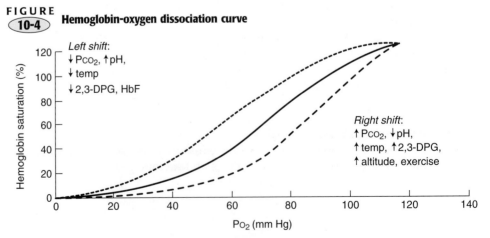

$2,3$-DPG=2,3-diphosphoglycerate; HbF=hemoglobin F; Pco_2=partial pressure of carbon dioxide; pH=hydrogen ion concentration; Po_2=partial pressure of oxygen; temp=temperature.

LYMPHOCYTE DIFFERENTIATION

T-helper (Th) lymphocytes express **MHC class II** and **CD4 proteins** on their membranes. They participate in the cellular response to **extracellular** antigens (e.g., bacteria). Cytotoxic T lymphocytes (T-cyt) **express MHC class I and CD8 proteins** on their membranes. T-cyt cells are involved in the immune response to **intracellular** antigens (e.g., viruses and obligate intracellular organisms such as *Chlamydiae* or *Rickettsiae*). Natural killer (NK) cells are a form of T lymphocytes that do not pass through the thymus for maturation. As one of the body's innate defenses, NK cells kill **tumor cells and viral infected cells** by secreting cytotoxins (perforins). They do not require antibodies to kill, but their potency is increased when antibody is present (i.e., antibody-dependent cellular cytotoxicity [ADCC]).

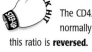 The CD4/CD8 ratio is normally 2:1. In AIDS, this ratio is **reversed.**

 Antibody-dependent cellular cytotoxicity (ADCC) is one of the mechanisms by which type II hypersensitivity reactions can occur. Other mechanisms are complement-fixing antibodies (e.g., Goodpasture's syndrome) and anti-cell surface receptor antibodies (e.g., Graves' disease).

● **T-cell differentiation (Figure 10-5)**

FIGURE 10-5 T-cell differentiation

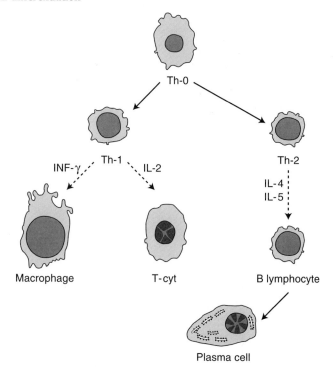

Th-0

Th-1

INF-γ   IL-2

Th-2

IL-4
IL-5

Macrophage

T-cyt

B lymphocyte

Plasma cell

IL=interleukin; *INF-γ*=interferon-γ; *T-cyt*=cytotoxic T lymphocytes; *Th*=T-helper lymphocytes.

IMMUNOGLOBULINS

I. Characteristics
A. Glycoproteins
B. Consist of **light (L) chain** and **heavy (H) chain**
C. Two identical H chains and two identical L chains linked by **disulfide bonds** in a "Y" shape
D. **Variable region** exists on both L and H chains
E. H chain composed of **Fc** and **Fab** fragment
F. L chain composed of Fab fragment only

II. Types (Table 10-2)

TABLE 10-2	Immunoglobulin (Ig) Properties				
	IgM	**IgG**	**IgE**	**IgA**	**IgD**
Percentage of total Ig	9%	75%	0.004%	15%	0.2%
Structure	Monomer or pentamer Pentamer held together by J chain	Monomer	Monomer	Monomer or dimer Dimer held together by J chain	Monomer
Function	Fixes complement Antigen receptor on B cell surface **Primary response**	Fixes complement Opsonizes **Crosses the placenta** Neutralizes bacterial toxins **Secondary response**	Allergic response **(type I hypersensitivity)** Binds to basophils and mast cells Antihelminthic	Found in **secretions** Prevents bacterial and viral attachment	Unknown May be antigen receptor on B cell surface

COMPLEMENT SYSTEM (Figure 10-6)

FIGURE 10-6 Complement pathway

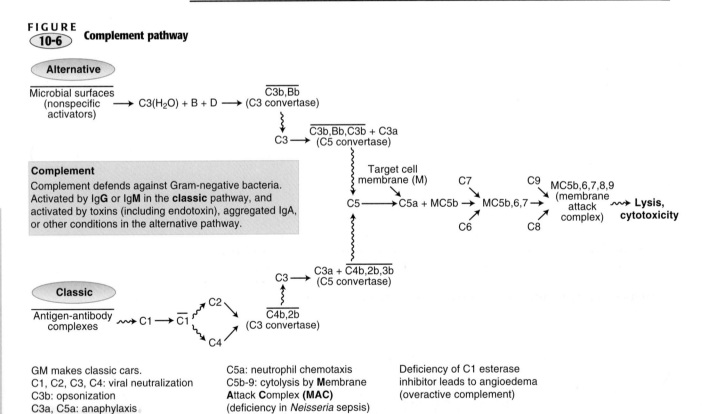

GM makes classic cars.
C1, C2, C3, C4: viral neutralization
C3b: opsonization
C3a, C5a: anaphylaxis

C5a: neutrophil chemotaxis
C5b-9: cytolysis by **M**embrane **A**ttack **C**omplex **(MAC)**
(deficiency in *Neisseria* sepsis)

Deficiency of C1 esterase inhibitor leads to angioedema (overactive complement)

(Adapted from Bhushan V, Le T, Amin C. First Aid for the USMLE Step 1. Stamford, CT: Appleton & Lange, 1999:207.)

I. Function of complement
A. Causes **lysis** of target cell
B. Defends against **Gram-negative bacteria**

II. Activation of pathways
A. IgG and IgM activate the **classic pathway.**
1. The activation is initiated by antigen-antibody complexes.
2. The first step of activation involves formation of complex by C1, C2, and C4.
B. Antigens activate the **alternative pathway.**
1. The activation is initiated by microbial surfaces and aggregated IgA.
2. The first step of activation involves C3.

III. Properties of complement cascade components
A. **C1:** only component not made in liver (made in gastrointestinal [GI] epithelium)
B. C1–C4: involved in viral neutralization
C. **C3b:** involved in opsonization
D. C3a: produces anaphylatoxin I
E. **C5a:** produces anaphylatoxin II, neutrophil and macrophage chemotaxis
F. **C5b–C9:** also known as the membrane attack complex (MAC)
G. **C1-inhibitor:** deficiency of this component leads to hereditary angioedema
H. Alteration in the complement cascade—complement deficiencies—are discussed in Table 10-3.

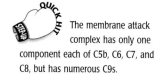

The membrane attack complex has only one component each of C5b, C6, C7, and C8, but has numerous C9s.

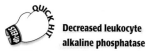

Decreased leukocyte alkaline phosphatase (LAP) is also seen in chronic myelogenous leukemia (CML).

TABLE 10-3 Complement Deficiencies

Disease	Defect	Significant Features
Hereditary angioedema	Decreased C1 inhibitor	Increased capillary permeability, edema
Paroxysmal nocturnal hemoglobinuria (PNH)	Deficiency of decay accelerating factor (DAF); increased complement activation	Complement-mediated hemolysis; brown urine in morning; **decreased leukocyte alkaline phosphatase (LAP)**

C1=first component of complement

IV. Deficiencies of C1, C3, C5, C6, C7, and C8 lead to increased bacterial infections. C3 defect causes increased susceptibility to *Staphylococcus aureus*. C6, C7, C8 deficiencies lead to *Neisseria gonorrhoeae* infection and meningitis. C2 and C4 deficiencies have manifestations resembling autoimmune diseases such as systemic lupus erythematosus (SLE). C2 deficiency is the most common complement deficiency.

V. Cytokines (Table 10-4)

Cytokines are hormones that have a low molecular weight and are involved in cell-to-cell communication.

TABLE 10-4 Cytokines		
Cytokine	**Secreted by**	**Function**
IL-1	Macrophages	Endogenous **pyrogen;** stimulates T cells
IL-2	T-helper cells	Activates T-helper and -cytotoxic cells
IL-4	T-helper cells	Stimulates growth of B cells; increases IgE and IgG
IL-5	T-helper cells	Differentiation of B cells; increases IgA
IL-10	T-helper cells	Inhibits development of Th-1 cells; inhibits INF-γ production
IL-12	Macrophages	Promotes Th-1 cell development; stimulates INF-γ production
INF-γ	T-helper cells	Stimulates macrophages and NK cells; increases MHC expression; stimulates phagocytosis and killing
Tumor necrosis factor	Macrophages	At low concentrations, activates neutrophils and increases IL-2 receptor synthesis; at high concentrations, mediates septic shock and results in tumor necrosis
Transforming growth factor	T cells, B cells, macrophages	Inhibits growth and activities of T cells; enhances collagen synthesis; dampens the immune response

Ig=immunoglobulin; *IL*=interleukin; *INF-γ*=interferon-γ; *MHC*=major histocompatibility complex; *NK*=natural killer

HYPERSENSITIVITY REACTIONS

I. There are four types of hypersensitivity reactions. They vary in onset of symptoms, severity, and mechanism (Table 10-5).

TABLE 10-5 Hypersensitivity Reactions	
Reaction Type	**Description**
Type 1 **(anaphylaxis)**	Mediated by **IgE** antibody bound to mast cells or basophils Antigens crosslink antibody Release **histamine,** SRS-A, eosinophilic chemotactic factor, and platelet-activating factor Results in asthma, **wheal,** and **flare**
Type 2 (cytotoxic)	Antibody-dependent cellular cytotoxicity Antibody produced to specific cell-surface antigens IgM- and IgG-mediated lysis via complement Examples: **Rh incompatibility, Goodpasture syndrome,** myasthenia gravis, hemolytic anemia, rheumatic fever, Graves disease
Type 3 (immune-complex)	**Antigen-antibody complexes** induce inflammatory response Deposition of complexes in tissue Examples: **Arthus reaction, serum sickness,** glomerulonephritis, rheumatoid arthritis, SLE, polyarteritis nodosum
Type 4 (delayed or cell-mediated)	**Helper (CD4) T lymphocyte-mediated** Response is delayed (from hours to days) Predominantly mononuclear cell infiltration Examples: **tuberculin (PPD) test, chronic transplant rejection,** contact hypersensitivity

Ig=immunoglobulin; *PPD*=purified protein derivative; *Rh*=rhesus (factor); *SLE*=systemic lupus erythematosus; *SRS-A*=slow-reacting substance of anaphylaxis

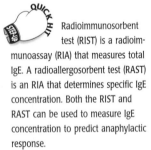

Radioimmunosorbent test (RIST) is a radioimmunoassay (RIA) that measures total IgE. A radioallergosorbent test (RAST) is an RIA that determines specific IgE concentration. Both the RIST and RAST can be used to measure IgE concentration to predict anaphylactic response.

Serum sickness is more common than an Arthus reaction.

II. Transplant rejection

III. Timeline (Figure 10-7)

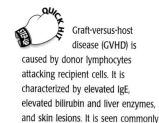

Graft-versus-host disease (GVHD) is caused by donor lymphocytes attacking recipient cells. It is characterized by elevated IgE, elevated bilirubin and liver enzymes, and skin lesions. It is seen commonly in bone marrow transplants.

FIGURE
10-7 **Transplant rejection timeline**

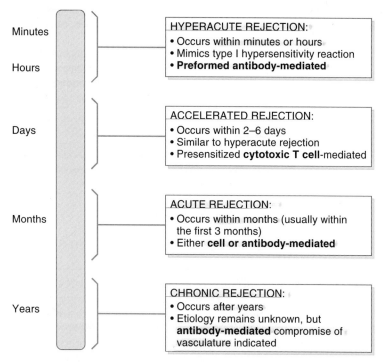

Minutes / Hours

HYPERACUTE REJECTION:
- Occurs within minutes or hours
- Mimics type I hypersensitivity reaction
- **Preformed antibody-mediated**

Days

ACCELERATED REJECTION:
- Occurs within 2–6 days
- Similar to hyperacute rejection
- Presensitized **cytotoxic T cell**-mediated

Months

ACUTE REJECTION:
- Occurs within months (usually within the first 3 months)
- Either **cell or antibody-mediated**

Years

CHRONIC REJECTION:
- Occurs after years
- Etiology remains unknown, but **antibody-mediated** compromise of vasculature indicated

IMMUNODEFICIENCIES

I. Diseases affecting the immune system leave the individual prone to infection. The immune system can be affected on any level or at any time, from its development to its most distal signaling mechanisms.

II. Congenital B-cell deficiencies (Table 10-6)

TABLE 10-6 Congenital B-Cell Deficiencies

Disease	Defect	Significant Features
X-linked agammaglobulinemia (of Bruton)	Lack of maturation of B cells, secondary to lack of tyrosine-kinase gene	Absence of plasma cells, serum IgG; recurrent **pyogenic infections** beginning after 6 months; one of most common congenital B cell diseases; lymphoid tissue has **poorly defined germinal centers**
Selective IgA deficiency	Lack of maturation of B cells; failure of gene switching in heavy chain	**Most common congenital B cell defect** 1/700; **pulmonary tract infections**
Common variable immunodeficiency	Failure of terminal B cell differentiation	See Table 10-8

Ig=immunoglobulin

(text continued on page 248)

III. Congenital T-cell deficiencies (Table 10-7)

Candida albicans causes thrush.

Treat hyper-IgM syndrome with pooled gamma-globulin.

Measles, a paramyxovirus, results in a T-cell deficiency.

TABLE 10-7 Congenital T-Cell Deficiencies		
Disease	**Defect**	**Significant Features**
Thymic aplasia (DiGeorge's syndrome)	Deficiency of development of third and fourth branchial pouches; T-cell defect	Defective development of the thymus, parathyroid glands, ear, mandible, aortic arch; leads to recurrent infections by **viral and fungal organisms; hypocalcemia** from low PTH leads to tetany
Chronic mucocutaneous candidiasis	Lack of T-cell response to *Candida*	Recurrent candidal skin and mucous membrane infections
Hyper IgM syndrome	Mutation in CD4⁺ helper T-cell interaction with CD40 on B cell prevents class switching	Increased IgM; decreased IgG, IgA, IgE; normal numbers of T and B cells

Ig=immunoglobulin; *PTH*=parathyroid hormone

IV. Congenital combined T- and B-cell deficiencies (Table 10-8)

Severe combined immunodeficiency (SCID) caused by adenosine deaminase (ADA) deficiency was one of the first diseases successfully treated with gene therapy.

TABLE 10-8 Congenital Combined T- and B-Cell Deficiencies		
Disease	**Defect**	**Significant Features**
Severe combined immunodeficiency (SCID)	**Autosomal recessive** (defect in tyrosine kinase ZAP-70, or adenosine deaminase deficiency); X-linked forms (IL-2 receptor defect)	Susceptible to recurrent bacterial, viral, fungal, and protozoal infections
Wiskott-Aldrich syndrome	IgM response to capsule polysaccharide (e.g., pneumococcus) is weak	**Eczema, thrombocytopenia, recurrent infections;** becomes notable in first year of life
Ataxia-telangiectasia	IgA deficiency and lymphopenia	**Autosomal recessive;** becomes noticeable in first 2 years of life; ataxia (cerebellar dysfunction), telangiectasia, recurrent infections, thymic aplasia

IL=interleukin; *ZAP*=zeta-associated protein

V. Plasma cell abnormalities (Table 10-9)

TABLE 10-9 Plasma Cell Abnormalities

Disease	Etiology	Clinical Features	Notes
Multiple myeloma	Clonal plasma cell tumor	**Lytic, punched-out bone lesions** especially in the skull; hyperglobulinemia; **Bence Jones proteinuria**	**Rouleaux formation** ("stack of coins" appearance)
Waldenström's macroglobu-linemia	Excessive production of IgM by lymphoid cells	Slowly progressive course; usually in men over 50 years of age; platelet function abnormal; hyperviscosity syndrome	No bone lesions (which differentiates this from multiple myeloma)
Benign monoclonal gammopathy	Increased production of monoclonal antibodies from an unknown origin	Asymptomatic; occurring in older individuals	Monoclonal spike without Bence Jones proteinuria (versus multiple myeloma)

Ig=immunoglobulin

VI. Phagocyte deficiencies (Table 10-10)

TABLE 10-10 Phagocyte Deficiencies

Disease	Defect	Significant Features
Chronic granulo-matous disease (CGD)	Neutrophils **lack NADPH oxidase**	**X-linked** (some autosomal recessive); no oxidative burst in macrophages; B and T cells normal; opportunistic infections (e.g., *Staphylococcus aureus, Aspergillus*, enteric Gram-negative rods)
Chédiak-Higashi syndrome	Failure of neutrophils to empty lysosomes	**Autosomal recessive;** recurrent pyogenic infections (e.g., *Staphylococcus, Streptococcus*)
Job's syndrome	T-helper lymphocytes fail to produce INF-γ	Eczema; increase in Th-2 (see Figure 10-5) leads to increase in IgE, causing increased histamine release
Leukocyte adhe-sion deficiency	Defect in adhesion protein LAF-1	Pyogenic infections early in life; poor phagocytosis

INF-γ=interferon-γ; *LAF-1*=leukocyte-activating factor; *NADPH*=reduced nicotinamide adenine dinucleotide phosphate

VII. Acquired immunodeficiencies (Table 10-11)

TABLE 10-11	Acquired Immunodeficiencies	
Disease	**Defect**	**Significant Features**
Common variable hypogamma-globulinemia	Acquired or congenital (unknown) B-cell defects	Recurrent pyogenic bacterial infections (e.g., pneumococcus, *Haemophilus influenzae*); decreased IgG production
AIDS	**HIV virus infects CD4 cells**	Opportunistic infections (e.g., ***Mycobacterium-avium intracellular,*** *Cryptococcus neoformans*, ***Pneumocystis carinii***, *Candida albicans*); increased tumors (e.g., Kaposi's)

AIDS=acquired immunodeficiency syndrome; *HIV*=human immunodeficiency virus

THROMBOSIS AND THE CLOTTING CASCADE (Figure 10-8)

Aspirin functions as an antithrombotic agent by permanently **acetylating cyclooxygenase** (COX), thereby inhibiting thromboxane A$_2$ (TXA$_2$) production. TXA$_2$ triggers the aggregation of platelets. Aspirin also inhibits prostaglandin formation, but unlike platelets, endothelium can synthesize new COX.

FIGURE 10-8 Thrombosis and the clotting cascade

Intrinsic System

HMW-K Kallikrein ← Pre-Kallikrein

Extrinsic System

XII → XIIa

VII

XI → XIa

Ca^{2+}

IX → IXa

Tissue Factor

VIII —IIa→ VIIIa | Ca^{2+},PL

VIIa + Tissue Factor

X ——————→ Xa

V —IIa→ Va | Ca^{2+},PL

Prothrombin II ——→ Thrombin (IIa) - - - - -

Fibrinogen I ——→ Fibrin (Ia)

XIIIa —IIa/Ca^{2+}→ XIII

Cross-linked Fibrin

Ca^{2+}=calcium; *HMW-K*=high-molecular-weight kininogen; *PL*=phospholipid.

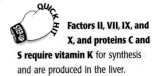

Factors II, VII, IX, and X, and proteins C and S require vitamin K for synthesis and are produced in the liver.

Thrombosis is the intravascular coagulation of blood and involves the interaction of platelets, coagulation proteins, and endothelial cells. With intact endothelium, a balance exists between prothrombotic (platelet-derived thromboxane A$_2$ [TXA$_2$]) and antithrombotic (endothelium-derived prostaglandin I$_2$ [PGI$_2$]) mediators. With damaged endothelium, exposed collagen causes adhesion of platelets through glycoprotein receptors and **von Willebrand's factor (vWf).** This adhesion triggers platelet release of adenosine diphosphate (ADP), serotonin, histamine, and platelet-derived growth factor (PDGF), resulting in primary plug formation and cessation of bleeding. Stabilization of the primary plug (formation of secondary plug) is mediated by fibrin and factor XIIIa, a result of activation of the clotting cascade.

Factor XIa in the presence of Ca^{2+} activates factor IX. Factor IXa requires Ca^{2+} and a phospholipid to activate factor X. Activated factor X requires Ca^{2+}, phospholipid, and factor Va to activate prothrombin to thrombin. Thrombin and Ca^{2+} inactivate factor XIII, which promotes the cross-linking of fibrin.

● Key Players in Inhibition of Coagulation

α-1-Antitrypsin	Inhibits factor XIa
α-2-Macroglobulin	Inhibits serine proteases
Antithrombin III	Inhibits factor Xa and thrombin
Inhibitor of first component of complement (C1 INH)	Inhibits factor XII and kallikrein
Heparin cofactor II	Inhibits thrombin
Protein C	Inactivates factors Va and VIIIa
Protein S	Is cofactor for protein C

ANTITHROMBOTIC THERAPEUTIC AGENTS

I. Platelet inhibitors (Figure 10-9)

Aspirin inhibits thromboxane-mediated platelet aggregation, ticlopidine and clopidogrel block platelet ADP receptors, and argatroban and hirudin inhibit thrombin directly.

FIGURE 10-9 Inhibition of platelet aggregation pathways

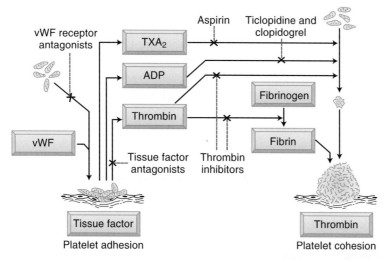

Aspirin inhibits thromboxane-mediated platelet aggregation, ticlopidine and clopidogrel block platelet ADP receptors, and argatroban and hirudin inhibit thrombin directly. *ADP*=adenosine diphosphate; *TXA₂*=thromboxane A2; *vWF*=von Willebrand factor.

A. Aspirin
   1. Irreversibly acetylates **platelet cyclooxygenase (COX)**
   2. Results in disruption of TXA_2-dependent platelet aggregation
   3. Leads to less platelet hemostasis
   4. Can be used in acute myocardial infarctions (MIs) or prophylactically to reduce the likelihood of platelet-mediated vascular occlusion

Partial thromboplastin time **(PTT)** measures the **intrinsic system.** Therapeutic drug monitoring of heparin is measured using PTT. Heparin overdose is treated with intravenous protamine sulfate.

Prothrombin time **(PT)** measures the **extrinsic system.** Therapeutic drug monitoring of warfarin is measured using PT. Warfarin overdose is treated with administration of vitamin K.

Factor VIII is the only clotting factor increased in liver disease.

Factor XIII is the only clotting factor that is not a serine protease.

Aspirin, ticlopidine, and clopidogrel work globally to reduce the risk of thrombo-occlusion and thromboembolism, regardless of the anatomic site.

   B. Ticlopidine and clopidogrel
      1. Irreversible **blockage of platelet ADP receptors**
      2. Can be used for the same clinical scenarios in which aspirin has failed
      3. Is at least as safe as aspirin in terms of side effects

II. Anticoagulants

   A. Heparin
      1. Binds to antithrombin III
      2. Greatly **enhances the ability of antithrombin III to inhibit coagulation proteases, primarily thrombin**
      3. Is useful in a variety of situations in which anticoagulation is necessary
         a. Deep venous thrombosis (DVT) or pulmonary embolism
         b. Brain attack (thrombotic occlusion)
         c. MI
         d. Others
      4. Leads to **heparin-induced thrombocytopenia or thrombosis,** a notable side effect, which occurs in 1%–3% of patients. A heparin-platelet factor 4 antibody is the cause.
   B. Warfarin
      1. **Impairs vitamin K metabolism**
         a. Low levels of vitamin K prevent γ-carboxylation of **clotting factors VII, IX,** and **X.**
         b. Lack of γ-carboxylation leads to **hypofunctional clotting factors VII, IX,** and **X.**
      2. Is used in a variety of clinical scenarios in which oral anticoagulation is required
         a. Atrial fibrillation
         b. Prosthetic valves
         c. DVT or pulmonary embolism
         d. Postoperative anticoagulation
         e. Hypercoagulable states
      3. Use requires care, because excessive anticoagulation can lead to hemorrhage.

III. Thrombolytics

   A. **Convert plasminogen to plasmin,** which disrupts vascular clot formation
   B. Are useful in acute MI, acute arterial thromboembolic occlusion, severe DVT, and pulmonary embolism
   C. Include tissue plasminogen activator (t-PA), streptokinase, urokinase, and anistreplase
      1. t-PA leads to the most rapid lysis of the clot and results in less systemic fibrinolysis.
      2. However, t-PA is also the most expensive.
   D. Require careful monitoring because of **increased risk of abnormal bleeding.**

IV. Direct thrombin inhibitors

   A. **Do not require anti-thrombin III for activity**
   B. Allow for more efficient inhibition of clot-bound fibrin
   C. Include hirudin and argatroban
   D. Are currently under study for use in venous thrombosis, heparin-induced thrombocytopenia, hemodialysis, arterial thrombosis (angioplasty, unstable angina), and other conditions

QUICK HIT Low-molecular weight heparins (LMWHs) such as enoxaparin and dalteparin are a recent advance in heparin therapy. Subcutaneous administration is much more convenient than standard intravenous heparin therapy, as it requires no PTT monitoring. Uses for LMWHs include postsurgical prophylaxis against deep venous thrombosis (DVT) and the treatment of venous thromboembolism.

QUICK HIT The effect of heparin is determined by measuring the activated partial thromboplastin time (aPTT). The effect of warfarin is determined by measuring the PT.

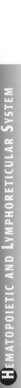

HEMATOPOIETIC AND LYMPHORETICULAR SYSTEM

V. Coagulation disorders (Table 10-12)

Abnormalities of the coagulation cascade, endothelial cells, or platelets can lead to inappropriate bleeding or clot formation. These coagulopathies can be manifested as symptomatology involving skin, joints, vasculature, or internal organs.

TABLE 10-12 Coagulation Disorders

Disease	Etiology	Clinical Features	Notes
Disseminated intra-vascular coagulation (DIC)	Multifactorial, causes include sepsis, trauma, and neoplasms	**Thrombocytopenia; diffuse hemorrhage;** microthrombus formation	Activation of factors V, VIII, and protein C
Von-Willebrand's (vWf) disease	**Autosomal dominant** disorder	Impaired platelet adhesion; **decreased factor VIII** (vWf binds factor VIII in the blood); **increased bleeding time**	**Most common hereditary bleeding disorder;** similar deficiency diseases include Bernard-Soulier disease and Glanzmann's thrombasthenia
Hemophilia A	**X-linked** factor VIII deficiency	Bleeding into muscle, subcutaneous tissues, and joints	**Most common type of hemophilia;** variable penetrance
Hemophilia B (Christmas disease)	**X-linked** factor IX deficiency	Bleeding into muscle, subcutaneous tissues, and joints	Presentation is identical to hemophilia A
Idiopathic thrombo-cytopenic purpura (ITP)	**Antiplatelet antibodies**	Thrombocytopenia	Follows URI in children and is self-limiting; chronic in adults
Thrombotic thrombocytopenic purpura (TTP)	Idiopathic systemic disease	Hyaline occlusions and microangiopathic hemolytic anemia leading to schistocytes and helmet cells	May cause neurologic abnormalities

URI=upper respiratory tract infection

VI. vWf deficiency versus hemophilia A (Table 10-13)

TABLE 10-13 vWF Deficiency Versus Hemophilia A

	vWf Deficiency	Hemophilia A
Factor VIII: coagulant activity	↓	↓
vWf level	↓	Normal
Ristocetin cofactor activity	↓	Normal
Ristocetin aggregation	↓	Normal
Bleeding time	↑	Normal
Inheritance	**Autosomal dominant**	**X-linked**

Ristocetin, an antibiotic not used for clinical disease, has platelet aggregation properties. *vWf*=von Willebrand factor

VII. Clotting time algorithm (Table 10-14)

TABLE 10-14	Clotting Time Algorithm	
	PT Normal	**PT Prolonged**
PTT Normal	Factor XIII deficiency	Factor VII deficiency
PTT Prolonged	Factor VIII, IX, XI deficiencies in patients with bleeding; factor XII, prekallikrein, HMW-K deficiencies in patients without bleeding	Common pathway deficiency: factor V, X, II, I; severe hepatic diseases; DIC

DIC=disseminated intravascular coagulation; *HMW-K*=high-molecular weight kininogen; *PT*=prothrombin time; *PTT*=partial thromboplastin time

LYMPHOMA

QUICK HIT

Staging of lymphoma (Ann Arbor System): (1) one node or organ affected; (2) two nodes or organs on same side of diaphragm affected; (3) both sides of diaphragm, spleen or other organ affected; (4) disseminated foci.

I. Tumors of the lymphoid system

II. Present as enlarged, firm, fixed, painless nodes

III. Are classified as Hodgkin's and non-Hodgkin's disease

IV. Comparison of Hodgkin's and non-Hodgkin's disease (Table 10-15)

TABLE 10-15	Hodgkin's Versus Non-Hodgkin's Disease
Hodgkin's Disease	**Non-Hodgkin's Disease**
Number of **Reed-Sternberg cells** (binucleated giant cells) proportional to severity	Malignant neoplasm of lymphocytes (85% B cell, 15% T cell) within lymph nodes (especially periaortic)
Causes inflammation, fever, diaphoresis (**night sweats**), **leukocytosis,** hepatosplenomegaly, pruritus	Causes painless peripheral lymphadenopathy
Usually affects **young men** (peak incidence in adolescents)	Usually affects white men under 65 years of age
Often curable. More reactive lymphocytes signal better prognosis	Nodular type has better prognosis than diffuse. Small cell type has better prognosis than large cell
Rye classifications (low-grade to high-grade): Lymphocytic predominance (least common, best prognosis) Mixed cellularity (most frequent) **Nodular sclerosis** (predominantly in **women;** fibrous bands in lymph nodes; lacunar cells; often found in the mediastinum) Lymphocytic depletion (worst prognosis; rare necrosis and fibrosis of lymphocytic tissue)	**Working classification** (low-grade to high-grade): Small lymphocytic cell (B cell; elderly; indolent course; CLL related) Follicular small cell (cleaved B cell; elderly; **most common non-Hodgkin's lymphoma t(14;18),** expression of *bcl-2* oncogene) Large cell (elderly and children; usually B cell) Lymphoblastic (T cell; children; **mediastinal mass** progressing to ALL) Small noncleaved [(**Burkitt's**) B cell, EBV infection; **"starry-sky"** appearance; related to B cell **ALL; t(8;14),** expression of *c-myc* oncogene] Cutaneous T cell (*Mycosis fungoides*, Pautrier's microabscesses, Sézary's syndrome, skin lesions)

ALL=acute lymphocytic leukemia; *CLL*=chronic lymphocytic leukemia; *EBV*=Epstein-Barr virus

LEUKEMIA (Table 10-16)

The symptoms of leukemia include fatigue, dyspnea on exertion, bleeding, pallor, and hepatosplenomegaly.

TABLE 10-16 Classification of Leukemia			
Acute Myeloblastic	**Acute Lymphoblastic**	**Chronic Myeloid**	**Chronic Lymphocytic**
Myeloblasts; defect in maturation beyond myeloblast or promyelocyte stage; **Auer rods;** predominantly affects **adults;** poor prognosis	Small lymphoblasts; decreased cytoplasm; predominantly affects **children;** responsive to therapy	t(9;22) results in **Philadelphia chromosome** (BCR-ABL); leukocytosis; **decreased LAP;** splenomegaly; onset at **35–55** years of age; ends in blastic crisis	Usually B cells; "smudge cells" in smear; warm autoimmune hemolytic anemia; hypogamma-globulinemia; lymphadenopathy; hepatosplenomegaly; more common in **men over 60** years of age

BCR=B-cell reactivity; *LAP*=leukocyte alkaline phosphatase

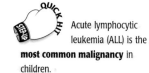

Acute lymphocytic leukemia (ALL) is the **most common malignancy** in children.

ANEMIA (Table 10-17)

Anemia, a decrease in circulating red blood cell mass, is usually defined as hemoglobin less than 12 g/dL in female patients and less than 14 g/dL in male patients.

TABLE 10-17 Classification of Anemia		
Microcytic (MCV < 80)	**Normocytic (MCV 80–100)**	**Macrocytic (MCV > 100)**
Iron deficiency	Aplastic anemia	Liver disease
Lead poisoning	Acute blood loss	Vitamin B_{12} deficiency
Sickle cell	Hemolytic anemia	Folate deficiency
Chronic disease		
Sideroblastic		
Thalassemia		

MCV=mean cell volume

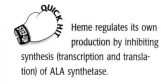

Heme regulates its own production by inhibiting synthesis (transcription and translation) of ALA synthetase.

Heme keeps the translational initiation complex active on the ribosome, which increases the production of globin.

I. Microcytic anemia

A. Iron deficiency
  1. **Most common anemia**
  2. **Total iron-binding capacity (TIBC) is increased, serum iron** and **bone marrow stores are low.**
  3. Occurs in menstruating or pregnant women, infants, and preadolescents
  4. Caused by dietary deficiency or bleeding (menorrhagia, GI bleeding, GI cancers, and inflammatory bowel disease)
  5. Pale, easy fatigability, dyspneic, may be associated with Plummer-Vinson syndrome (characterized by glossitis, esophageal web)

B. Lead poisoning
  1. Inhibits heme synthesis (Δ-ala dehydratase and ferrochelatase)
  2. **Basophilic stippling** of RBCs is seen microscopically.
  3. Finger, wrist, and foot drop occur from neurotoxicity.
  4. Renal lesions, GI colic, and gingival lead lines occur.
  5. Treatment is with ethylenediamine tetraacetic acid (EDTA).

In sickle cell disease, the sixth amino acid of the β chain of hemoglobin is changed from glutamate to valine. Sickling only occurs when the RBCs are **deoxygenated.** Oxygenated HbS RBCs function normally.

C. Sickle cell disease (sickle cell hemoglobin or hemoglobin S [HbS])
1. Primarily seen in **African-Americans**
2. The homozygous form is most severe.
3. Severe hemolytic anemia is seen.
4. Leads to painful crises; organ infarction (**autosplenectomy**); strokes
5. Aplastic crises occur, usually provoked by viral infection (usually parvovirus B19).
6. Patients are especially susceptible to infection by **encapsulated bacteria** (*Streptococcus pneumoniae* and *Haemophilus influenzae*) and osteomyelitis caused by salmonella.
7. Sickle cells and Howell-Jolly bodies are seen in peripheral blood smear.
8. Treatment is with **hydroxyurea** to increase HbF.

D. Chronic disease
1. Second most common anemia
2. **TIBC is reduced (ferritin is increased).**
3. Low serum iron, but high iron stores in the bone marrow

E. Sideroblastic anemia
1. Iron stain reveals ringed sideroblasts.
2. TIBC is reduced, and serum iron is increased.
3. RBC count is reduced.

F. Thalassemia
1. This is a group of genetic disorders, all in some way deficient in α or β globin chain synthesis.
2. **β-Thalassemia is more common** (especially in people of Mediterranean origin).
3. The homozygous form, called thalassemia major (also known as Mediterranean or Cooley's anemia), causes splenomegaly, bone distortions, hemosiderosis, and increased HbF, and is fatal in childhood.
4. The heterozygous form of β-thalassemia (thalassemia minor) causes a minor anemia, but has no effect on life span.
5. α-Thalassemia is caused by a deletion in one or more of the four α globin genes; loss of all four genes is not compatible with life.

II. Normocytic anemias

A. Aplastic anemia
1. Dysfunctional or deficient multipotent myeloid stem cells leads to pancytopenia.
2. Caused by viruses, chemicals, radiation, or renal failure (via decreased erythropoietin) or may be idiopathic
3. Drugs causing aplastic anemia include nonsteroidal anti-inflammatory drugs (**NSAIDs), benzene,** and **chloramphenicol.**
4. Symptoms include fatigue, pallor, mucosal bleeding, and petechia owing to thrombocytopenia.
5. Neutropenia occurs, leading to frequent infections.
6. **Fat infiltration** into hypocellular marrow occurs.

B. Anemia caused by acute blood loss
1. Leads to a **transient normocytic** anemia
2. May appear macrocytic because of increased reticulocyte release from bone marrow 7–10 days later

C. Hemolytic anemias
1. Increased red blood cell destruction leads to an increase in unconjugated bilirubin, hemoglobinemia, hemoglobinuria, hemosiderosis, and decreased serum haptoglobin.
2. Increase in reticulocytes occurs because of additional erythropoiesis.
3. Extracorpuscular (acquired) hemolytic anemias

a. Warm autoimmune hemolytic immunoglobulin (AIHI) (IgG): associated with lymphoma, spherocytosis, **positive direct Coombs' test**

b. Cold AIHI (IgM): associated with lymphoid neoplasm, anti-I antibodies, ABO incompatibility, **Raynaud's phenomenon**

c. Erythroblastosis fetalis (hemolytic diseases of the newborn): usually caused by Rh blood group incompatibility; can result in kernicterus and death

d. Caused by infections including bartonellosis, clostridia, malaria

4. Intracorpuscular (genetic) hemolytic anemias

a. Hereditary ovalocytosis (elliptocytosis): **autosomal dominant**

b. Hereditary spherocytosis: **autosomal dominant, spectrin** deficiency

c. Paroxysmal nocturnal hemoglobinuria: deficiency of decay accelerating factor (DAF), decreased leukocyte alkaline phosphatase (LAP)

d. Glucose-6-phosphate dehydrogenase deficiency (G-6-PD): **X-linked;** more common in Mediterraneans and African-Americans; precipitated by oxidative stress (primaquine therapy); **Heinz bodies** are seen.

e. Pyruvate kinase deficiency: **autosomal recessive,** chronic

III. Macrocytic anemias

A. Liver disease—usually cirrhosis

1. Excess lipid is added to RBC membrane in diseased liver.

2. Hypersplenism occurs.

3. Spur cells are present.

B. Vitamin B_{12} (cobalamin) deficiency

1. **Megaloblastic anemia,** characterized by **hypersegmented neutrophils,** pancytopenia, achlorhydria

2. Decreased DNA synthesis

3. Most common form is **pernicious anemia.**

a. Caused by a deficiency of intrinsic factor secondary to destruction of parietal cells

b. Associated with increased incidence of gastric carcinoma

4. Other etiologies for vitamin B_{12} deficiency anemia include strict vegetarian diet, distal ileum pathology, bacterial overgrowth, *Diphyllobothrium latum* infection; type A gastritis

5. **Neurologic symptoms** caused by demyelination of posterior and lateral columns, ataxia, and paresthesia in distal extremities

C. Folate deficiency

1. Megaloblastic anemia

2. Hematologic findings are identical to vitamin B_{12} deficiency.

3. **No neurologic** deficits are present.

4. Folate deficiency can mask vitamin B_{12} deficiency.

5. Etiologies include dietary deficiency, sprue, *Giardia lamblia* infection, oral contraceptives, **antineoplastics** (methotrexate), and pregnancy.

MYELOPROLIFERATIVE DISORDERS

I. Polycythemia vera

A. Chronic increase in the number of red cells caused by bone marrow hyperplasia of unknown etiology

B. Clinical manifestations

1. Presents in middle age

2. Symptoms are headache, vertigo, splenomegaly, and pruritus.

C. Differential diagnosis

1. Absolute polycythemia vera

a. Primary polycythemia—**low or absent erythropoietin levels**

b. Secondary polycythemia

ABO transfusion reactions are almost always a result of clerical (human) error.

Hemolytic disease of the newborn (HDNB) can be prevented with **RhoGAM** (anti-D antibody), which neutralizes the mother's immunogenic response to fetal RBCs, which carry the D antigen.

Spherocytes are characterized by osmotic fragility in hypotonic solution.

Spur cells occur in liver disease and are caused by the reticuloendothelial system "biting" the RBCs.

Schilling's test is used to diagnose the etiology of pernicious anemia.

(1) Elevated erythropoietin levels

(2) Appropriate: response to hypoxia

(3) Inappropriate: secondary to an inappropriate secretion of erythropoietin owing to a cyst or tumor

2. Relative polycythemia vera (e.g., dehydration) is often caused by a decrease in extracorpuscular volume, thus causing a relative increase in the hematocrit level.

D. Diagnosis

1. Major diagnostic criteria

a. Increased red blood cell mass (hematocrit)

b. Normal arterial oxygen saturation (>92%)

c. Splenomegaly

2. Minor diagnostic criteria

a. Thrombocytosis

b. Leukocytosis

c. Elevated LAP

d. Elevated serum vitamin B_{12}

3. Diagnosis requires all three major criteria or increased red blood cell mass, normal arterial oxygen saturation, and at least two minor criteria including leukocytosis and thrombocytosis.

II. Myelofibrosis

A. Generalized fibrosis of bone marrow characterized by pancytopenia in the face of increased megakaryocytes in the marrow

B. Clinical manifestations

1. Presents in the late 50s

2. **Tear-drop deformity** of RBCs occcurs, along with splenomegaly and extramedullary hematopoiesis.

3. "Dry tap" seen on bone biopsy.

C. **Differential diagnosis**

1. Primary myelofibrosis

a. Marrow fibrosis

b. Extramedullary hematopoiesis

2. Secondary myelofibrosis

a. Infections: tuberculosis, osteomyelitis

b. Metastatic carcinoma

c. Paget's disease

III. Essential thrombocythemia

A. A primary disorder of unknown etiology resulting in increased platelets

B. Clinical manifestations

1. Thrombocytosis

2. Megakaryocytic hyperplasia

3. Splenomegaly

4. Hemorrhage and thrombosis

5. Increased bone marrow reticulin and absence of *bcr/abl* gene

Myelodysplastic syndromes also exist: refractory anemia; refractory anemia with ringed sideroblasts; refractory anemia with excess blasts; refractory anemia with excess blasts in transformation; and chronic myelomonocytic leukemia.

Drug Index

The therapeutic agents shown in boldface type are those which are often emphasized in the classroom and the clinic. Particular attention should be paid to the information about these agents.

Therapeutic Agent (common name, if relevant) [Trade name, where appropriate]	Class—Pharmacology and Pharmacokinetics	Indications	Side or Adverse Effects	Contraindications or Precautions to Consider; Notes
Acarbose [Precose]	Hypoglycemic agent—inhibits α-glucosidase; delays absorption of glucose from gut	Oral treatment for NIDDM (type II diabetes)	Flatulence, cramps, diarrhea; may reduce absorption of iron	
Acebutolol [Sectral]	Antiarrhythmic (class II)—antihypertensive; β blocker	Hypertension; PVCs		Cardioselective
Acetaminophen [Tylenol]	**Analgesic, antipyretic—unknown mechanism; not anti-inflammatory**	**Pain; fever**	**Liver toxicity in high doses**	**Overdose treated with N-acetylcysteine**
Acetazolamide [Diamox]	Diuretic—carbonic anhydrase inhibitor on PCT and DCT; decreases production of aqueous humor in the eye	Glaucoma; high altitude; alkalinization of urine	Metabolic acidosis; renal calculi	
Acetylcholine	Muscarinic agonist	Eye surgery (miotic)	Increased parasympathetic/cholinergic stimulation	
Acetylsalicylic acid (aspirin)	**Anti-inflammatory, antipyretic, analgesic—acetylates COX irreversibly**	**Articular, musculoskeletal pain; chronic pain; acute gout**	**Irritates GI; inhibits platelet aggregation; causes hypersensitivity reactions**	**Contraindicated for patients with peptic ulcer, asthma, hyperthyroidism, or Parkinsonism** Contraindicated for children with the flu or chicken pox (leads to Reye's syndrome), gouty patients
ACTH (corticotropin)	Increases production of steroids by the adrenal cortex			
Acyclovir [Zovirax]	Antiviral—guanosine analog; inhibits DNA polymerase	Herpes, varicella, EBV, CMV (at high doses)	GI disturbances; CNS; renal problems; headache; tremor; rash	
Adenosine [Adenocard]	Antiarrhythmic—short duration; decreases conduction velocity; prolongs refractory period	Supraventricular tachycardia	Flushing; chest pain; hypotension	
Albendazole [Albenza]	Antihelminthic	*Ascaris* (roundworm), *Ancylostoma* (hookworm), *Trichuris* (whipworm), *Strongyloides*	Teratogenic; embryotoxic	Contraindicated in pregnant patients
Albuterol [Proventil, Ventolin]	Bronchodilation—β$_2$ agonist	Asthma	Tremor, tachycardia	
Alcohol (EtOH)	Acts at GABA$_a$ receptor	Sedative; hypnotic; depressive action on brain		

Therapeutic Agent (common name, if relevant) [Trade name, where appropriate]	Class–Pharmacology and Pharmacokinetics	Indications	Side or Adverse Effects	Contraindications or Precautions to Consider; Notes
Alendronate [Fosamax]	Bone stabilizer—pyrophosphate analog; reduces hydroxyapatite crystal formation, growth, and dissolution, which reduces bone turnover	Hypercalcemia of malignancy; Paget's disease; osteoporosis; hyperparathyroidism	Pill-induced esophagitis	
Allopurinol [Zyloprim]	Antigout—competitive inhibitor of xanthine oxidase	Chronic gout (caused by renal obstruction or impairment or overproduction); rheumatic arthritis	Rash; fever; GI problems; hepato-toxicity; inhibition of the metabolism of other drugs; enhance effect of azathioprine	
Alprazolam [Xanax]	Antianxiety—benzodiazepine	Panic attack	Sedation	
Alprostadil [Vasoprost]	Impotency therapy; prostaglandin E_1 agonist	Impotency; maintain patent ductus arteriosus	Penile pain; prolonged erection; flushing, bradycardia, tachycardia, hypotension, apnea	
Aluminum hydroxide	Antacid	Gastric irritability/constipation		Constipation
Amantadine [Symmetrel]	Antiviral—antiparkinsonian; inhibits fusion of lysosomes; inhibits uncoating; increases release of endogenous dopamine	Influenza A; Parkinson's disease	Anticholinergic; nervousness; insomnia; drowsiness; GI disturbances	
Amicar (EACA)	Competitive inhibition of plasminogen activation	Inhibits fibrinolysis; promotes thrombosis		Oral administration
Amikacin [Amikin]	Antibiotic—aminoglycoside; binds 30S ribosome subunits; bacteriostatic at low concentration; bactericidal at high concentration	Proteus, Pseudomonas, Enterobacter	Ototoxicity; neurotoxicity	
Amiloride [Midamor]	Diuretic—K^+ sparing; inhibits Na^+ transport in the DCT	Diuresis	Hyperkalemia	
Aminoglutethimide [Cytadren]	Antineoplastic—aromatase inhibitor; inhibits adrenal steroid synthesis	Cancer		
Aminoglycosides	Antibiotic—binds 30S ribosome subunits; bacteriostatic at low concentration; bactericidal at high concentration	Broad-spectrum: Gram-positive and -negative; good for bone infections	Auditory, vestibular, renal toxicity; nausea; vomiting; vertigo; allergic skin rash; superinfections	Examples include gentamycin, neomycin, streptomycin

Drug	Class/Action	Clinical Application	Side Effects/Toxicity	Notes
Amiodarone [Cordarone]	**Antiarrhythmic (class III)—K⁺-channel blocker**	Ventricular/supraventricular arrhythmias	Bradycardia; heart block/failure; pulmonary fibrosis; photodermatitis	Also functions as class IA, II, and IV
Amitriptyline [Elavil]	**Antidepressant—TCA; blocks 5-HT and NE reuptake**	**Sedative; antidepressant; prophylaxis for migraines**		
Amobarbital [Amytal sodium]	Sedative—hypnotic; barbiturate; prolongs IPSP duration	Antiepileptic; cerebral edema; anesthetic		
Amodiaquine	Antimalarial—uncertain mechanism	Suppression and treatment of acute attacks	Headache; GI and visual disturbances; pruritus; prolonged therapy may lead to retinopathy	
Amoxicillin + Clavulanic acid [Augmentin]	**Antibiotic—clavulanic acid inhibits β-lactamase; synergistic with penicillins**			
Amphetamine	**Stimulant—releases NE, 5-HT, dopamine**	Narcolepsy; attention-deficit disorder; weight reduction	Psychosis; hallucinations	
Amphotericin B [Fungizone]	**Antifungal—binds to cell membrane sterols (esp. ergosterol); forms pores in membrane; fungicidal**	*Candida, Histoplasma, Cryptococcus, Sporothrix*	**Hypersensitivity; flushing; chills; fever; headache; pain; hypotension; convulsions; thrombophlebitis; anemia; vomiting; impairment of renal function**	
Amrinone [Inocor]	Inotropic agent—phosphodiesterase inhibitor; increases contractility via increase in intracellular Ca^{2+}	CHF	Thrombocytopenia	
Anistreplase (APSAC) [Eminase]	Thrombolytic—plasminogen activator	Lysis of clots	Hemorrhage	Active compound via deacylation by esterase
Anthraquinones	Laxative—reduces absorption of electrolytes and water from gut	Stimulant laxative		
α₂-Antiplasmin	Inhibits fibrinolysis	Inhibits fibrinolysis		
Antiprogesterone [RU-486, Mifepristone]	Abortive agent—progesterone receptor blocker	Abortion		
Aprotinin [Trasylol]	Hemostatic agent—antiplasmin activator	Inhibits fibrinolysis; promotes thrombosis		
Asparaginase [Elspar]	Antineoplastic—deprives cells of asparagine	Cancer	Fever, mental depression; coma; hepatotoxicity	
Atenolol [Tenormin]	**Antihypertensive—β₁ blocker**	**Hypertension, angina**		**Cardioselective**
Atorvastatin [Lipitor]	**Lipid-lowering agent—inhibits HMG-CoA reductase; lowers LDL**	Hyperlipidemia (esp. type II)	**Liver toxicity; myopathy; mild GI disturbances**	**Contraindicated in pregnant or lactating women and children**
Atracurium [Tracrium injection]	Nondepolarizing neuromuscular blocker			Minimal histamine release

Therapeutic Agent (common name, if relevant) [Trade name, where appropriate]	Class—Pharmacology and Pharmacokinetics	Indications	Side or Adverse Effects	Contraindications or Precautions to Consider; Notes
Atropine	**Cholinergic muscarinic blocker**	**Dries salivary secretions; Parkinson's disease; peptic ulcer; diarrhea; GI spasm; bladder spasm; COPD; asthma; cholinomimetic poisoning; antidiarrheal; antiemetic; high dose: vasodilation as a result of histamine release**	**Dry mouth; hyperthermia; mydriasis; tachycardia; hot and flushed skin; agitation; delirium**	**Contraindicated in patients with glaucoma and elderly men with BPH**
Aurothioglucose [Solganal]	Antirheumatic—gold salt	Rheumatic arthritis	Skin eruption; itching; toxic nephritis; bone marrow suppression	
Aurothiomalate	Antirheumatic—gold salt	Rheumatic arthritis	Skin eruption; itching; toxic nephritis; bone marrow suppression	
Azathioprine [Imuran]	**Immunosuppressant—purine antagonist; inhibits nucleic acid metabolism; blocks both CMI and humoral response**	**Transplant (esp. kidney); acute glomerulonephritis; renal component of lupus; rheumatoid arthritis**	**Bone marrow depression; rash; fever; nausea; vomiting; hepatotoxicity; malignancy; GI intolerance**	**Metabolized by xanthine oxidase**
Azlocillin	Antibiotic—β-lactam	*Pseudomonas; Proteus*		
Aztreonam [Azactam]	Antibiotic—inhibits transpeptidase and cell wall synthesis; monocyclic β-lactam	Gram-negative bacteria		IV
Bacitracin	Antibiotic—inhibits cell wall formation; bactericidal	Gram-positive bacteria	Nephrotoxic	Topical only
Baclofen [Lioresal]	Skeletal muscle relaxant—GABA mimetic; works at the GABA_b receptor	Muscle spasms; tetanus contractions; orthopedic manipulation		
BCNU (carmustine)	Antineoplastic—DNA alkylation	Cancer	Delayed bone marrow suppression; lung and kidney damage	
Benserazide	Antiparkinsonian—inhibits decarboxylase (L-DOPA to dopamine) in periphery	Parkinson's disease		
Benztropine [Cogentin]	Antiparkinsonian—muscarinic blocker; H_1 blocker	Parkinson's disease		
Bephenium hydroxynaphthoate	Antihelmintic—cholinergic agonist causing contraction, then relaxation in worm	*Necator* and *Ancylostoma* (hookworms)	Vomiting	

Drug	Action	Clinical use	Toxicity	Notes
Bethanechol [Urecholine, Duvoid]	Muscarinic agonist	Atony of bladder; paralytic ileus		Contraindicated in patients with peptic ulcer, asthma, hyperthyroid, Parkinson's
Bis-chloroethylamines (nitrogen mustards) [Mustargen]	Antineoplastic—DNA alkylation and cross-linking	Cancer	Nausea; vomiting; bone marrow suppression; alopecia; teratogenicity; carcinogenicity	
Bismuth (colloidal) [Pepto-Bismol]	Antiulcer, antidiarrheal—cytoprotective	Bactericidal for *Helicobacter pylori* (with ranitidine and clarithromycin)		
Black widow spider venom	Presynaptic neuromuscular junction blocker—overstimulates ACh release			
Bleomycin [Blenoxane]	Antineoplastic—binds, intercalates, and cuts DNA	Cancer	Fever; blistering; stomatitis; pulmonary fibrosis	
Botulinum [Botox, Dysport]	Neuromuscular blocker—presynaptic neuromuscular junction blocker; prevents ACh release			
Bretylium [Bretylol]	Antiarrhythmic (class III)—K$^+$-channel blocker	Arrhythmias; orthostatic hypotension; nausea; vomiting		
Bromocriptine [Parlodel]	Antiparkinsonian—agonist at D$_2$; partial antagonist at D$_1$	Parkinson's disease; acromegaly (paradoxical effect—releases growth hormone from normal pituitary)	Inhibits prolactin release	
Buclizine	Antiemetic	Sedation; Parkinsonism		
Bumetanide [Bumex]	Loop diuretic—inhibits Na$^+$/K$^+$/Cl$^-$ reabsorption in the Loop of Henle	CHF; diuresis	Ototoxicity; hyperuricemia; acute hypovolemia; hypokalemia; metabolic alkalosis; hyperglycemia	
α-Bungarotoxin	Postsynaptic neuromuscular junction blocker; irreversibly binds nicotinic receptor			
Bupivacaine	Anesthetic—blocks Na$^+$ channel intracellularly	Local anesthetic	Sleepiness; light-headedness; visual/audio disturbances; restlessness; nystagmus; shivering; tonic-clonic convulsions; death	
Buprenorphine [Buprenex]	Opioid analog—mixed agonist/antagonist action	Treatment of opioid/cocaine dependence		
Bupropion [Wellbutrin, Zyban]	Antidepressant—agonist at D$_2$, 5-HT	Depression; smoking cessation		Decreased sexual dysfunction compared with other SSRIs

Therapeutic Agent (common name, if relevant) [Trade name, where appropriate]	Class—Pharmacology and Pharmacokinetics	Indications	Side or Adverse Effects	Contraindications or Precautions to Consider; Notes
Buspirone [BuSpar]	Antidepressant—benzodiazepine-like agonist	Depression		
Caffeine [NoDoz]	Stimulant—phosphodiesterase inhibitor, resulting in increased cAMP; stimulates CNS and cardiac muscle; relaxes smooth muscle; produces diuresis; increases cerebrovascular resistance	Acute migraine attack		
Calcitonin [Calcimar, Miacalcin]	Hypocalcemic agent—antiosteoporotic agent; lowers plasma Ca^{2+} and phosphate; inhibits bone and kidney reabsorption	Hypercalcemia; Paget's disease; osteoporosis		
Calcium carbonate [Caltrate]	Dietary Ca^{2+} supplement	Ca^{2+} deficiency		
Calcium citrate	Dietary Ca^{2+} supplement	Ca^{2+} deficiency		
Calcium gluconate	Dietary Ca^{2+} supplement	Ca^{2+} deficiency		
Calcium lactate	Dietary Ca^{2+} supplement	Ca^{2+} deficiency		
Captopril [Capoten]	Antihypertensive heart failure agent; post-MI agent; vasodilator; ACE inhibitor	CHF	Postural hypotension; renal insufficiency; hyperkalemia; persistent dry cough	Contraindicated in pregnancy
Carbachol [Isopto carbachol]	Antiglaucoma agent—muscarinic agonist	Miotic; glaucoma		Contraindicated in patients with peptic ulcer, asthma, hyperthyroid, and Parkinson's disease
Carbamazepine [Tegretol]	Antiepileptic—Na^+-channel blocker; decreases glutamate (and other excitatory neurotransmitters)	Epilepsy (partial and tonic-clonic); trigeminal neuralgia	Agranulocytosis	Induces cytochrome P-450
Carbidopa [Sinemet]	Antiparkinsonian—inhibits decarboxylase (L-DOPA to dopamine) in periphery	Parkinson's disease; used with levodopa as Sinemet		
Carboplatin [Paraplatin]	Antineoplastic—cross-links DNA	Cancer	Bone marrow and renal toxicity; cystitis; peripheral neuropathy; ototoxicity; alopecia (severe)	Contains platinum
Carboprost [Prostin]	Abortive agent—$PGF_{2\alpha}$	Therapeutic abortion	Nausea; vomiting; diarrhea	

Drug	Action/Mechanism	Clinical Use	Side Effects	Notes
Castor oil	Laxative—reduces absorption of electrolytes and water from gut; active component is ricinoleic acid	Stimulant laxative		
Cephalosporins	**Antibiotic—inhibits transpeptidase and cell wall synthesis**	**Third-generation cephalosporins are used for meningitis, *Klebsiella*, Lyme disease, and Gram-negative bacteria**	**Allergic reactions; pain at injection site; thrombophlebitis; bleeding disorders**	**First-generation: cefazolin, cephalexin; second-generation: cefaclor, cefoxitin, cefuroxime; third-generation: ceftriaxone; fourth-generation: cefepime**
Chloral hydrate	Anesthetic agent	Sedative; hypnotic		Inexpensive
Chlorambucil [Leukeran]	Antineoplastic—DNA alkylation and cross-linking	Cancer	Nausea; vomiting, bone marrow suppression (mild), alopecia, teratogenicity, carcinogenicity, pulmonary fibrosis	
Chloramphenicol [Chloromycetin]	**Antibiotic—binds 50S ribosome subunits; bacteriostatic, but bactericidal versus *Haemophilus influenzae* and *Neisseria meningitidis***	**Broad-spectrum versus Gram-negatives; typhoid fever; *Salmonella*; Rocky Mountain spotted fever in children**	**Red cell anemia; bone marrow aplasia; gray baby syndrome**	**Interactions with phenytoin, warfarin, or coumarin; inhibits cytochrome P-450**
Chlordiazepoxide [Libritabs]	Antianxiety—benzodiazepine; enhances GABA; increases IPSP amplitude	Sedative; hypnotic; antianxiety; antiepileptic		
Chlorguanide	**Antimalarial—inhibits dihydrofolate reductase**	**Prophylaxis for falciparum malaria; suppression of vivax malaria**	**Minor GI upset**	
Chloroquine phosphate [Aralen]	**Anti-malarial—uncertain mechanism**	**Suppression of malaria and treatment of acute attack; amebiasis; *Clonorchis*; rheumatoid arthritis; SLE**	**Headache; GI disturbances; visual disturbances; pruritus; prolonged therapy may lead to retinopathy**	
Chlorpheniramine [Chlor-Trimeton]	Antihistamine—H_1 blocker	Allergies; motion sickness	Sedation; CNS depression; atropinelike effects; allergic dermatitis; blood dyscrasias; teratogenicity; acute antihistamine poisoning	
Chloroprocaine	Anesthetic—block Na^+ channel intracellularly	Local anesthetic	Sleepiness; light-headedness; visual/audio disturbances; restlessness; nystagmus; shivering; tonic-clonic convulsions, death	
Chlorpromazine [Thorazine]	Antiemetic, antipsychotic—blocks D_2 receptors	Antipsychotic; antiemetic; hiccups	Parkinsonism; tardive dyskinesia; orthostatic hypotension; anticholinergic effects; sedation; jaundice; photosensitivity; teratogenic	

Therapeutic Agent (common name, if relevant) [Trade name, where appropriate]	Class—Pharmacology and Pharmacokinetics	Indications	Side or Adverse Effects	Contraindications or Precautions to Consider; Notes
Chlorpropamide [Diabinese]	Hypoglycemic agent—sulfonylurea; reduces K$^+$ efflux, increases Ca^{2+} influx, increases secretion of insulin	Oral treatment for NIDDM (type II diabetes)	Hypoglycemia; GI disturbances; muscle weakness; mental confusion	
Cholestyramine [Questran]	Lipid-lowering agent—impedes fat absorption; lowers LDL; binds cholesterol metabolites	Reduction of cholesterol	Steatorrhea; constipation; impairment of absorption of drugs/vitamins	Inhibits warfarin absorption
Chorionic gonadotropin [Pregnyl]	Infertility therapy—LH-like in action	Treat infertility; induces ovulation; induces masculinization in infertile men; diagnostic for cryptorchidism in young boys		
Cimetidine [Tagamet]	H$_2$ blocker	Inhibition of gastric acid secretion	Gynecomastia; rare: headache, dizziness, fatigue, CNS, weak antiandrogenic effect, leukopenia, reduced sperm count	Inhibits metabolism or absorption of some drugs; inhibits cytochrome P-450
Ciprofloxacin [Cipro]	Quinolone antibiotic—blocks DNA synthesis by inhibiting DNA gyrase	Gram-negative infections (esp. UTI and bone): *Pseudomonas, Enterobacteriaceae, Neisseria;* Gram-positive infections; intracellular: *Legionella*	GI disturbances; headache; dizziness; phototoxicity; cartilage damage	May elevate theophylline to toxic levels causing seizure
Cisapride [Propulsid]	GI stimulant—agonist at 5-HT$_4$; prokinetic	Increases stomach motility		Arrhythmias; taken off the market
Cisplatin [Platinol]	Antineoplastic—cross-links DNA	Cancer	Bone marrow and renal toxicity; cystitis; peripheral neuropathy; ototoxicity; alopecia (severe)	
Clavulanic acid	β-lactamase inhibitor; synergistic with penicillins			
Clindamycin [Cleocin]	Antibiotic—binds to 50S subunits; bacteriostatic or bactericidal	Gram-positive bone infections; anaerobic infections	Severe diarrhea; potentially fatal pseudomembranous colitis caused by *Clostridium difficile*	
Clofazimine [Lamprene]	Antibiotic—antileprosy; unknown mechanism	*Mycobacterium leprae*	Turns skin red-brown or black	
Clofibrate [Atromid-S]	Lipid-lowering agent—lowers VLDL, TG, cholesterol; increases activity of LPL; inhibits lipolysis; increases HDL	Hyperlipidemia (esp. type III)	Increased risk of GI and liver cancer; potentiates anticoagulant drugs; myositis; gallstones; mild GI disturbances	LDL may rise, thus no change in total cholesterol

Drug	Mechanism	Use	Side effects	Notes
Clomiphene [Clomid]	Ovulation stimulant—partial estrogen receptor agonist; decreases estrogen feedback inhibition of GnRH; leads to increase in gonadotropin secretion	Stimulates ovulation in infertility	Ovarian enlargement	Increased incidence of multiple gestations
Clonazepam [Klonopin]	Antiepileptic—benzodiazepine	Epilepsy (absence seizures)		
Clonidine [Catapres]	Antihypertensive—α_2 agonist	Hypertension; smoking withdrawal; heroin and cocaine withdrawal	Drowsiness; dry mouth; rebound hypertension after abrupt withdrawal	
Clotrimazole [Lotrimin, Mycelex]	Antifungal—inhibit ergosterol synthesis, so cell membrane cannot form	Topical use against dermatophytes, ringworm, fungi, mold, and oral candidiasis in AIDS		
Cloxacillin [Cloxapen]	Antibiotic—β-lactam; penicillinase-resistant	Staphylococcus infections		
Clozapine [Clozaril]	Antipsychotic—blocks D_2 and $5\text{-}HT_2$ receptors; also blocks dopamine$_4$	Antipsychotic	Orthostatic hypotension; sedation; agranulocytosis	Weekly CBCs
Cocaine	CNS stimulant—blocks NE, 5-HT, and dopamine reuptake	Local anesthetic	Vasoconstriction; hypertension; nasal mucus ischemia	
Codeine	Opioid agonist	Good antitussive; moderate for pain		
Colchicine	Antigout—inhibits phagocytosis and secretion of inflammatory mediators; decreases LTB_4	Acute gout	Nausea; diarrhea; vomiting; abdominal cramps	Contraindicated in elderly and feeble patients and in patients with GI disturbances, cardiac anomalies, or renal problems
Colestipol [Colestid]	Lipid-lowering agent—impedes fat absorption; lowers LDL; binds cholesterol metabolites	Reduction of cholesterol	Steatorrhea; constipation; impaired absorption of drugs and vitamins	
Corticotropin-releasing hormone (CRH)	Increases ACTH production by anterior pituitary	Used in diagnosis of Cushing's syndrome		
Cortisol (hydrocortisone) [Hydrocortone, Nutracort]	Glucocorticoid—induces new protein synthesis; increases gluconeogenesis and lipolysis; reduces peripheral glucose use; catabolic effect on muscle, bone, skin, fat, lymph tissue; anti-inflammatory; immunosuppressant	Adrenal insufficiency; congenital adrenal hyperplasia; diagnosis of pituitary-adrenal disorder; reduces inflammation (esp. chronic); leukemia; decreases hypercalcemia	Iatrogenic Cushing's syndrome; redistribution of fat; acne; insomnia; weight gain; hypokalemia; decrease in skeletal muscle; osteoporosis; hyperglycemia; ulcers; psychosis; cataracts; increased susceptibility to infections; growth suppression in children	

Therapeutic Agent (common name, if relevant) [Trade name, where appropriate]	Class—Pharmacology and Pharmacokinetics	Indications	Side or Adverse Effects	Contraindications or Precautions to Consider; Notes
Cosyntropin [Cortrosyn]	ACTH analog—increases production of steroids by adrenal	Used in diagnosis of adrenocortical insufficiency		
Cromolyn [Nasalcrom, Gastrocrom]	**Antiasthmatic—antiallergic; inhibits histamine release from mast cells**	**Prophylaxis for asthma**	**Laryngeal edema (rare)**	
Cyanocobalamin (Anacobin)	Supplies vitamin B_{12}	B_{12} deficiency		
Cyclobenzaprine [Flexeril]	Centrally acting muscle relaxant	Muscle spasms; tetanus contractions; orthopedic manipulation	Antimuscarinic effects	
Cyclophosphamide [Cytoxan]	**Immunosuppressant—alkylating agent; destroys proliferating lymphoid cells; alkylates resting cells**	**Transplant rejection; rheumatic arthritis**	**GI and bone marrow toxicity; hemorrhagic cystitis**	
Cycloserine [Seromycin]	Antibiotic—analog of D-alanine; interferes with cell wall synthesis	Mycobacterium	Psychotic reactions	
Cyclosporine [Sandimmune]	**Immunosuppressant—inhibits T-helper cell activity; inhibits IL-2, IL-3, and IFN-γ formation by T-helper cells**	**Transplant rejection**	**Nephrotoxic; hepatotoxic; hypertension; increased incidence of viral infection and lymphoma**	
Cyproheptadine [Periactin]	Antihistamine—antipruritic; 5-HT_3 agonist; histamine blocker	Decreases diarrhea in carcinoid tumors; decreases dumping syndrome	Weight gain	
Cytosine arabinoside [Cytosar-U]	Antineoplastic—inhibits DNA replication and RNA polymerization; competitive inhibitor of dCTP; inhibits chain elongation	Cancer; AML	Severe myelosuppression; stomatitis; alopecia	
Dacarbazine [DTIC-Dome]	Antineoplastic—DNA alkylation; strand breakage; inhibits nucleic acid and protein synthesis	Cancer		
Dactinomycin [Cosmegen]	Antineoplastic—cross-links DNA; intercalates into DNA	Cancer	Skin eruptions; hyperkeratosis	
Danazol [Danocrine]	**Testosterone derivative—weak agonist for androgen, progesterone, and glucocorticoid receptors**	**Endometriosis and fibrocystic disease**	**Masculinization in females; gynecomastia in males**	

Drug	Action/Class	Use	Side Effects/Toxicity	Notes
Dantrolene [Dantrium]	Non-centrally acting muscle relaxant—decreases Ca²⁺ from sarcoplasmic reticulum	Malignant hypertension	Hepatotoxic	
Dapsone [Dapsone]	Antibiotic—related to sulfonamides	*Mycobacterium leprae*	GI disturbances; hemolysis; methemoglobinemia	
Daunorubicin [DaunoXome, Cerubidine]	Antineoplastic—oxidizes free radicals; breaks DNA; intercalates into DNA; affects plasma membrane	Cancer	Cardiac changes resulting in cumulative cardiotoxicity	
Deferoxamine [Desferal]	Metal chelator	Acute toxicity of iron	Hypotensive shock; neurotoxic if long-term use	
Desflurane [Suprane]	Anesthetic	General anesthetic	Irritating to airway	
Desipramine [Norpramin]	Antidepressant—TCA; blocks NE, 5-HT, muscarinic, α_1, and histamine receptors	Depression	Tremors (NE block); anorexia (5-HT block); anticholinergic (muscarinic block); hypotension (α_1 block); drowsiness (histamine block)	
Desmopressin (DDAVP)	Antidiuretic—recruits water channels to luminal membrane in collecting duct	Antidiuresis; central diabetes insipidus	Overhydration; allergic reaction; larger doses result in pallor, diarrhea, hypertension; coronary constriction; chronic rhinopharyngitis	Synthetic analog to vasopressin; intranasal administration
Dexamethasone [Decadron, Maxidex]	Corticosteroid—reduces lymph node and spleen size; inhibits cell cycle activity of lymphoid cells; lyses T cells; suppresses antibody, prostaglandin, and leukotriene synthesis; blocks monocyte production of IL-1	Antiemetic; autoimmune disorders; allergic reactions; asthma; organ transplant (esp. during rejection crisis); test for etiology of hypercortisolism	Insomnia; epigastric disturbances; Cushingoid reaction; psychosis; glucose intolerance; infection; hypertension; cataracts	
DHEA	Androgen and estrogen precursor		Acne; hair loss; hirsutism; deepening of voice	
Diazepam [Valium]	Antianxiety, benzodiazepine—enhances GABA; increases IPSP amplitude	Sedative; hypnotic; antianxiety; antiepileptic (status epilepticus, grand mal)	Sedation	
Diazepam binding inhibitor (DBI)	Benzodiazepine receptor antagonist			
Diclofenac [Cataflam, Voltaren]	NSAID—enteric coated			
Dicloxacillin [Dynapen, Pathocil]	Antibiotic—β-lactam; penicillinase-resistant	*Staphylococcus* infections		

Therapeutic Agent (common name, if relevant) [Trade name, where appropriate]	Class—Pharmacology and Pharmacokinetics	Indications	Side or Adverse Effects	Contraindications or Precautions to Consider; Notes
Dicyclomine [Bentyl]	Antimuscarinic	Bladder/GI spasm; decreases acid in ulcer		
Dideoxyinisine [ddI], Didanosine [ddA] [Videx]	**Antiviral—reverse transcriptase inhibitors**	**AIDS**	**Abdominal cramps; diarrhea; peripheral neuropathy; acute pancreatitis**	
Diethylcarbamazine [Hetrazan]	Antihelmintic—sensitizes helminths to phagocytosis by macrophages	Filariasis	Headache, malaise; joint pain; anorexia; death of filaria causes: swelling and edema of skin, enlarged lymph nodes, hyperpyrexia, tachycardia	
Digitoxin [Crystodigin]	Inotropic agent—cardiac glycoside; increases cardiac contractility	Severe left ventricular systolic dysfunction; antiarrhythmic	Progressive dysrhythmia; anorexia; nausea; vomiting; headache; fatigue; confusion; blurred vision; altered color perception; halos around dark objects	Contraindicated in patients with right-sided heart failure, diastolic failure; Wolf-Parkinson-White syndrome; ECG changes: increases PR, decreases QT, depresses ST, inverts T
Digoxin [Lanoxin]	**Inotropic agent—cardiac glycoside; increases cardiac contractility**	**Severe left ventricular systolic dysfunction; antiarrhythmic**	**Progressive dysrhythmia; anorexia; nausea; vomiting; headache; fatigue; confusion; blurred vision; altered color perception; haloes around dark objects**	**Contraindicated in patients with right-sided heart failure, diastolic failure; ECG changes: increases PR, decreases QT, depresses ST, inverts T**
Diiodohydroxyquin [Yodoxin]	Antiprotozoal—direct action	Amebae	Subacute myelo-optic neuropathy	
Diltiazem [Cardizem, Dilacor]	**Antiarrhythmic (class IV)—Ca^{2+} blocker**	**Angina; AV nodal arrhythmia; decreases blood pressure**		
Dimenhydrinate [Dramamine]	Antivertigo—antiemetic; H$_1$ blocker	Emesis; dizziness		
Dimercaprol [British antilewisite]	Metal chelator	Arsenic, mercury, or cadmium poisoning	Hypertension; tachycardia; headaches; nausea; vomiting; pain at injection site	
Dinoprostone [Cervidil, Prepidil]	Antihemorrhagic (oxytocin agonist)—PGE$_2$; increases collagenase	Softening, ripening, dilation of cervix (induces labor)		
Diphenhydramine [Benadryl]	**Antihistamine—antiemetic; muscarinic blocker; H$_1$ blocker**	**Allergic reactions; asthma; motion sickness; antiemetic**	**Sedation; CNS depression; atropinelike effects; allergic dermatitis; blood dyscrasias; teratogenicity; acute antihistamine poisoning**	**Rarely used as antiparkinsonian agent**
Disopyramide [Norpace]	Antiarrhythmic (class IA)—Na$^+$-channel blocker	Wolf-Parkinson-White	Heart failure	Contraindicated in patients with sick sinus syndrome

Drug	Mechanism/Class	Clinical Use	Side Effects/Toxicity	Notes
Disulfiram [Antabuse]	Antialcoholic agent—inhibits aldehyde dehydrogenase	Alcohol ingestion	Tachycardia; hyperventilation; nausea	
Dobutamine [Dobutrex]	Inotropic agent—β agonist; positive inotropic effects on the heart and vasodilation	Acute heart failure; increases cardiac output		
Doxazosin [Cardura]	Antihypertensive—α_1-blocker	Hypertension		
Doxepin [Sinequan]	Antidepressant, antianxiety—TCA; blocks NE, 5-HT, muscarinic, α_1, histamine receptors	Antidepressant	Tremors (NE block); anorexia (5-HT block); anticholinergic (muscarinic block); hypotension (α_1 block); drowsiness (histamine block)	
Doxorubicin [Adriamycin]	Antineoplastic—oxidizes free radicals; breaks DNA; intercalates into DNA; affects plasma membrane	Cancer	Cardiac changes resulting in cumulative cardiotoxicity	
Dronabinol [Marinol]	Antiemetic—unknown mechanism; binds opiate receptors and directly inhibits vomiting center in medulla	Antiemetic	Dry mouth; dizziness; inability to concentrate; disorientation; anxiety; tachycardia; depression; paranoia; psychosis	THC derivative
Echothiophate [Phospholine Iodide]	Antiglaucoma—inhibits cholinesterase; nicotinic receptor stimulator; irreversible	Closed-angle glaucoma	Open-angle glaucoma	
Edetate calcium disodium (calcium EDTA) [Calcium disodium versenate]	Metal chelator	Lead toxicity	Nephrotoxic	
Edrophonium [Enlon, Tensilon]	Cholinesterase inhibitor	Diagnosis of myasthenia gravis; emergency anesthetic		
Emetine	Antiprotozoal—causes degeneration of nucleus and reticulation of cytoplasm; directly lethal	Severe amebic infection	Diarrhea; nausea; vomiting; abdominal pain; cardiac effects: hypotension, precordial pain, ECG changes	
Enalapril [Vasotec]	Antihypertensive—vasodilator; ACE inhibitor	CHF	Postural hypotension; renal insufficiency; hyperkalemia; persistent dry cough	Pregnancy
Encainide	Antiarrhythmia (class IC)—Na^+-channel blockers	Wolf-Parkinson-White syndrome		No antimuscarinic action; no effect on action potential
Enflurane [Ethrane]	Anesthetic agent	General anesthetic	Seizure	Abnormal ECG or seizures
Ephedrine	Bronchodilation—mixed adrenergic agonist	Stimulates NE release; antitussive; myasthenia gravis	Increases BP	

Therapeutic Agent (common name, if relevant) [Trade name, where appropriate]	Class–Pharmacology and Pharmacokinetics	Indications	Side or Adverse Effects	Contraindications or Precautions to Consider; Notes
Epinephrine	Adrenergic agonist	Acute asthma; anaphylactic shock		Activates both α and β receptors, but is preferential for β
Epoprostenol [Flolan]	Prostacyclin—increases cardiac index, stroke volume; decreases pulmonary vascular resistance and mean systemic pressure	Pulmonary hypertension		
Ergotamine [Ergomar]	Antimigraine—vasoconstriction	Acute attack of migraine	Gangrene as a result of vasoconstriction	Contraindicated in pregnant patients or patients with cardiovascular disease or coronary artery disease
Erythromycin [E-Mycin]	Antibiotic—binds to the 23S RNA of the 50S ribosome subunits	First choice for cell wall–deficient bugs: *Mycoplasma, Rickettsia, Chlamydia, Legionella; Corynebacterium diphtheria*		
Erythropoietin (EPO) [Procrit, Epogen]	Colony-stimulating factor	Anemia; renal defects; AIDS	Hypertension	
Esmolol [Brevibloc]	Antiarrhythmic (class II)—β blocker	Block effect of catecholamines on heart; decrease activity of nodal tissue; slow sinus rate; depress AV conduction	Asthma; negative inotropic agent	
Estrogen [Estratab, Premarin]	Growth and development of female organs; linear bone growth; epiphyseal closure; endometrial growth; maintains responsiveness of breasts, uterus, and vagina; inhibits bone resorption; increases hepatic production of α_2-globulins, coagulation factors II, VII, IX, and X, and HDL; decreases antithrombin III and cholesterol	Osteoporosis; contraception; can be used in combination with progesterone	May lead to sodium and water retention; nausea; breast tenderness; hyperpigmentation; increased risk of bleeding, gallbladder disease, migraines, hypertension	
Ethacrynic acid [Edecrin]	Loop diuretic—inhibits $Na^+/K^+/Cl^-$ reabsorption in Loop of Henle	Diuresis	Ototoxicity; metabolic alkalosis; hypokalemia; hyperglycemia; hyperuricemia	
Ethambutol [Myambutol]	Antibiotic—unknown mechanism	*Mycobacterium*	Visual disturbances; tolerance develops	

Drug	Class / Mechanism	Clinical use	Side effects / Toxicity	Notes
Ethosuximide	Antiepileptic—decrease Ca²⁺ conduction	Epilepsy (absence seizures)		
Ether	**Anesthetic agent**	**General anesthetic**		
Etidocaine [Duranest]	Anesthetic agent—blocks Na⁺ intracellularly	Local anesthetic	Sleepiness; light-headedness; visual/audio disturbances; restlessness; nystagmus; shivering; tonic-clonic convulsions; death; greater toxicity than other local anesthetics	
Etidronate [Didronel]	Bone stabilizer—pyrophosphate analog; reduces hydroxyapatite crystal formation, growth, and dissolution, which reduces bone turnover	Hypercalcemia of malignancy; Paget's disease; osteoporosis; hyperparathyroidism		
Etomidate [Amidate]	Anesthetic agent	Induces stage 3 anesthesia	Painful injection; myoclonic movements	
Etretinate	Vitamin A analog	Severe acne; psoriasis		
Famotidine [Pepcid]	**H₂ blocker**	**Inhibits gastric acid secretion (esp. ulcer)**	**Gynecomastia; rare: headache, dizziness, fatigue, CNS, leukopenia, reduced sperm count**	**Inhibits metabolism or absorption of some drugs**
Fentanyl [Duragesic]	**Opioid agonist**	**Analgesic; general anesthetic**	Prolonged recovery; nausea	
Fexofenadine hydrochloride [Allegra]	Antihistamine			
Finasteride [Proscar]	**Androgen hormone inhibitor—inhibits 5-α-reductase**	**Benign prostatic hyperplasia**		
Flecainide [Tambocor]	**Antiarrhythmic (class IC)—Na⁺-channel blocker**			
Fluconazole [Diflucan]	**Antifungal—inhibits ergosterol synthesis, preventing cell membrane formation**	**Cryptococcal meningitis; oral candidiasis in AIDS**	**Abdominal pain; nausea**	
Flucytosine [Ancobon]	Antifungal—competitive inhibitor of thymidylate synthetase; impairs DNA synthesis	*Candida; Cryptococcus; Aspergillus*	Nausea; vomiting; diarrhea; rash; bone marrow and liver toxicity; enterocolitis	Imported in the fungus via permease
Fludrocortisone [Florinef]	Mineralocorticoid—aldosterone analog	Used with cortisol in adrenal insufficiency		
Flumazenil [Romazicon]	Benzodiazepine receptor antagonist	Alcohol abuse; anxiety	IV only	
Flunarizine [Sibelium]	Weak Ca²⁺-channel blocker	Prophylaxis for migraine		

Therapeutic Agent (common name, if relevant) [Trade name, where appropriate]	Class–Pharmacology and Pharmacokinetics	Indications	Side or Adverse Effects	Contraindications or Precautions to Consider; Notes
Fluoride	Stabilizes hydroxyapatite crystal structure; stimulates new growth of bone (unknown mechanism)		Nausea; vomiting; neurologic symptoms; arthralgias; arthritis	Stains teeth in toxic amounts
5-Fluorouracil (5-FU)	**Antineoplastic—inhibits thymidylate synthetase; inhibits RNA synthesis**	**Colon and breast cancer**	**Delayed toxicity: nausea, oral and GI ulcers, bone marrow depression**	
Fluoxetine [Prozac]	**Antidepressant—antianxiety; SSRI**	**Depression; anxiety; obsessive-compulsive disorder**	**Agitation; tremors; mania; preoccupation with suicide; nausea; headache; insomnia**	
Fluphenazine [Prolixin]	Antipsychotic—blocks D_2 receptors	Psychosis	Parkinsonism; tardive dyskinesia	
Flurazepam [Dalmane]	Benzodiazepine—enhances GABA; increases IPSP amplitude	Sedative; hypnotic; antianxiety; antiepileptic		
Flutamide [Eulexin]	**Antineoplastic—competitive androgen receptor blocker**	**Metastatic prostate cancer**		
Fluvastatin [Lescol]	Lipid-lowering agent—inhibits HMG-CoA reductase; lowers LDL	Hyperlipidemia (esp. type II)	Liver toxicity; myopathy; mild GI disturbances	Contraindicated in pregnant or lactating women or children
Fluvoxamine [Luvox]	Antidepressant—SSRI	Anxiety; obsessive-compulsive disorder		
Foscarnet [Foscavir]	Antiviral—nonnucleoside inhibitor of DNA polymerase	CMV, herpes in AIDS	Hypocalcemia; CNS, cardiac, and renal toxicity; anemia	
Fosinopril [Monopril]	Antihypertensive—ACE inhibitor; vasodilator	CHF	Postural hypotension; renal insufficiency; hyperkalemia; persistent dry cough	Contraindicated in pregnant women
Furosemide [Lasix]	**Loop diuretic—inhibits $Na^+/K^+/Cl^-$ reabsorption in the Loop of Henle**	**CHF; diuresis**	**Ototoxicity; hyperuricemia; acute hypovolemia; hypokalemia; metabolic alkalosis; hyperglycemia**	
Gabapentin [Neurontin]	Antiepileptic—blocks Na^+ channels	Add-on drug for epilepsy		
Ganciclovir [Cytovene]	**Antiviral—guanosine analog; inhibits DNA polymerase**	**CMV (esp. CMV retinitis in AIDS)**	**Bone marrow suppression; renal impairment; seizures**	
Gemfibrozil [Lopid]	**Lipid-lowering agent—lowers VLDL, TG, cholesterol; increases activity of LPL; inhibits lipolysis; increases HDL**	**Hyperlipidemia**	**Potentiates anticoagulant drugs; myositis; gallstones; mild GI disturbances**	**Contraindicated in patients with impaired renal or hepatic function, and in pregnant or lactating women**

Drug	Mechanism	Clinical Use	Side Effects	Notes
Gentamicin [Garamycin]	Antibiotic—aminoglycoside; binds 30S ribosome subunits; bacteriostatic at low concentration; bactericidal at high	Gram-negative meningitis		Contraindicated in neonates; peak and trough levels must be measured
Glipizide [Glucotrol]	Hypoglycemic agent—sulfonylurea; reduces K^+ efflux, increases Ca^{2+} influx, increases secretion of insulin	Oral treatment for NIDDM (type II diabetes)	Hypoglycemia; GI disturbances; muscle weakness; mental confusion	
Glyburide [DiaBeta, Micronase]	Hypoglycemic agent—sulfonylurea; reduces K^+ efflux, increases Ca^{2+} influx, increases secretion of insulin	Oral treatment for NIDDM (type II diabetes)	Hypoglycemia; GI disturbances; muscle weakness; mental confusion	
Glyceryl guaiacolate [Fenesin]	Expectorant—increases bronchial secretions	Promotes cough		
Glycopyrrolate [Robinul]	Antimuscarinic	Bladder/GI spasm; decreases acid in ulcer		
GnRH	Controls release of FSH, LH	Stimulates pituitary function		
Gonadorelin [Lutrepulse]	Analog of GnRH—controls release of FSH, LH	Stimulates pituitary function		
Griseofulvin [Fulvicin, Grifulvin, Grisactin]	Antifungal—inhibits cell mitosis by disrupting mitotic spindles; binds to tubulin	Dermatophytes (esp. *Trichophyton rubrum*)	Headache; lethargy; mental confusion; fever; rash; nausea; vomiting; diarrhea; hepatotoxic; photosensitivity	
Growth hormone (somatotropin) [Somatrem]	Causes liver to produce insulin-like growth factors (somatomedins)	Replacement therapy in children and burn victims		
Growth hormone-releasing hormone (GH-RH)	Stimulates release of GH	Dwarfism	Pain at injection	
Guanethidine [Ismelin]	Antihypertensive—interferes with NE release	Severe hypertension	Postural hypotension; impotence	Contraindicated in patients taking TCAs
Haloperidol [Haldol]	Antipsychotic—blocks D_2 receptors	Psychosis	Parkinsonism; tardive dyskinesia	
Haloprogin [Halotex]	Antifungal—unknown mechanism; fungistatic	Topical for tinea pedis		
Halothane	Anesthetic agent	General anesthetic	Hepatotoxic; malignant hyperthermia (with succinylcholine); arrhythmia	Contraindicated in adults

Therapeutic Agent (common name, if relevant) [Trade name, where appropriate]	Class—Pharmacology and Pharmacokinetics	Indications	Side or Adverse Effects	Contraindications or Precautions to Consider; Notes
Heparin	Increases PTT by joining with antithrombin III	Deep vein thrombosis; pulmonary thrombosis	Overdose reversed by IV protamine sulfate; osteoporosis	Fast-acting; does not cross placenta
Heroin	Metabolized to morphine			More lipid-soluble than morphine
Hexamethonium	Nicotinic ganglionic blocker	Hypertensive emergency		
Hydralazine [Apresoline]	Antihypertensive—vasodilator	CHF, hypertension	Lupus-like reaction	Used in pregnancy
Hydrochlorothiazide [Esidrix, HydroDIURIL]	Diuretic—decreases Na^+ reabsorption in the distal tubule by inhibiting the Na^+/Cl^- transport	Hypertension, CHF, Nephrogenic diabetes insipidus, idiopathic hypercalciuria	Hypokalemia; hyperuricemia; hypovolemia; hyperglycemia (especially in diabetics); hypersensitivity	
Hydrocodone [Bancap-HC]	Opioid agonist	Antitussive; analgesic		
Hydromorphone [Dilaudid]	Opioid agonist	Antitussive; analgesic		
Hydroxychloroquine [Plaquenil]	Antiprotozoal—antirheumatic	Rheumatic arthritis; malaria	Ocular toxicity (blurred vision)	Contraindicated in patients with psoriasis
Hydroxyurea [Hydrea]	Antineoplastic—binds ribonucleotide reductase; inhibits formation of DNA	Melanoma; chronic myelogenous leukemia; sickle cell disease	Nausea; vomiting; bone marrow suppression	
Ibuprofen [Advil, Motrin]	NSAID	Inflammation; pain	GI side effects, fewer than aspirin	
Ibutilide [Convert]	Antiarrhythmic (class III)—K^+-channel blocker	Terminate atrial fibrillation and flutter	Prolongs QT interval	
Idazoxan	Antihypertensive—α_2 blocker			
Idoxuridine [Herplex Liquifilm]	Antiviral—thymidine analog; inhibits DNA polymerase; inhibits DNA synthesis	Topical for HSV keratitis	Local irritation; allergic contact keratitis	
Ifosfamide [IFEX]	Antineoplastic—DNA alkylation and cross-linking	Cancer	Cystitis; nephrotoxicity; nausea; vomiting; bone marrow suppression; alopecia; teratogenicity; carcinogenicity	
Imipenem [Primaxin]	Antibiotic—inhibits transpeptidase and cell wall synthesis; monocyclic β-lactam	Dormant bacteria	Seizure	

Drug	Class/Mechanism	Use	Notes/Side effects
Imipramine [Tofranil]	Antidepressant—TCA; blocks NE, 5-HT, muscarinic, α₁, histamine receptors; antiarrhythmic (class IA)	Antidepressant; bed-wetting	Tremors (NE block); anorexia (5-HT block); anticholinergic (muscarinic block); hypotension (α₁ block); drowsiness (histamine block)
Indecainide	Antiarrhythmic (class IC)—Na⁺-channel blockers		No antimuscarinic action; no effect on action potential
Indinavir [Crixivan]	Antiviral—protease inhibitor	AIDS	
Indomethacin [Indocin]	NSAID	Closes PDA; gout	
Interferon alfa-2a (Roferon A), alfa-2b (Intron A), and alfa-n3 (Alferon-N)	Antiviral—decreases protein synthesis	Genital warts; chronic hepatitis B and C; AIDS-related Kaposi's sarcoma; laryngeal papillomatosis; hairy cell leukemia	Flulike symptoms; tachycardia; fever; neutropenia; headache; somnolence; malaise
Ipratropium [Atrovent]	Bronchodilator—antimuscarinic	Bronchodilates for asthma	
Isocarboxazid [Marplan]	Antidepressant—MAO inhibitor; nonselective but isoenzyme A most important; irreversible	Depression	
Isoflurane	Anesthetic	General anesthetic	Best muscle relaxer; most widely used
Isoniazid [INH, Nydrazid]	Antibiotic—inhibits synthesis of mycolic acids	*Mycobacterium* (*M. tuberculosis* and *M. kansasii*) treatment	Peripheral and CNS effects as a result of pyridoxine deficiency; liver damage; hemolytic anemia in G-6-PD deficiency
Isoproterenol [Isuprel]	Bronchodilator—β agonist (nonselective)	Asthma	
Isosorbide dinitrate [Isordil]	Antianginal—stimulates synthesis of cGMP leading to muscle relaxation via NO formation; vasodilator	Angina; CHF	Headache; orthostatic hypotension; syncope; Long-acting
Isotretinoin [Accutane]	Vitamin A analog	Severe acne; psoriasis	Keratinization; teratogenic
Itraconazole [Sporanox]	Antifungal—inhibits ergosterol synthesis, preventing cell membrane formation	Oral for fungal infections (esp. dermatophytoses and onychomycosis)	GI disturbances; hepatotoxicity
Kanamycin [Kantrex]	Antibiotic—aminoglycoside; binds 30S ribosome subunits; bacteriostatic at low concentration; bactericidal at high	Reduction of gut flora	Ototoxicity; neurotoxicity
Ketamine [Ketalar]	Anesthetic agent	General anesthetic	Dissociative anesthesia; catatonia; hallucinations

Therapeutic Agent (common name, if relevant) [Trade name, where appropriate]	Class—Pharmacology and Pharmacokinetics	Indications	Side or Adverse Effects	Contraindications or Precautions to Consider; Notes
Ketoconazole [Nizoral]	Antifungal—inhibits ergosterol synthesis, preventing cell membrane formation; inhibits adrenal and gonadal steroid synthesis	Chronic mucocutaneous candidiasis; blastomycosis; histoplasmosis; prostate carcinoma	Nausea; vomiting; diarrhea; rash; headache; anorexia; thrombocytopenia; gynecomastia; hepatotoxic	Inhibits cytochrome P-450
Labetalol [Normodyne, Trandate]	Antihypertensive—β and α₁ blocker	Hypertension		
Lactulose [Chronulac]	Osmotic laxative	Decreases ammonia in hepatic encephalopathy		
Lamivudine [Epivir]	Antiviral—reverse transcriptase inhibitor	AIDS		
Lamotrigine [Lamictal]	Antiepileptic—blocks Na⁺ channels	Add-on drug for epilepsy		
Leucovorin	Allows stem cells to bypass the inhibition of dihydrofolate reductase caused by methotrexate	Treat acute toxicity of methotrexate		
Leuprolide [Lupron]	GnRH antagonist—suppression of FSH, LH when given continuously	Prostate cancer; polycystic ovary disease; uterine fibroids; endometriosis; precocious puberty		
Levamisole [Ergamisol]	Antihelminthic—immunostimulatory to host; helps rid host of parasite	Ascaris (roundworm); Ancylostoma (hookworm); therapy for immunodeficiency	GI disturbances; rashes; neutropenia	
Levodopa [Larodopa]	Antiparkinsonian agent—precursor of dopamine; administered with carbidopa (most often) or benserazide to inhibit carboxylase deactivation of levodopa in periphery	Parkinson's disease		Inhibited by vitamin B₆; do not give with MAOI or pyridoxine
Levofloxacin [Levaquin]	Quinolone antibiotic—blocks DNA synthesis by inhibiting DNA gyrase	Gram-negative infections (esp. UTI and bone): Pseudomonas, Enterobacteriaceae, Neisseria; Gram-positive infections; intracellular: Legionella	GI disturbances; headache; dizziness; phototoxicity; cartilage damage	May elevate theophylline to toxic levels causing seizure
Levomethadyl	Opioid agonist	Long-lasting maintenance therapy for heroin addiction		

Drug	Class / Mechanism	Clinical Use	Side Effects	Notes
Levothyroxine (T$_4$) [Levothroid]	Synthetic analog of thyroid hormone T$_4$	Replacement therapy for thyroid hormone		
Lidocaine [Xylocaine]	Antiarrhythmic (class IB), anesthetic agent—blocks Na$^+$ channels intracellularly	Local anesthetic; ventricular tachycardia	Sleepiness; light-headedness; visual/audio disturbances; restlessness; nystagmus; shivering; tonic-clonic convulsion; death	Given with epinephrine to maintain locality and increase duration of anesthetic properties via epinephrine-mediated vasoconstriction
Lisinopril [Prinivil, Zestril]	Antihypertensive—vasodilator; ACE inhibitor	CHF	Postural hypotension; renal insufficiency; hyperkalemia; persistent dry cough	Pregnancy
Lithium carbonate [Eskalith, Lithobid, Lithotabs, Lithonate]	Antimanic agent	Manic-depression; cluster headache	Diabetes insipidus; ataxia; tremors; confusion; seizures	
Loperamide [Imodium]	Antidiarrheal—similar to opioid agonist	Oral antidiarrheal		
Loratadine [Claritin]	Antihistamine	Seasonal allergies	Gynecomastia; rare: headache, dizziness, fatigue, CNS, weak antiandrogenic effect, leukopenia, reduced sperm count	Inhibits metabolism or absorption of some drugs
Lorazepam [Ativan]	Antianxiety—benzodiazepine; enhances GABA; increases IPSP amplitude	Sedative; hypnotic; antianxiety; antiepileptic; panic attack		
Losartan [Cozaar]	Antihypertensive—angiotensin II receptor antagonist	Hypertension	Dizziness; upper respiratory infection; headache	
Lovastatin [Mevacor]	Lipid-lowering agent—inhibits HMG-CoA reductase; lowers LDL	Hyperlipidemia (esp. type II)	Liver toxicity; myopathy; mild GI disturbances	Contraindicated in pregnant or lactating women or children
α$_2$-Macroglobulin	Inhibits fibrinolysis			
Magnesium hydroxide [Milk of Magnesia]	Laxative—antacid	Constipation		Diarrhea
Magnesium salts	Osmotic laxative			
Malathion	Organophosphate—inhibits cholinesterase	Least toxic organophosphate		
Mannitol [Osmitrol]	Osmotic diuretic—affects the PCT	Diuresis		
Mebendazole [Vermox]	Antihelminthic—irreversible; inhibits glucose uptake	Hookworm; roundworm; threadworm; some cestodes		
Mecamylamine [Inversine]	Antihypertensive—nicotinic ganglionic blocker	Hypertension emergency; smoking cessation	Decreases GI motility; cycloplegia; hypotension; xerostomia	

Therapeutic Agent (common name, if relevant) [Trade name, where appropriate]	Class—Pharmacology and Pharmacokinetics	Indications	Side or Adverse Effects	Contraindications or Precautions to Consider; Notes
Mechlorethamine (nitrogen mustard) [Mustargen]	Antineoplastic—DNA alkylation and cross-linking	Cancer	Nausea; vomiting; bone marrow suppression; alopecia; teratogenicity; carcinogenicity	
Meclizine [Antivert, Bonine]	Antiemetic agent—H_1 blocker	Emesis; vertigo	Teratogenic	
Mefloquine [Lariam]	Antimalarial—uncertain mechanism	Treatment of acute attack of chloroquine-resistant organisms	CNS: dizziness, disorientation, hallucinations, seizure, depression; GI disturbances; nausea; vomiting; abdominal pain	
Melatonin	Promotes sleep			
Melphalan [Alkeran]	Antineoplastic—DNA alkylation and cross-linking	Cancer	Nausea; vomiting; bone marrow suppression (serious); alopecia; teratogenicity; carcinogenicity; pulmonary fibrosis; hypersensitivity	
Menotropin [Pergonal]	Mixture of FSH and LH	Secondary hypogonadism with infertility		
Meperidine [Demerol]	**Opioid agonist**	**Analgesic; acute migraine attacks**	**CNS excitation at high doses; histamine release**	**Contraindicated in patients with MAOI (results in hyperpyrexia)**
Mephenesin	Centrally acting muscle relaxant	Muscle spasms; tetanus contractions; orthopedic manipulation	Sedation	
Mepivacaine [Isocaine]	Anesthetic agent—blocks Na^+ channels intracellularly	Local anesthetic	Sleepiness; light-headedness; visual/audio disturbances; restlessness; nystagmus; shivering; tonic-clonic convulsion; death	
Mercaptopurine [Purinethol]	Antineoplastic—inhibits purine synthesis; disrupts DNA and RNA synthesis	Childhood leukemias	Bone marrow suppression	
Metformin [Glucophage]	Hypoglycemic agent—decreases glucose production in liver; increases glucose uptake	Oral treatment of NIDDM (type II)	Lactic acidosis	
Methadone [Dolophine]	**Opioid agonist—synthetic**	**Maintenance therapy for heroin addiction**		

Drug	Action/Class	Use	Side Effects/Toxicity	Notes
Methicillin	Antibiotic—β-lactam; penicillinase-resistant	*Staphylococcus* infections		
Methimazole [Tapazole]	**Thyrotoxic agent—inhibits peroxidase enzyme in thyroid; decreases synthesis of thyroid hormone**	**Hyperthyroidism**	**Agranulocytosis**	
Methohexital [Brevital]	Anesthetic agent—barbiturate; prolongs IPSP duration	Antiepileptic; cerebral edema; anesthetic (stage 3 anesthetic)		Ultrashort acting
Methotrexate [Rheumatrex]	**Antineoplastic—dihydrofolate reductase inhibitor; immunosuppressant**	**Rheumatic arthritis; bone marrow transplant; acute lymphocytic and myelogenous leukemia; choriocarcinoma; lung cancer**	**Oral and GI ulceration; bone marrow suppression; thrombocytopenia; leukopenia; hepatotoxic**	**Leucovorin is given as an adjuvant after treatment**
Methoxyflurane [Penthrane]	Anesthetic agent	General anesthetic	Nephrotoxic	
Methylcellulose [Citrucel]	Dietary fiber	Laxative		
Methyldopa [Aldomet]	**Antihypertensive—inhibits sympathetic outflow; centrally acting**	**Hypertension**	**Hemolytic anemia**	**Positive Coombs' test**
Methylphenidate [Ritalin]	CNS stimulant—amphetamine; releases neurotransmitter from synapse	Stimulant; treatment of choice for attention-deficit hyperactivity disorder		
Methysergide [Sansert]	**Antimigraine—5-HT antagonist and weak vasoconstrictor**	**Prophylaxis of migraine**	**GI distress; inflammatory fibrosis of kidney, lung, and cardiac valves**	**Contraindicated in patients with peripheral vascular disease, coronary artery disease, and pregnancy; patient placed on a drug holiday to prevent side effects**
Metoclopramide [Reglan]	**GI stimulant—stimulates ACh (D_2 and 5-HT_3 antagonists); prokinetic**	**Antiemetic; relief of nausea from migraine; increases stomach motility**	**Sleepiness; fatigue; headache; insomnia; dizziness; nausea**	
Metocurine [Metubine Iodide]	**Nondepolarizing neuromuscular blocker**			
Metolazone [Mykrox, Zaroxolyn]	Diuretic—decreases Na^+ reabsorption in the distal tubule by inhibiting the Na^+/Cl^- cotransporter; reduced peripheral resistance	Hypertension, CHF	Hypokalemia; hyperuricemia; hypovolemia; hyperglycemia (especially in diabetics); hypercalcemia; hypersensitivity reaction; Na^+ excretion in advanced renal failure	
Metoprolol [Toprol XL]	Antihypertensive, antiarrhythmic (class II)—β blocker	Hypertension; angina; MI		

Therapeutic Agent (common name, if relevant) [Trade name, where appropriate]	Class–Pharmacology and Pharmacokinetics	Indications	Side or Adverse Effects	Contraindications or Precautions to Consider; Notes
Metronidazole [Flagyl]	Antibiotic—penetrates cell membrane and gives off nitro moiety; reacts with DNA; inhibits replication; bactericidal	*Bacteroides fragilis* (esp. for endocarditis and CNS); amebiasis; giardiasis	Nausea; vomiting; disulfiram-like reaction to alcohol; metallic taste; paresthesia; stomatitis; carcinogenic and mutagenic	Contraindicated in pregnancy
Metyrapone [Metopirone]	Inhibits cortisol synthesis	Diagnosis of pituitary dysfunction		
Mevastatin	Lipid-lowering agent—inhibits HMG-CoA reductase; lowers LDL	Hyperlipidemia (esp. type II)	Liver toxicity; myopathy; mild GI disturbances	Contraindicated in pregnant or lactating women or children
Mexiletine [Mexitil]	Antiarrhythmic (class IB)—Na^+-channel blocker			
Mezlocillin [Mezlin]	Antibiotic—β-lactam	*Pseudomonas; Proteus*		IV
Miconazole [Monistat IV]	Antifungal—inhibits ergosterol synthesis, preventing cell membrane formation	Broad-spectrum, including yeasts and dermatophytes	Burning, itching, and redness when used topically; thrombophlebitis; nausea; vomiting; anaphylaxis when used IV	
Milrinone [Primacor]	Inotropic agent—phosphodiesterase inhibitor; increases contractility via increase in intracellular Ca^{2+}	CHF		
Mineral oil [Fleet Mineral Oil Enema]	Laxative	May interfere with absorption of fat-soluble vitamins		
Minoxidil [Loniten, Rogaine]	Antihypertensive—hair growth stimulant; vasodilator	CHF, hypertension	Hypertrichosis (hair growth)	
Misoprostol [Cytotec]	Antiulcer—PGE_1	Protects against ulcers	Diarrhea; nausea; miscarriages	
Molindone [Moban]	Antipsychotic—blocks D_2 receptors	Psychosis	Parkinsonism; tardive dyskinesia	
Moricizine [Ethmozine]	Antiarrhythmic (class IC)—Na^+-channel blockers	Ventricular arrhythmia	Dizziness; nausea	
Morphine [Astramorph, Duramorph, Infumorph, Kadian, MS Contin, Oramorph, MSIR, Roxanol]	Opioid agonist—converted to more potent morphine-6-glucose	Severe pain; general anesthetic; antitussive; antidiarrheal	Histamine release; constipation; nausea	
Muromonab (OKT3)	Immunosuppressant—monoclonal antibody against CD3 on T lymphocytes	Acute rejection of renal transplants		

Drug	Mechanism/Class	Clinical Use	Side Effects	Contraindicated in patients with peptic ulcer, asthma, hyperthyroid, Parkinson's disease
Muscarine	Muscarinic agonist		Abdominal pain; diarrhea; bronchoconstriction	
Nabilone [Cesamet]	Antiemetic—unknown mechanism; binds opiate receptors and directly inhibits vomiting center in medulla	Emesis	Dry mouth; dizziness; inability to concentrate; disorientation; anxiety; tachycardia; depression; paranoia; psychosis	THC derivative
***N*-Acetylcysteine [Mucomyst]**	Mucolytic—replenishes glutathione	Overdose of acetaminophen; liquefy sputum to assist expulsion		
Nadolol [Corgard]	Antihypertensive—antianginal; β blocker	Hypertension; angina		
Nafcillin [Unipen]	Antibiotic—β-lactam; penicillinase-resistant	*Staphylococcus* infections		
Naftifine [Naftin]	Antifungal—inhibits squalene-2,3-epoxidase	Topical for tinea cruris and tinea corporis		
Nalbuphine [Nubain]	Mixed agonist/antagonist of opioids	Similar to pentazocine		
Nalidixic acid [NegGram]	Antibiotic—urinary antiseptic; unknown mechanism of action	Coliform UTIs		
Nalorphine	Mixed agonist/antagonist of opioids	Antagonizes effects of morphine	Respiratory depression; analgesia	
Naloxone [Narcan]	Antagonist of all opioids	Drug of choice for opioid antagonism	Ineffective to use against barbiturate overdose, but safe	
Naltrexone [ReVia]	Antagonist of all opioids	Longer action than naloxone; can be used orally		
Naproxen [Naprosyn]	NSAID	Inflammation; pain	GI side effects, fewer than aspirin	
Natamycin [Natacyn]	Antifungal—binds to cell membrane sterols (esp. ergosterol); forms pores in membrane; fungicidal	Topical for fungal keratitis (eye)		
Nefazodone [Serzone]	Antidepressant—postsynaptic 5-HT$_2$ antagonist	Depression		
Nelfinavir	Antiviral—protease inhibitor	AIDS		
Neomycin [Mycifradin, Neosporin]	Antibiotic—lipid-lowering agent; lowers LDL; inhibits resorption of cholesterol and bile acids; aminoglycoside; binds 30S ribosome subunits; bacteriostatic at low concentration; bactericidal at high	Hyperlipidemia; reduction of gut flora		Inhibits absorption of digitalis

Therapeutic Agent (common name, if relevant) [Trade name, where appropriate]	Class—Pharmacology and Pharmacokinetics	Indications	Side or Adverse Effects	Contraindications or Precautions to Consider; Notes
Neostigmine [Prostigmin]	**Inhibits cholinesterase**	**Paralytic ileus; neurogenic bladder; myasthenia gravis**		
Niclosamide [Niclocide]	Antihelminthic—inhibits anaerobic metabolism	Tapeworms: *Taenia solium, Taenia saginata, Hymenolepis nana*		
Nicotine [Habitrol Nicoderm, Nicotrol]	**Nicotinic agonist**	**Stop smoking**		
Nifedipine [Adalat, Procardia]	**Antianginal—Ca²⁺-channel blocker**	**Angina, hypertension**	**Dizziness; nausea; headache; gingival problems**	
Niridazole	Antihelminthic—induces breakdown of glycogen; inhibits glucose uptake	Schistosomes	CNS; inhibits spermatogenesis; ECG changes; GI disturbances	Contraindicated in patients with hepatosplenic form of disease—more likely to cause CNS problems
Nitrofurantoin [Furadantin]	Antibiotic—urinary antiseptic; unknown mechanism of action	Gram-positive and -negative bacteria		Contraindicated in patients with renal insufficiency
Nitroglycerin [Deponit]	**Antianginal—stimulates synthesis of cGMP leading to muscle relaxation via NO formation**	**Angina**	**Headache; orthostatic hypotension; syncope**	**Monday disease; short-acting**
Nitrosoureas	Antineoplastic—alkylating agent; lipid-soluble	CNS tumors		
Nitrous oxide	Anesthetic agent	General anesthetic	Hypoxia	
Nizatidine [Axid]	H₂ blocker	Inhibits gastric acid secretion (esp. ulcer)	Gynecomastia; rare: headache, dizziness, fatigue, CNS, weak antiandrogenic effect, leukopenia, reduced sperm count	Inhibits metabolism or absorption of some drugs
Nortriptyline [Pamelor]	Antidepressant—TCA; blocks NE, 5-HT, muscarinic, α₁, histamine receptors	Depression	Tremors (NE block); anorexia (5-HT block); anticholinergic (muscarinic block); hypotension (α₁ block); drowsiness (histamine block)	
Nystatin [Mycostatin]	**Antifungal—binds to cell membrane sterols (esp. ergosterol); forms pores in membrane; fungicidal**	**Mucosal candida infections (skin, vaginal, GI)**	**Few**	

Octreotide [Sandostatin]	Analog of somatostatin—decreases release of GH, gastrin, secretin, VIP, CCK, glucagon, insulin	Acromegaly; glucagonoma; insulinoma; carcinoid syndrome	Nausea; cramps; gallstones
Ofloxacin [Floxin]	Quinolone antibiotic—blocks DNA synthesis by inhibiting DNA gyrase	Gram-negative infections (esp. UTI and bone): *Pseudomonas, Enterobacteriaceae, Neisseria*; Gram-positive infections; intracellular: *Legionella*	GI disturbances; headache; dizziness; phototoxicity; cartilage damage	May elevate theophylline to toxic levels causing seizure
Olanzapine [Zyprexa]	Antipsychotic	Psychosis	
Omeprazole [Prilosec]	Antiulcer—proton pump inhibitor; blocks H^+/K^+ ATPase	Reduce gastric acid secretion		Inhibits cytochrome P-450; given with clarithromycin and amoxicillin for *Helicobacter pylori*
Ondansetron [Zofran]	Antiemetic—5-HT$_3$ blocker	Emesis (caused by cancer therapy)	Headache; constipation; dizziness
Oxacillin [Bactocill]	Antibiotic—β-lactam; penicillinase-resistant	*Staphylococcus* infections	
Oxaprozin [Daypro]	NSAID—mildly uricosuric	Acute gout		Contraindicated in patients with kidney stones
Oxazepam [Serax]	Antianxiety—benzodiazepine; enhances GABA; increases IPSP amplitude	Sedative; hypnotic; antiepileptic	
Oxybutynin [Ditropan]	Antimuscarinic	Bladder/GI spasm; decrease acid in ulcer	
Oxytocin [Syntocinon]	Stimulates uterine contraction; contraction of breast myoepithelial cells; milk letdown reflex	Induce labor	
Paclitaxel [Taxol]	Antineoplastic—polymerizes tubules	Ovarian and breast cancer	
Pamidronate [Aredia]	Bone stabilizer—pyrophosphate analog; reduces hydroxyapatite crystal formation, growth and dissolution, which reduces bone turnover	Hypercalcemia of malignancy; Paget's disease; osteoporosis; hyperparathyroidism	
Pancuronium [Pavulon]	Nondepolarizing neuromuscular blocker			Minimal histamine release
Paroxetine [Paxil]	Antidepressant—SSRI	Depression; anxiety	Nausea; headache; insomnia
Penicillamine [Cuprimine, Depen]	Antiarthritis—antigold medicine; not specific; unknown mechanism; arthritis relief	Rheumatic arthritis; copper poisoning; metal chelator	Decreases vitamin B$_6$; bone marrow suppression; proteinuria; autoimmune syndrome

Therapeutic Agent (common name, if relevant) [Trade name, where appropriate]	Class—Pharmacology and Pharmacokinetics	Indications	Side or Adverse Effects	Contraindications or Precautions to Consider; Notes
Penicillin	**Antibiotic—inhibits transpeptidase and cell wall synthesis**	**Gram-positive bacteria: aerobic, some anaerobic, and spirochetes**	**Allergic reactions; platelet aggregation problems; direct CNS toxicity; superinfections**	
Pentazocine [Talwin]	Mixed agonist/antagonist of opioids	Analgesia		Only mixed agonist/antagonist available orally
Pentobarbital [Nembutal sodium]	Barbiturate—prolongs IPSP duration	Cerebral edema; anesthetic		
Pergolide [Permax]	Antiparkinsonian—dopamine agonist; inhibits prolactin release	Treat breast engorgement; inhibits lactation		
Phenazocine	Opioid agonist			
Phenobarbital	**Barbiturate—prolongs IPSP duration**	**Antiepileptic (partial and tonic-clonic); cerebral edema; anesthetic**		
Phenolphthalein [Ex-Lax]	Laxative—reduces absorption of electrolytes and water from gut	Stimulant laxative	Tumorigenic	
Phenoxybenzamine [Dibenzyline]	Antihypertensive—α blocker; long-acting; irreversible	Pheochromocytoma	Nasal congestion; miosis; orthostatic hypotension	
Phentolamine [Regitine]	**Antihypertensive—α blocker**	Diagnosis of pheochromocytoma; hypertension (especially tyrosine-induced)		
Phenylbutazone [Butazolidin]	**NSAID**	Rheumatic arthritis; acute gout	**Agranulocytosis; aplastic anemia**	
Phenylephrine [Neo-Synephrine, Nostril]	Nasal decongestant—α₁-agonist	Tachycardia		
Phenylzin	Antidepressant—MAOI; nonselective but isoenzyme A most important; irreversible	Depression		
Phenytoin [Dilantin]	Antiepileptic—decreases Na$^+$ flux	Epilepsy (partial and tonic-clonic); digitalis-induced arrhythmia	Decreases folic acid; gingival hyperplasia; hirsutism; nystagmus	Induces cytochrome P-450
Physostigmine [Eserine]	Inhibits cholinesterase	Intestinal or bladder atony; glaucoma		
Pilocarpine [Ocusert]	Antiglaucoma—muscarinic agonist	Xerostomia; narrow- and open-angle glaucoma	Focusing problems; nausea; abdominal pain; sweating; high dose: bradycardia, hypotension	Contraindicated in patients with peptic ulcer, asthma, hyperthyroid, Parkinson's disease

Drug [brand]	Classification / Mechanism	Clinical use	Side effects	Notes
Pindolol [Visken]	Antihypertensive antiarrhythmic (class II)—β blocker	Hypertension		
Piperacillin [Pipracil]	Antibiotic—β-lactam	*Pseudomonas; Proteus*		IV
Piperazine [Entacyl]	Antihelminthic—causes flaccid paralysis in worm	Ascariasis (roundworm); Oxyuriasis (pinworm)	GI disturbances; urticaria; minor CNS	
Piroxicam [Feldene]	NSAID			Long-acting; contraindicated in the elderly
Platelet-activating factor [PAF]	Activation of platelets and PMN aggregation; increases vascular permeability			
Plicamycin [Mithracin]	Antineoplastic—inhibits DNA-directed RNA synthesis; decreases protein synthesis needed for bone reabsorption	Paget's disease; hypercalcemia		
Polymyxins [Aerosporin]	**Antibiotic—disrupts cell membranes; bactericidal**	**Gram-negative bacteria: *Pseudomonas* and coliforms; topical only; intrathecal for *Pseudomonas* meningitis**	**Neurotoxic; nephrotoxic**	
Potassium iodide [Thyro-Block]	Expectorant—increases bronchial secretions; high doses decrease release of thyroid hormone	Promote cough; hyperthyroidism		
Pralidoxime [Protopam]	**Acetylcholinesterase reactivator**	**Overdose of malathion/parathion organophosphates; must be used before aging occurs**		
Pravastatin [Pravachol]	Lipid-lowering agent—inhibits HMG-CoA reductase; lowers LDL	Hyperlipidemia (esp. type II)	Liver toxicity; myopathy; mild GI disturbances	Contraindicated in pregnant or lactating women or children
Praziquantel [Biltricide]	Antihelminthic—increases membrane permeability causing loss of Ca^{2+}	Schistosomes; flukes	GI disturbances; headache; fever; urticaria	
Prazosin [Minipress]	**Antihypertensive—α_1 blocker**	**Pheochromocytoma; hypertension**	**Postural hypotension**	
Prednisone [Deltasone]	**Glucocorticoid—inhibits protein synthesis; reduces lymph node and spleen size; inhibits cell cycle activity of lymphoid cells; lyses T cells; suppresses antibody, prostaglandin, and leukotriene synthesis; blocks monocyte production of IL-1**	**Rheumatic arthritis; autoimmune disorders; allergic reaction; asthma; organ transplant (esp. during rejection crisis)**	**Osteoporosis; cushingoid reaction; psychosis; glucose intolerance; infection; hypertension; cataracts**	

Therapeutic Agent (common name, if relevant) [Trade name, where appropriate]	Class—Pharmacology and Pharmacokinetics	Indications	Side or Adverse Effects	Contraindications or Precautions to Consider; Notes
Prilocaine [Citanest]	Anesthetic agent—blocks Na$^+$ channels intracellularly	Local anesthetic	Sleepiness; light-headedness; visual/audio disturbances; restlessness; nystagmus; shivering; tonic-clonic convulsion; death	
Primaquine phosphate [Primaquine Phosphate]	Antimalarial—unknown mechanism	Cures vivax malaria; prophylaxis for falciparum malaria	GI disturbances; mild anemia; marked hemolysis in G-6-PD-deficient individuals; prolongs QT interval	
Probenecid [Benemid]	Antigout—small dose inhibits uric acid secretion; large dose inhibits uric acid reabsorption (e.g., promotes excretion) of uric acid	Chronic gout	Rash; GI disturbances; drowsy	Acute gout
Probucol [Bifenabid, Lesterol]	Lipid-lowering agent—lowers HDL and LDL; mechanism unknown	Hyperlipidemia	Prolongs QT interval; GI disturbances	Contraindicated in patients with heart disease
Procainamide [Pronestyl, Procanbid]	Antiarrhythmic (class IA)—Na$^+$-channel blocker	Ventricular arrhythmia	Lupuslike syndrome	
Procaine [Novocain]	Anesthetic agent—blocks Na$^+$ intracellularly	Local anesthetic	Sleepiness; light-headedness; visual/audio disturbances; restlessness; nystagmus; shivering; tonic-clonic convulsion; death	
Procarbazine [Matulane]	Antineoplastic—DNA alkylation and strand breakage; inhibits nucleic acid and protein synthesis	Cancer		
Prochlorperazine [Compazine]	Antiemetic—D$_2$ receptor antagonist	Counteract nausea of migraine; antiemetic	Teratogenic	
Progesterone [Progestasert]	Hormone—secretory changes in endometrium and breast; necessary to maintain pregnancy	Treat primary hypogonadism; relief of menopause; decrease osteoporosis; suppress dysmenorrhea and excess androgen secretion by ovary; used in combination with estrogen for oral contraception	Long-lasting suppression of menses; endometriosis; hirsutism; bleeding disorders; nausea; breast tenderness; hyperpigmentation; gallbladder disease; migraines; hypertension	
Prolactin	Hormone—stimulates lactation of breast			

Drug	Description	Use	Side effects	
Promethazine [Phenergan]	Antihistamine—antiemetic; D$_2$ receptor antagonist; H$_1$ blocker	Counteract nausea of migraine; allergies; motion sickness	Sedation; CNS depression; atropinelike effects; allergic dermatitis; blood dyscrasias; teratogenicity; acute antihistamine poisoning	
Propafenone [Rythmol]	Antiarrhythmic (class IC)—Na$^+$-channel blocker			
Propofol [Diprivan]	Anesthetic agent	General anesthetic; fast-acting for ambulatory or outpatients	Seizure	
Propranolol [Inderal]	**Antihypertensive; antianginal; antiarrhythmic (class II)—antimigraine; β blocker**	**Hypertension; angina; MI; arrhythmias; prophylaxis of migraine**	**Reduces renin secretion**	
Propylthiouracil [PropylThyracil]	**Inhibits peroxidase enzyme in thyroid; decreases synthesis of thyroid hormone**	**Hyperthyroidism**	**Agranulocytosis**	
Protriptyline [Vivactil]	Antidepressant—TCA; blocks NE, 5-HT, muscarinic, α$_1$, and histamine receptors	Depression	Tremors (NE block); anorexia (5-HT block); anticholinergic (muscarinic block); hypotension (α$_1$ block); drowsiness (histamine block)	
Psyllium [Per diem Fiber]	Laxative—dietary fiber	Constipation		
PTH	Increases plasma Ca^{2+} levels by increasing reabsorption in kidney; activates vitamin D, which aids in Ca^{2+} absorption from gut; resorbs Ca^{2+} from bone; decreases phosphate reabsorption by kidney	Used to distinguish between hypoparathyroidism and pseudohypoparathyroidism		
Pyrantel [Antiminth, Reese's Pinworm Medicine]	Antihelminthic—depolarizing neuromuscular blocker causing spastic paralysis in worms	*Ascaris* (roundworm); *Ancylostoma* (hookworm); Threadworm		
Pyrazinamide	Antibiotic	*Mycobacterium*	Impairs liver function	
Pyridostigmine [Mestinon]	**Inhibits cholinesterase**	**Myasthenia gravis**		
Pyrimethamine [Daraprim]	Antimalarial—inhibits dihydrofolate reductase	Malaria	Large doses cause megaloblastic anemia	
Quetiapine	**Antipsychotic**	**Psychosis**		
Quinacrine [Atabrine]	Antiprotozoal—unknown mechanism	*Giardia*	Headache; nausea; vomiting; blood dyscrasias; yellow staining of skin; exfoliative dermatitis; retinopathy	
Quinapril [Accupril]	Antihypertensive—vasodilator; ACE inhibitor	CHF	Postural hypotension; renal insufficiency; hyperkalemia; persistent dry cough	Contraindicated in pregnancy

Therapeutic Agent (common name, if relevant) [Trade name, where appropriate]	Class–Pharmacology and Pharmacokinetics	Indications	Side or Adverse Effects	Contraindications or Precautions to Consider; Notes
Quinidine [Quinaglute]	Antiarrhythmic (class IA)—Na^+-channel blocker	Arrhythmias; acute malarial infection	May precipitate arrhythmias at high doses; nausea; vomiting; diarrhea; cinchonism: tinnitus, headache, nausea, disturbed vision; renal damage; hemolytic anemia; purpura; agranulocytosis	Torsades des pointes
Quinine	Antimalarial—unknown mechanism	Suppression and treatment of acute attack of chloroquine-resistant organism; leg cramps	Cinchonism: tinnitus, headache, nausea, disturbed vision; renal damage; hemolytic anemia; purpura; agranulocytosis	
Quinolones	Antibiotic—blocks DNA synthesis by inhibiting DNA gyrase	Gram-negative infections (esp. UTI and bone): *Pseudomonas, Enterobacteriaceae, Neisseria;* Gram-positive infections; intracellular: *Legionella*	GI disturbances; headache; dizziness; phototoxicity; cartilage damage	May elevate theophylline to toxic levels causing seizure
Radioiodide [I-131]	Destroys thyroid gland	Hyperthyroidism	Hypothyroidism	
Ranitidine [Zantac]	H_2 blocker	Inhibits gastric acid secretion (esp. ulcer)	Gynecomastia; rare: headache, dizziness, fatigue, CNS, leukopenia, reduced sperm count	Inhibits metabolism or absorption of some drugs
Reserpine [Reserfia]	Antihypertensive—prevents storage of monoamines in synaptic vesicle	Hypertension	Mental depression	
RhoGAM	Rh immunoglobulin	Prevents hemolytic disease of the newborn		
Ribavirin	Antiviral—guanosine analog	RSV in children; hepatitis C when given with interferon	Headache; rash; fatigue; dyspnea	
Rifampin [Rifadin]	Antibiotic—inhibits DNA-dependent RNA polymerase	*Mycobacterium*	Orange body fluids	Interferes with birth control pills by increasing estrogen metabolism; induces cytochrome *P-450*
Risperidone [Risperdal]	Antipsychotic—blocks D_2 and $5-HT_2$ receptors	Psychosis		
Ritodrine [Yutopar]	$β_2$ agonist	Inhibits preterm labor; relaxes uterus		
Ritonavir [Norvir]	Antiviral—protease inhibitor	AIDS		

Drug	Mechanism/Category	Clinical use	Side effects/Toxicity
Ropivacaine	Anesthetic agent—blocks Na$^+$ intracellularly	Local anesthetic	Sleepiness; light-headedness; visual/audio disturbances; restlessness; nystagmus; shivering; tonic-clonic convulsion; death
Saquinavir [Invirase]	Antiviral—protease inhibitor	AIDS	
Sarin/Soman	Inhibits cholinesterase	Rapidly fatal	
Scopolamine [Transderm Scop]	Cholinergic blocker	Motion sickness; Parkinson's disease; antiemetic	
Scorpion toxin	Presynaptic neuromuscular junction blocker; overstimulates ACh release		
Secobarbital [Seconal]	Antiepileptic—anesthetic agent; barbiturate; prolongs IPSP duration	Epilepsy; cerebral edema	
Selegiline [Eldepryl]	Antiparkinsonian—increases dopamine by inhibiting MAO$_b$ irreversibly	Parkinson's disease	
Sertraline [Zoloft]	Antidepressant—SSRI	Depression	Nausea; headache; insomnia
Sevoflurane [Sevorane, Ultrane]	Anesthetic agent	General anesthetic	
Sildenafil [Viagra]	**Phosphodiesterase type 5 inhibitor (cGMP-specific)**	**Erectile dysfunction**	**Abnormal vision; UTIs; cardiovascular events; priapism; dyspepsia**
Simvastatin [Zocor]	Lipid-lowering agent—inhibits HMG-CoA reductase; lowers LDL	Hyperlipidemia (esp. type II)	Liver toxicity; myopathy; mild GI disturbances
Sodium nitroprusside	Antianginal—antihypertensive; vasodilator (arterial dilation)	CHF; hypertensive emergency	Cyanide toxicity; hypotension
Somatostatin [Zecnil]	**Hormone—decreases release of GH, gastrin, secretin, VIP, CCK, glucagon, insulin**	**Acromegaly; glucagonoma; insulinoma**	**Nausea; cramps; gallstones**
Sotalol [Betapace]	Antiarrhythmic (class III)—K$^+$-channel blocker	Torsades de pointes	
Spectinomycin [Trobicin]	Antibiotic—aminoglycoside; binds 30S ribosome subunits; bacteriostatic at low concentration; bactericidal at high	Used to treat gonorrhea in those allergic to penicillin	Contraindicated in pregnant or lactating women or children
Spironolactone [Aldactone]	**K$^+$-sparing diuretic; aldosterone antagonist acts at DCT**	**Diuresis**	**Hyperkalemia; gynecomastia; impotence; GI disturbances**
Streptokinase [Streptase]	**Thrombolytic—plasminogen activator**	**Lysis of clots**	**Hemorrhage**

Therapeutic Agent (common name, if relevant) [Trade name, where appropriate]	Class–Pharmacology and Pharmacokinetics	Indications	Side or Adverse Effects	Contraindications or Precautions to Consider; Notes
Streptomycin	**Antibiotic—aminoglycoside; binds 30S ribosome subunits; bacteriostatic at low concentration; bactericidal at high**	**Tuberculosis and other mycobacteria**		
Strychnine	Acts on the postsynaptic Renshaw cell; binds to glycine receptor (mimics effect of tetanus)	Depression		
Succinylcholine [Anectine]	**Depolarizing neuromuscular blocker**	**Rapid-sequence intubation**	**Increases intraocular pressure; succinylcholine apnea in genetically defective pseudocholinesterase; malignant hyperthermia if given with halothane**	**Contraindicated in patients with glaucoma, antibiotics**
Sucralfate [Carafate]	Antiulcer—protective coating of GI lining	Reduces effect of gastric acid on mucosa	Constipation	
Sulfinpyrazone [Anturane]	Antigout—uricosuric (similar to probenecid)	Chronic gout	GI irritation; hypersensitivity reaction; agranulocytosis	
Sulfonamides	**Antibiotic—competitive inhibitor of dihydropteroate synthetase (blocks folic acid synthesis)**	**Broad-spectrum; Gram-positive UTI; *Chlamydia* infection of genital tract and eye; treatment of nocardiosis**	**Form crystals in kidney and bladder causing damage, nausea, vomiting, headache**	
Sulindac [Clinoril]	Anti-inflammatory—prodrug sulfide	Chronic inflammation (arthritis)		
Sumatriptan [Imitrex]	**Antimigraine—agonist at 5-HT$_{1d}$ receptors**	**Acute attack of migraine**		
Syrup of Ipecac [Quelidrine]	Expectorant—increases bronchial secretions	Promotes cough		
Tacrine [Cognex]	**Alzheimer's agent—noncompetitive cholinesterase inhibitor; muscarinic agonist**	**Alzheimer's disease**	**Hepatotoxicity**	
Tacrolimus (FK506) [Prograf]	**Immunosuppressant—blocks activation of T-cell transcription factors; involved in interleukin synthesis**	**Transplant rejection**	**Nephrotoxic; neurotoxic; hyperglycemia; GI disturbances**	
Tamoxifen [Nolvadex]	**Antineoplastic—competitive estrogen receptor blocker**	**Treats estrogen-dependent breast cancer in postmenopausal women; reduces contralateral breast cancer**	**May increase risk of other cancer; hot flashes; flushing**	

Drug	Mechanism/Class	Indication	Side Effects/Notes
Temazepam [Restoril]	Benzodiazepine—enhances GABA; increases IPSP amplitude	Sedative; hypnotic; antianxiety; antiepileptic	
Terazosin [Hytrin]	Antihypertensive—α_1 blocker	Pheochromocytoma; hypertension; benign prostatic hyperplasia	Postural hypotension
Terbinafine [Lamisil]	Antifungal—inhibits squalene-2,3-epoxidase	Orally for onychomycosis; topically for dermatophytes	
Terbutaline [Brethine, Bricanyl, Brethaire]	**Bronchodilator—β_2 agonist**	**Bronchodilates to treat asthma; inhibits preterm labor; relaxes uterus**	
Tetanus toxin	**Acts at the presynaptic Renshaw cell; prevents glycine release**		
Tetracaine [Pontocaine]	Anesthetic agent—blocks Na^+ channels intracellularly	Local anesthetic	Sleepiness; light-headedness; visual/audio disturbances; restlessness; nystagmus; shivering; tonic-clonic convulsion; death
Tetracycline [Achromycin, Sumycin, Topicycline]	**Antibiotic—binds 30S ribosome subunits; bacteriostatic**	**Broad-spectrum including Chlamydia, Rickettsia, and Mycoplasma**	**Liver toxicity; depression of bone/teeth development; phototoxic reactions; superinfections owing to broad-spectrum; Fanconi's syndrome. Contraindicated in pregnancy and children**
THC (active ingredient in marijuana)	Unknown mechanism; binds opiate receptors and directly inhibits vomiting center in medulla	Antiemetic	Dry mouth; dizziness; inability to concentrate; disorientation; anxiety; tachycardia; depression; paranoia; psychosis
Theobromine	Unknown mechanism; stimulates CNS, cardiac muscle; relaxes smooth muscle; produces diuresis; increases cerebral vascular resistance		
Theophylline [Aerolate, Elixophyllin, Respbid, Slo-bid, Slo-Phyllin, Theo-24, Theo-Dur, Theolair, T-Ohyl, Uniphyl]	**Bronchodilator—unknown mechanism; stimulates CNS, cardiac muscle; relaxes smooth muscle; produces diuresis; increases cerebral vascular resistance**	**Asthma**	**Tolerance develops**
Thiabendazole [Mintezol]	**Antihelminthic**	***Strongyloides; Ancylostoma* (hookworm); *Enterobius* (pinworm); *Trichuris* (whipworm)**	**Vomiting; diarrhea; dizziness; bradycardia; hypotension; paresthesias; yellow vision; angioneurotic edema; perianal rashes**
6-Thioguanine	Antineoplastic—inhibits purine synthesis; disrupts DNA and RNA synthesis	Adult leukemias	Bone marrow suppression

Therapeutic Agent (common name, if relevant) [Trade name, where appropriate]	Class–Pharmacology and Pharmacokinetics	Indications	Side or Adverse Effects	Contraindications or Precautions to Consider; Notes
Thiopental [Pentothal]	Anesthetic agent—barbiturate; prolongs IPSP duration	Antiepileptic; cerebral edema; anesthetic (stage 3 anesthetic)	Laryngospasm during stage 3 induction	
Thioridazine [Mellaril]	Antipsychotic—blocks D_2 receptors	Psychosis	Orthostatic hypotension; anticholinergic effects; sedation	
Thiotepa [Thioplex]	Antineoplastic—unknown mechanism	Cancer		
Thiothixene [Navane]	Antipsychotic—blocks D_2 receptors	Psychosis	Anticholinergic effects	
Ticarcillin [Ticar]	Antibiotic—β-lactam	*Pseudomonas; Proteus*		IV; given with clavulanic acid
Ticlopidine [Ticlid]	**Inhibits ADP-induced platelet aggregation; acts on ADP receptor**	**Transient ischemic attack; stroke**		
Timentin	Inhibits β-lactamase; synergistic with penicillins			
Timolol [Betimol, Blocadren, Timoptic]	Antiglaucoma—antihypertensive; β blocker	Hypertension; MI; glaucoma	Asthma	
Tizanidine [Zanaflex]	Centrally acting muscle relaxant—presynaptic inhibition of motor neurons; acts like clonidine on α_2	Muscle spasms from spinal cord injury; multiple sclerosis		
Tobramycin [Tobrex]	Antibiotic—binds 30S ribosome subunits; bacteriostatic at low concentration; bactericidal at high	Similar to gentamicin		
Tocainide [Tonocard]	Antiarrhythmic (class IB)—Na^+-channel blocker			
Tolazamide [Tolinase]	Hypoglycemic agent—sulfonylurea; reduces K^+ efflux, increases Ca^{2+} influx, increases secretion of insulin	Oral treatment for NIDDM (type II diabetes)	Hypoglycemia; GI disturbances; muscle weakness; mental confusion	
Tolbutamide [Orinase]	Hypoglycemic agent—sulfonylurea; reduces K^+ efflux, increases Ca^{2+} influx, increases secretion of insulin	Oral treatment for NIDDM (type II diabetes)	Hypoglycemia; GI disturbances; muscle weakness; mental confusion	
Tolnaftate [Tinactin, Desenex]	Antifungal—unknown mechanism; bactericidal	Topical against *Trichophyton rubrum*, *Trichophyton tonsurans*, *Trichophyton versicolor*, *Trichophyton mentagrophytes*		
Topiramate [Topamax]	Antiepileptic—blocks Na^+ channels	Add-on drug for epilepsy		

Drug	Mechanism	Use	Adverse effects	Notes
Torsemide [Demadex]	Loop diuretic; inhibits Na⁺/K⁺/Cl⁻ channel	Diuresis	Ototoxicity; metabolic alkalosis; hypokalemia; hyperglycemia; hyperuricemia	
tPA [Activase]	**Thrombolytic—plasminogen activator**	**Lysis of clots**	**Hemorrhage**	
Tramadol [Ultram]	Analgesic—similar to opioid agonist	Chronic pain of osteoarthritis		
Tranexamic acid (AMCHA) [Cyklokapron]	Thrombotic agent—competitive inhibitor of plasminogen activation	Inhibits fibrinolysis; promotes thrombosis		
Tranylcypromine [Parnate]	Antidepressant—MAOI; nonselective, but isoenzyme A most important; reversible	Depression		Only reversible MAOI
TRH (protirelin) [Relefact TRH]	Stimulates TSH, prolactin, release	Diagnosis of thyroid disease		
Triamterene [Dyrenium]	Diuretic—K⁺-sparing diuretic; decreases K⁺ secretion and Na⁺ resorption in DCT	Diuresis	Hyperkalemia	
Triazolam [Halcion]	Benzodiazepine—enhances GABA; increases IPSP amplitude	Sedative; hypnotic; antianxiety; antiepileptic	Paranoia; violent behavior	
Trientine	Metal chelator	Copper poisoning; Wilson's disease		
Trifluridine [Viroptic]	Antiviral—thymidine derivative; inhibits DNA polymerase; inhibits DNA synthesis	DNA viruses		
Trihexyphenidyl [Artane]	Antiparkinsonian—muscarinic blocker	Parkinson's disease		
Trimethaphan [Arfonad]	Antihypertensive—nondepolarizing nicotinic blocker	Hypertension (short term)		
Trimethoprim [Proloprim, Trimpex]	**Antibiotic—competitive inhibition of dihydrofolate reductase (blocks folic acid synthesis)**	**Gram-negative UTI; combined with sulfonamides to treat UTI, otitis media, chronic bronchitis, shigellosis, and PCP**		
Trovafloxacin [Trovan]	Quinolone antibiotic—blocks DNA synthesis by inhibiting DNA gyrase	Gram-negative infections (esp. UTI and bone): *Pseudomonas, Enterobacteriaceae, Neisseria*; Gram positive infections; intracellular: *Legionella*	GI disturbances; headache; dizziness; phototoxicity; cartilage damage in children	May elevate theophylline to toxic levels causing seizure
TSH (thyrotropin) [Thyrogen]	**Increases output of thyroid hormone**	**Assess thyroid function; increase uptake of I-131 in thyroid carcinoma**		
d-Tubocurarine [Tubarine]	Nondepolarizing neuromuscular blocker			

Therapeutic Agent (common name, if relevant) [Trade name, where appropriate]	Class–Pharmacology and Pharmacokinetics	Indications	Side or Adverse Effects	Contraindications or Precautions to Consider; Notes
Undecylenic acid [Desenex]	Antifungal—unknown mechanism; fungistatic	Topical for dermatophytes (esp. tinea pedis)		
Urofollitropin [Metrodin]	FSH analog	Infertility		
Urokinase [Abbokinase]	Thrombolytic agent— plasminogen activator	Lysis of clots	Hemorrhage	
Valacyclovir [Valtrex]	Antiviral—guanosine analog; inhibits DNA polymerase	Herpes; varicella; EBV and CMV at high doses	GI disturbances; CNS and renal problems; headache; tremor; rash	Longer-lasting than acyclovir
Valproic acid [Depakene]	Antiepileptic—blocks Na$^+$ channels and increases GABA	Epilepsy: partial, absence, and tonic-clonic	Liver toxicity; pancreatitis; potentially fatal	
Vancomycin [Vancocin]	Antibiotic—disrupts cell wall and cell membrane; bactericidal	Serious infections by Gram-positive bacteria: *Streptococcus, Staphylococcus, Pneumococcus,* and some anaerobes (esp. *Clostridium difficile*)	Ototoxicity; nephrotoxicity; "red man syndrome"; caused by histamine release	
Vasopressin [Pitressin]	Antidiuretic—recruits water channels to luminal membrane in collecting duct	Antidiuresis; treats central diabetes insipidus	Overhydration; allergic reaction; larger doses: pallor, diarrhea, hypertension; coronary constriction; chronic rhinopharyngitis	Also known as ADH, AVP
Vecuronium [Norcuron]	Nondepolarizing neuromuscular blocker			
Verapamil [Calan, Isoptin]	Antiarrhythmic (class IV)—Ca^{2+} blocker	Atrial tachyarrhythmia; decreases reperfusion injury	AV block; constipation; hypotension; GI distress	
Vidarabine [Vira-A]	Antiviral—adenosine analog; inhibits DNA polymerase	Herpes (also topical for HSV keratitis); varicella	GI disturbances; CNS, bone marrow suppression; liver and kidney dysfunction	
Vinblastine [Velban]	Antineoplastic—depolymerizes microtubules	Hodgkin's disease	Peripheral neuritis	
Vincristine [Oncovin]	Antineoplastic—depolymerizes microtubules	Acute leukemia	Peripheral neuritis	
Vitamin A (Retinol) [Aquasol A]	Vitamin	Night blindness, xerophthalmia	Hyperkeratosis	

Vitamin B₁ (thiamine)	**Vitamin**	**Alcoholics (prophylaxis for Wernicke-Korsakoff)**		**Decrease results in beriberi**
Vitamin B₁₂ [Anacobin, Cyanocobalamin, Shovite]	Vitamin	**Megaloblastic anemia**		
Vitamin B₂ (riboflavin)	Vitamin—component of flavin compounds: FMN, FAD			Inhibits chlorpromazine; decrease results in skin, oral, ocular lesions
Vitamin B₃ (nicotinic acid, niacin)	Vitamin—component of nicotinic compounds: NAD, NADH	Maintains integrity of skin; decreases VLDL and LDL		Decrease results in dermatitis, diarrhea, dementia, death
Vitamin B₅ (pantothenic acid)	Vitamin—component of CoA			
Vitamin B₆ (pyridoxine)	Vitamin	Protein metabolism; neurotransmitter synthesis	Neuritis; convulsions	Isoniazid decreases amount
Vitamin C (ascorbic acid)	Vitamin	Maintains collagen; oxidation-reduction reactions		Decrease results in scurvy
Vitamin D (calcitriol) [Rocaltrol]	**Vitamin—binds to receptors in cytoplasm; alters gene expression and protein synthesis; increases bone resorption of Ca²⁺; increases renal and intestinal absorption of Ca²⁺ and phosphate**	**Rickets; osteomalacia; hypocalcemia; hypoparathyroidism; osteoporosis**		
Vitamin E	Vitamin—antioxidant	**Prophylaxis for heart disease**		**Decrease results in abortion, creatinuria, ceroid pigment**
Vitamin K (Mephyton)	Vitamin—enhances clotting factors	Bleeding disorders		**Decreased in children of mothers taking phenytoin or phenobarbital**
Vitamin M (folic acid) [Folvite]	Vitamin—one carbon carrier Nucleic acid synthesis; given to	pregnant mothers		**Decrease results in neural tube defects in utero; decreased in pregnancy or with use of phenytoin, isoniazid**
Warfarin (Coumadin)	Anticoagulant—inhibits potassium epoxide regeneration	Thrombosis	Bleeding	**Contraindicated in pregnancy, patients with liver, CNS, hemostatic disease; 99% exists protein bound; extremely sensitive to cytochrome P-450 system**
Yohimbine	Impotence therapy—α_2 antagonist			
Zafirlukast [Accolate]	Antiasthma agent—blocks leukotriene receptors (LTD_4)	Reduces bronchoconstriction and inflammatory cell infiltrate in asthma		

Therapeutic Agent (common name, if relevant) [Trade name, where appropriate]	Class—Pharmacology and Pharmacokinetics	Indications	Side or Adverse Effects	Contraindications or Precautions to Consider; Notes
Zidovudine [Retrovir, AZT]	Antiviral—thymidine analog; reverse transcriptase inhibitor	AIDS	Nausea; headache; bone marrow suppression; myalgias	
Zileuton	Antiasthma agent— 5-lipoxygenase inhibitor	Improves asthma		
Zolpidem [Ambien]	Binds to benzodiazepine receptor, but is not a benzodiazepine	Hypnotic		

5-HT=5-hydroxytryptamine (serotonin); *ACE*=angiotensin-converting enzyme; *ACh*=acetylcholine; *ACTH*=adrenocorticotropic hormone; *ADP*=adenosine diphosphate; *AML*=acute myelocytic leukemia; *ATPase*=adenosine triphosphatase; *AV*=atrioventricular; *BP*=blood pressure; *BPH*=benign prostatic hypertrophy; *CCK*=cholecystokinin; *cGMP*=cyclic guanosine monophosphate; *CBC*=complete blood count; *CHF*=congestive heart failure; *CMI*=cell-mediated immunity; *CMV*=cytomegalovirus; *CNS*=central nervous system; *CoA*=coenzyme A; *COPD*=chronic obstructive pulmonary disease; *COX*=cyclooxygenase; *DCT*=distal convoluted tubule; *dCTP*=deoxycytidine triphosphate; *DHEA*=dehydroepiandrosterone; *EBV*=Epstein-Barr virus; *ECG*=electrocardiogram, electrocardiography; *FAD*=flavin adenine dinucleotide; *FMN*=flavin mononucleotide; *FSH*=follicle-stimulating hormone; *GABA*=γ-aminobutyric acid; *GH*=growth hormone; *GI*=gastrointestinal; *GnRH*=gonadotropin-releasing hormone; *HDL*=high-density lipoprotein; *HMG-CoA*=3-hydroxy-3-methylglutaryl coenzyme A; *IFN*=interferon; *IPSP*=inhibitory postsynaptic potential; *LDL*=low-density lipoprotein; *L-DOPA*=levodopa (levo-3, 4-dihydroxyphenylalanine); *LH*=luteinizing hormone; *LPL*=lipoprotein lipase; *LTB₄*=leukotriene B₄; *MAO*=monoamine oxidase; *MAO*ᵦ=monoamine oxidase B; *MAOI*=monoamine oxidase inhibitor; *MHC*=major histocompatibility complex; *MI*=myocardial infarction; *NAD*=nicotinamide adenine dinucleotide; *NADH*=reduced nicotinamide adenine dinucleotide; *NE*=norepinephrine; *NIDDM*=non–insulin-dependent diabetes mellitus; *NO*=nitric oxide; *NSAID*=nonsteroidal anti-inflammatory drug; *PCP*=phencyclidine; *PCT*=proximal convoluted tubule; *PDA*=patent ductus arteriosus; *PGE₁*=prostaglandin E₁; *PGE₂*=prostaglandin E₂; *PGF₂ₐ.*=prostaglandin F₂ₐ; *PMN*=polymorphonuclear; *PTH*=parathyroid hormone; *PTT*=partial thromboplastin time; *Rh*=rhesus [factor]; *RSV*=respiratory syncytial virus; *SLE*=systemic lupus erythematosus; *SSRI*=selective serotonin reuptake inhibitor; *TCA*=tricyclic antidepressant; *TG*=triglycerides; *THC*=tetrahydrocannabinol; *TSH*=thyroid-stimulating hormone; *UTI*=urinary tract infection; *VIP*=vasoactive intestinal peptide; *VLDL*=very low density lipoprotein

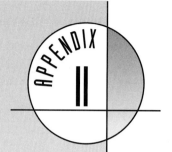

APPENDIX

II

Bug Index

Bacteria

Name	Morphology	Pathogenesis	Description of Disease	Laboratory Findings, Notes	Transmission	Prevention and Therapy
Actinomyces israelii	Gram +; filamentous; anaerobic	Unknown	Actinomycosis—abscesses with draining sinus tracts	Forms filaments; sulfur granules	Dental disease or trauma	Penicillin and drainage
Bacillus anthracis	Gram +; rod with square ends; capsule of D-glutamate (only protein capsule); nonmotile; spore-former; aerobic	Anthrax toxin—edema factor (exotoxin); protective antigen for cell entry; lethal factor (mode of action unknown)	Anthrax—cutaneous eschar (malignant pustules), pulmonary disease, septicemia	Medusahead colonies; catalase +	Spores from animals (usually cattle)	Attenuated strain human vaccine; penicillin; ciprofloxacin; doxycycline
Bacillus cereus	Gram +; rod; spore-former; aerobic	Spores germinate when rice is reheated; enterotoxins—emetic toxin, diarrheal toxin	Food poisoning—early vomiting and late diarrhea		Enter through the GI tract via reheated rice	Avoid refried rice and beans; treatment is symptomatic; cephalosporin
Bacteroides fragilis	Gram –; bacilli; anaerobic; capsulated; no endotoxin	Capsule; weak endotoxin	Sepsis; peritonitis; bacteremia; foul-smelling abscess	Mixed infections	Deep penetrating wounds; wound débridement	Metronidazole; clindamycin
Bordetella pertussis	Gram –; coccobacilli; capsule	Noninvasive infection of bronchial epithelium; pertussis toxin (2 subunits)—A subunit ADP ribosylates adenylate cyclase increasing cAMP, while B subunit causes attachment	Whooping cough	Culture nasopharynx onto 10%–15% blood agar (Bordet-Gengou agar); slide agglutination test	Droplet nuclei	Acellular pertussis vaccine (at 2, 4, and 6 months) or whole inactive cells; erythromycin
Borrelia burgdorferi	Spirochete; microaerophilic; flagella	Invasion and replication in the bloodstream	Lyme disease—erythema chronicum migrans with involvement of the heart, joints, and CNS	Common in the Northeast, Midwest, and Western U.S.	Deer ticks	Avoid ticks, wear long pants in wooded areas; doxycycline and penicillin
Brucella species	Gram –; coccobacillus; facultative intracellular	Catalase; LPS; inhibits release of peroxidase in macrophages	Undulant fever—macrophages engulf and then re-release into the bloodstream; granulomas		Contaminated milk and cheese	Pasteurization of dairy products; tetracycline plus streptomycin
Campylobacter jejuni	Gram –; comma-shaped bacilli; motile	Enterotoxin with antigenic diversity stimulates cAMP	Gastroenteritis—blood and pus in stool	Microaerophilic; Campy plate; diarrhea in college students; oxidase +	Milk, water, poultry	Symptomatic

Name	Morphology	Pathogenesis	Description of Disease	Laboratory Findings, Notes	Transmission	Prevention and Therapy
Chlamydia psittaci	Obligate intracellular	Unknown	Psittacosis—dry cough with CNS symptoms	Giemsa stain; inactive form extracellular (elementary body) and metabolically active form intracellular (reticulate body)	Aerosol of dried bird feces	Tetracycline
Chlamydia trachomatis	Obligate intracellular	Unknown	Strains A–C—blindness; strains D–K: nongonococcal urethritis, cervicitis; strains L1–L3: lymphogranuloma venereum	Leading cause of preventable blindness in the world; inactive form extracellular (elementary body) and metabolically active form intracellular (reticulate body)	Sexual contact or via birth canal	Tetracycline
Clostridium botulinum	Gram +; rod; spore-former; anaerobic	Botulinum toxin inhibits release of acetylcholine; exotoxins A, B, and E	Botulism (weakness and respiratory paralysis); food, wound, and infant types; floppy baby syndrome; dysphagia; constipation	Toxin	Spores from contaminated food	Sterilization of canned foods; cook to inactivate toxin; trivalent antitoxin; respiratory support
Clostridium difficile	Gram +; rod; spore-former; anaerobic	Exotoxins A and B—A (cholera-like) causes fluid release, B (diphtheria-like) damages mucosa and causes pseudomembrane formation	Antibiotic-associated pseudomembranous colitis; bloody diarrhea	ELISA detects toxin B in the stool sample	Hospital workers	Withdraw causative antibiotics (usually clindamycin); oral metronidazole; oral vancomycin
Clostridium perfringens	Gram +; rod; spore-former; anaerobic	α-Toxin (damages cell membranes); γ-toxin (tissue necrosis and hemolysis); cholera-like heat-labile enterotoxin (food poisoning—watery diarrhea)	Gas gangrene; food poisoning; anaerobic cellulitis	Large rods found in food; double-zone of hemolysis	Grows in traumatized tissue (muscle); spores in food and soil germinate in reheated foods	Clean and débride wounds; cook food well
Clostridium tetani	Gram +; rod; spore-former (tennis racquet–shaped); anaerobic	Tetanus toxin (exotoxin)—blocks release of inhibitory neurotransmitters	Tetanus: lockjaw (trismus), spastic paralysis (opisthotonos), sardonic grin (risus sardonicus)	Usually not recovered by culture	Spore entry via wound (e.g., a rusty nail)	Toxoid vaccine (2, 4, 6, 18 months) booster every 10 years; tetanus immunoglobulin (passive immunity); penicillin

Organism	Characteristics	Toxin/Virulence	Lab ID	Disease	Transmission	Treatment/Vaccine
Corynebacterium diphtheriae	Gram +; rod; club-shaped; arranged in V or L; non–spore-former	Exotoxin—A ADP ribosylates EF-2 and B binds toxin to the cell; phage conversion	Tellurite plate (Löffler's medium) grows black colonies	Diphtheria—pseudomembrane forms in the throat; bull neck; systemic toxemia	Airborne droplets	Inactivated toxoid vaccine; antitoxin (neutralizes unbound toxin); penicillin; erythromycin
Coxiella burnetii	Obligate intracellular	Unknown	Only rickettsia not transmitted to humans by an arthropod vector	Q fever	Inhalation of aerosols of urine, feces; transplacental	Tetracycline
Entercoccus faecalis	Gram +; cocci	Lipoteichoic acid	Catalase-negative; bacitracin-resistant; variable hemolysis; grows in 6.5% NaCl/Lancefield group D	Urinary, biliary, and cardiovascular infections; endocarditis	Normal flora of gut gaining access to blood	Penicillin and an aminoglycoside
Escherichia coli	Gram –; bacilli	Endotoxin—septic shock; heat-labile (LT) enterotoxin: increased cAMP leads to diarrhea; heat-stable (ST) stimulates guanylate cyclase to cause diarrhea; pili: adhere to epithelium especially in UTIs; Verotoxin (O157:H7): shigella-like toxin in EHEC that inhibits 28S rRNA to cause bloody diarrhea	Oxidase –	UTIs; sepsis; neonatal meningitis; enteropathogenic *E. coli* (EPEC): traveler's diarrhea; enterotoxigenic *E. coli* (ETEC): watery diarrhea; enteroinvasive *E. coli* (EIEC): dysentery; enterohemorrhagic *E. coli* (EHEC): bloody diarrhea, hemolytic uremic syndrome	Transplacental; fecal-oral route	UTIs: trimethoprim-sulfamethoxazole; sepsis: cephalosporins; traveler's diarrhea: rehydration
Francisella tularensis	Gram –; rod; intracellular	Capsule; intracellular within macrophages	Cysteine agar	Painful lymph nodes; glandular and ocular ulcers	Zoonotic via rabbits	Live attenuated vaccine; streptomycin; thorough cooking of meat
Gardnerella vaginalis	Gram variable; bacillus; anaerobic	Unknown	Clue cells	Vaginosis—watery discharge, fishy odor	Sexually transmitted	Metronidazole
Haemophilus ducreyi	Gram –; bacilli	Virulence via pili	Lesions similar to those of syphilis; lymphadenopathy	Chancroid with pain and purulent exudate	Sexually transmitted	Nafcillin; erythromycin
Haemophilus influenzae	Gram –; coccobacilli; polysaccharide capsule (poly-ribitol phosphate)	IgA protease degrades antibody and attaches to respiratory tract; capsule (type B) prevents phagocytosis	Needs heme (factor X) and NAD (factor V) to grow; chocolate agar; check CSF	Infantile meningitis; epiglottitis; otitis media	Respiratory droplets	Hib vaccine (B type capsule conjugated to diphtheria toxoid as a carrier protein); ceftriaxone

Name	Morphology	Pathogenesis	Description of Disease	Laboratory Findings, Notes	Transmission	Prevention and Therapy
Helicobacter pylori	Gram −; bacilli; motile; flagella	Urease results in ammonia production and subsequent gastric damage	Peptic ulcers (type B gastritis)	Microaerophilic; Campy plate; urea breath test; urease +	Ingestion	Triple therapy regimens— (1) bismuth, tetracycline, metronidazole, omeprazole; (2) amoxicillin, omeprazole, clarithromycin
Klebsiella pneumoniae	Gram −; bacilli; capsule; + quellung reaction	Large capsule hinders phagocytosis	Pneumonia particularly in malnourished alcoholics; UTI; bacteremia	Currant-jelly sputum	Aspiration of respiratory droplets	Cephalosporins
Legionella pneumophila	Gram −; bacilli	Endotoxin affects smokers, alcoholics, and those older than 55 years of age	Legionnaire's disease (atypical pneumonia)	Dieterle silver stain; cysteine required for culture	Aerosol from environmental water sources	Erythromycin
Listeria monocytogenes	Gram +; rod; arranged in V or L; tumbling motility; non-spore-former	Grows intracellularly in macrophages; listeriolysin-O cytotoxic	Meningitis and sepsis in newborns and immunocompromised	Small gray colonies; β-hemolysis; motility	Transferred to humans by animals or their feces; unpasteurized milk; contaminated vegetables	Ampicillin
Mycobacterium avium-intracellulare (MAC)	Acid-fast bacilli	Unknown	Tuberculosis-like disease in the immunocompromised		From the soil and water to the immunocompromised individuals	Amikacin plus doxycycline
Mycobacterium leprae	Acid-fast; bacilli; obligate intracellular	Tuberculoid: cell-mediated response causes damage; lepromatous: anergy of CD8 cells leads to uncontrolled replication	Leprosy—tuberculoid and lepromatous; lesions in cool parts of body	Cannot be grown in culture but is harvested in the footpads of armadillos; acid-fast stain of infected areas	Prolonged contact, especially with the lepromatous form	Dapsone and rifampin for tuberculoid form; clofazimine, dapsone, rifampin for lepromatous form; 2-year treatment
Mycobacterium tuberculosis	Acid-fast bacilli; aerobic; high lipid cell walls (mycolic acids and wax D)	Cord factor; granulomas and caseation	Tuberculosis	Ziehl-Neelsen stain; slow-growing (3–8 weeks) on Lowenstein-Jensen medium; niacin +; PPD + if >10 cm after 48 hours	Droplets from coughing	BCG vaccine with live, attenuated organisms (rarely used in the U.S.); isoniazid, rifampin, pyrazinamide for 6–9 months
Mycoplasma pneumoniae	Obligate intracellulare; not seen on a Gram's stain; smallest free-living organism; only bacteria with cholesterol in membrane (no cell wall)	Hydrogen peroxide and lytic enzymes resulting in damage to the respiratory tract	Walking pneumonia; bullous myringitis (inflamed tympanic membrane); common in young adults (college)	Positive cold-agglutinin; highest incidence in 5- to 15-year-olds	Respiratory droplets	Erythromycin

Organism	Characteristics	Virulence/Pathogenesis	Disease	Laboratory Identification	Transmission	Treatment/Prevention
Neisseria gonorrhoeae (gonococcus)	Gram –; cocci; coffee bean–shaped pairs; no polysaccharide capsule	Endotoxin (lipid A); pili with variation; proteins I, II, III (porin, adhesin, autoagglutination); deficiencies in late-acting complement components	Urethral and vaginal infections; discharge; salpingitis and PID; neonatal conjunctivitis; septic arthritis	Thayer-Martin agar; only glucose fermentation; oxidase +; also check for chlamydia caused by common coinfection	Sexual contact; newborns; symptomatic in men but not usually in women	Condoms; erythromycin or silver nitrate in neonates; ceftriaxone; spectinomycin and tetracycline
Neisseria meningitidis (meningococcus)	Gram –; diplococci; coffee bean–shaped pairs; polysaccharide capsule (antiphagocytic)	Endotoxin (LPS) contains lipid A; capsule; IgA protease; pili variation; deficiencies in late-acting complement components; asplenic patients	Meningitis; petechial rash; pharyngitis	Glucose and maltose fermentation; oxidase +; lumbar puncture with high protein and low glucose; grows on Thayer-Martin agar	Respiratory droplets	Vaccine, rifampin; penicillin G
Nocardia asteroides	Acid-fast; bacillus; aerobic	Unknown; immunocompromised at risk	Nocardiosis—lung, heart, and brain abscesses	Forms filaments	Airborne particles	Sulfonamides
Pseudomonas aeruginosa	Gram –; coccobacilli	Pili; A/B toxin similar to diphtheria; flagella; hemolysin	UTI; septicemia; burn infections	Fruity smell; green, water-soluble pigment	Water; environment; opportunistic: catheters, leukemia patients, burns, cystic fibrosis	Very resistant to antibiotics; requires combination therapy
Rickettsia prowazekii	Obligate intracellular	Invasion of the endothelial lining; possible endotoxin	Epidemic typhus		Human-to-human spread	Tetracycline
Rickettsia rickettsii	Obligate intracellular	Invasion of endothelial lining	Rocky Mountain spotted fever: vasculitis, rash spreads from periphery inward	Weil-Felix reaction (agglutination when patient's serum mixed with OX strain of *Proteus vulgaris*)	*Dermacentor* ticks	Tetracycline
Rickettsia typhi	Obligate intracellular	Invasion of endothelial lining; possible endotoxin	Endemic typhus—rash spreads from the trunk outward		Spread by fleas	Tetracycline
Salmonella species	Gram –; rod; multiple flagella; anaerobic	Invades mucosa of GI tract; flagellor proteins	Typhoid fever; gastroenteritis; sepsis	Lactose –; polysaccharide somatic O antigens and protein flagellor H antigens; encapsulated	Fecal-oral	Chloramphenicol; amoxicillin; trimethoprim-sulfamethoxazole
Shigella species	Gram –; rod; nonmotile; non-spore-formers	Invades mucosa; ulceration and PMN infiltrate; Shiga toxin (A/B toxin) works on 28S ribosome and removes the base; low infective dose	Bacterial dysentery (shigellosis): ulcerative colitis of large intestine, fever, chills, cramps, tenesmus, bloody stool	Rectal swab; three types: *dysenteriae* (rare), *sonnei* (most common, daycare), *flexneri* (gay men)	Fecal-oral route	Public health measures; significant resistance; fluids; ampicillin

Name	Morphology	Pathogenesis	Description of Disease	Laboratory Findings, Notes	Transmission	Prevention and Therapy
Staphylococcus aureus	Gram +; cocci; capsule; protein A in the cell wall; yellow, creamy, grapelike clusters on culture	Rapid growth; protein A (antiphagocytic); enterotoxin (watery diarrhea); toxic shock syndrome toxin; exfoliation; α-toxin; coagulase	Abscesses; pyogenic infections (endocarditis, osteomyelitis); food poisoning; toxic shock syndrome; scalded skin syndrome	Coagulase +; catalase +; β-hemolytic; novobiocin-sensitive; ferment mannitol	Via the hands from the skin, nasal mucosa	Hand washing; 80% penicillin-resistant (make β-lactamase); vancomycin; cephalosporin
Staphylococcus epidermidis	Gram +; cocci; white, creamy, grapelike clusters on culture	Surface glycocalyx	Endocarditis; infection on catheters and implant sites; sepsis in neonates	Coagulase; catalase +; no hemolysis; novobiocin-sensitive	On skin; IV drug users	Vancomycin
Staphylococcus saprophyticus	Gram +; cocci; creamy, grapelike clusters	Selectively adheres to transitional epithelium	UTIs in young women	Coagulase; catalase +; no hemolysis; novobiocin-resistant	Many sexual partners	Quinolones
Streptococcus agalactiae	Gram +; cocci; diploid	Capsular antigen	Neonatal sepsis and meningitis	Catalase −; bacitracin-resistant; β-hemolysis; Lancefield group B	Genital tract of some women	Ampicillin before delivery; penicillin G
Streptococcus pneumoniae	Gram +; cocci; lancet-shaped; in pairs; polysaccharide capsule (85 different types)	Capsule prevents phagocytosis; IgA protease; adheres to mucosa	Pneumonia; meningitis; bacteremia; upper respiratory infection; otitis media	Catalase −; α-hemolysis; bile soluble; inhibited by Optochin; quellung reaction (capsular swelling)	Noncommunicable	Polysaccharide capsular vaccine available for high-risk groups; penicillin and erythromycin
Streptococcus pyogenes	Gram +; cocci; chains or pairs; rough or smooth hyaluronic acid capsule	M protein (pili); streptokinase (dissolves fibrin); DNase; hyaluronidase; hemolysins: erythrogenic toxin (scarlet fever rash); streptolysin O and S; exotoxin A (superantigen causing TSS-like syndrome)	Pharyngitis; cellulitis; rheumatic fever; acute glomerulonephritis; TSS-like syndrome	Catalase −; bacitracin (A disk)-sensitive; (β-hemolytic; antistreptolysin-O for serotyping; Lancefield group A	Normal flora of skin, throat causing disease when in blood	Penicillin G
Treponema pallidum	Spirochete	Multiplication followed by blood vessel involvement	Syphilis—primary with painless sores, purulent exudate, and induration; secondary with a rash; tertiary (rare) includes CNS involvement and aortitis	Darkfield microscopy; RPR (or VDRL) test for cardiolipin; systemic illness can occur with treatment (Jarisch-Herxheimer reaction)	Sexually transmitted; transplacental	Penicillin

Tropheryma whippelii	Gram +; rod	Foamy macrophages found in the lamina propria of the jejunum	Whipple's disease—steatorrhea, lymphadenopathy, fever, and cough	Visualization of the organism in a biopsy of the small bowel	Unknown	Trimethoprim-sulfamethoxazole
Vibrio cholerae	Gram –; comma-shaped rod; polar flagella	Pili adhere to gut mucosa; phage-coded cholera toxin: 2 A active subunits and 5 B binding units (A subunit ADP ribosylates G protein increasing cAMP and causing movement of ions and water out of the cell)	Rice-water stools		Fecal-oral route via water and food	Vaccine not effective; rehydration, tetracycline
Vibrio parahaemolyticus	Gram –; comma-shaped rod	Toxin	Explosive diarrhea; cramps; nausea	High infective dose required	Shellfish	Self-limiting
Yersinia pestis	Gram –; bacillus; intracellular	V and W antigens (active within macrophages); fibrinolysin; F1 protein inhibits phagocytosis	Bubonic plague (with lymph node swelling and bubo); fever; conjunctivitis	Cultures are hazardous and precautions must be taken	Zoonotic via rat fleas	Vaccine; streptomycin

ADP=adenosine diphosphate; *bCG*=bacille Calmette-Guérin; *cAMP*=cyclic adenosine monophosphate; *CNS*=central nervous system; *CSF*=cerebrospinal fluid; *DNase*=deoxyribonuclease; *EHEC*=enterohemorrhagic *Escherichia coli*; *EIEC*=enteroinvasive *Escherichia coli*; *ELISA*=enzyme-linked immunosorbent assay; *EPEC*=enteropathogenic *Escherichia coli*; *ETEC*=enterotoxigenic *Escherichia coli*; *GI*=gastrointestinal; *Hib*= *Haemophilus influenza* type B; *IV*=intravenous; *LPS*=lipopolysaccharide; *NAD*=nicotinamide-adenine dinucleotide; *PID*=pelvic inflammatory disease; *PMN*=polymorphonuclear neutrophils; *PPD*=purified protein derivative; *RPR*=rapid plasma reagin; *TSS*=toxic shock syndrome; *UTI*=urinary tract infection; *U.S.*=United States; *VDRL*=Venereal Disease Research Laboratory.

Viruses

Name	Morphology	Pathogenesis	Description of Disease	Laboratory Findings, Notes	Transmission	Prevention; Therapy
Adenovirus	Non-enveloped DNA virus; double-stranded	Pharyngitis or pneumonia; acute gastroenteritis	Infects the epithelium of the eyes, respiratory tract, and GI tract	Complement fixation	Respiratory droplets; hand-to-eye; also fecal-oral	Live vaccine to high-risk populations; no treatments
Coxsackie B virus	Non-enveloped RNA virus; single-stranded; linear; + polarity	Myocarditis, pericarditis	Replicates in the pharynx and GI tract and spreads to other tissues	Isolating virus in cell culture; rise in convalescent antibody	Fecal-oral and respiratory	No therapy or prevention
Cytomegalovirus	Enveloped DNA virus; linear; double-stranded	Pneumonia, retinitis, and hepatitis in immunocompromised; mononucleosis in transplant patients; cytomegalic inclusion disease of fetus	Infects the oropharynx initially; involves lymphocytes	"Owl's eye" nuclear inclusions	Human body fluids; transplacental, organ transplant	Ganciclovir
Ebola virus	Enveloped RNA virus; single-stranded; linear; − polarity	African hemorrhagic fever—often rapidly fatal	Viral replication in all organs leads to necrosis	Virus isolation; rise in antibody titer	Contact with blood and body secretions	None
Epstein-Barr virus	Enveloped DNA virus; linear; double-stranded	Infectious mononucleosis; causes Burkitt's lymphoma	Spreads via the lymph nodes and bloodstream to the liver and spleen from the pharyngeal epithelium	Atypical lymphocytes; + heterophil antibody (Monospot test); common infection of college students	Saliva	None
Hanta virus	Enveloped, RNA virus; single-stranded; circular-circular, segmented; − polarity	Hanta pulmonary syndrome—influenza-like followed by acute respiratory failure	Invasion of the respiratory epithelium	PCR assay of viral RNA from lung tissue	Airborne (inhalation of rodent urine and feces); found in southwestern U.S.	None
Hepatitis A virus	Non-enveloped RNA virus; single stranded; + polarity	Hepatitis A	Replicates in the GI tract; spreads to the liver; hepatocellular injury via cytotoxic T-cell response	Detect IgM antibody	Fecal-oral route	Killed viral vaccine; immune globulin during the incubation period may hinder disease
Hepatitis B virus	Enveloped DNA virus; incomplete circular double-stranded; polymerase in virion (virion called the Dane particle); surface antigen (HbsAg); capsid antigen (HbcAg)	Hepatitis B; arthritis; rash; glomerulonephritis; may result in carcinoma of the liver	Immune response (CD8 cells) to the virus results in hepatocellular injury; Ag-Ab complexes form	Serologic tests for Hb-sAg, HbsAb, and HbcAb	Blood, sexual, and transplacental	Vaccine; interferon-α; lamivudine inhibit HBV DNA synthesis

Virus	Characteristics	Disease	Diagnosis	Transmission	Treatment
Hepatitis C virus	Enveloped RNA virus; single-stranded; + polarity	Hepatitis C; possible predisposition to hepatocellular carcinoma	Cytotoxic T cells result in hepatocellular injury	Serologic; currently the most common cause of transfusion-related hepatitis	Blood, transplacental, sexual	Interferon-α; ribavirin
Hepatitis D virus (Delta virus)	Enveloped defective RNA virus; single-stranded; − polarity; no polymerase	Hepatitis D	Cytotoxic T cells result in hepatocellular injury; uses hepatitis B surface antigen as a protein coat and can only replicate in hosts already infected with hepatitis B virus	Serologic testing for delta antigen	Blood, transplacental, sexual	Interferon-α; prevention of hepatitis B
Herpes simplex virus type 1	Enveloped DNA virus; linear; double-stranded	Herpes labialis (fever blisters and cold sores); keratitis; encephalitis	Lesions on the mouth and face initially; travels retrograde and becomes latent in the trigeminal ganglion; recurrences induced by sunlight, stress, fever	Multinucleated giant cells on Tzanck smear; immunofluoresence of infected cells; in-situ hybridization defects viral DNA	Saliva; direct contact with the lesion	Acyclovir; trifluorothymidine for keratitis
Herpes simplex virus type 2	Enveloped DNA virus; linear; double-stranded	Herpes genitalis; meningitis	Vesicular lesions on the genitalia; retrograde passage through the axon and latency in the sacral ganglion; stress-induced recurrences	Multinucleated giant cells on Tzanck smear; immunofluoresence of infected cells; in-situ hybridization defects viral DNA	Sexual, transplacental	Acyclovir
Human herpes virus 6	Enveloped DNA virus; linear; double-stranded	Roseola infantum (exanthem subitum)—common disease of children characterized by high fever and rash	Infects T and B cells	PCR or acute and convalescent antibody titers	Saliva	Symptomatic
Human immunodeficiency virus	Enveloped RNA virus; diploid; single-stranded; + polarity; reverse transcriptase	AIDS	Infects and kills helper T cells via the CD4 receptors and gp120 protein	Screen with ELISA; Western blot test confirms	Sexual, body fluids, transplacental; products blood	AZT to HIV-infected mothers and newborns; AZT, ddI, ddC; treat opportunistic infections like pneumonia or Kaposi's sarcoma
Influenza virus	Enveloped RNA virus; segmented; single-stranded; − polarity; polymerase in virion	Influenza	Infects the epithelium of the respiratory tract via hemagglutinin and neuraminidase on surface spikes; antigenic shift and drift of surface spikes lead to epidemics	Cell culture; hemagglutination inhibition; complement fixation; H and N protein spikes	Respiratory droplets; vaccine composed of inactivated strains of current virus which causes disease	Amantadine for both prevention and treatment; vaccine composed of inactivated strains of current virus which causes disease

Name	Morphology	Pathogenesis	Description of Disease	Laboratory Findings, Notes	Transmission	Prevention; Therapy
Measles virus	Enveloped RNA virus; single-stranded; − polarity; polymerase in virion	Measles; subacute sclerosing panencephalitis (SSPE)	Infection spreads via the bloodstream from the upper respiratory tract to the organs; maculopapular rash caused by an immune response (koplik spots)	Usually not done	Respiratory droplets	Attenuated vaccine; no treatment
Mumps virus	Enveloped RNA virus; single-stranded; − polarity; polymerase in virion	Mumps; sterility owing to bilateral orchitis	Spreads from the upper respiratory tract to the organs (parotid glands, testes, ovaries, CNS) via the bloodstream	Cell culture and hemadsorption; rise in antiviral antibody	Respiratory droplets	Attenuated vaccine; no treatment
Norwalk virus	Non-enveloped; RNA virus; single-stranded; linear; + polarity	Gastroenteritis	Immune response to viral invasion results in the destruction of the small intestinal epithelium	Not performed	Fecal-oral	Symptomatic treatment
Papillomavirus	Non-enveloped DNA virus; circular; double-stranded	Papillomas (warts); condylomata acuminata; cervical and penile carcinoma	E6 and E7 early viral genes inhibit activity of p53 and rb tumor suppressor genes	Koilocytes (squamous cell with perinuclear clearing) in lesions; in-situ DNA hybridization to define type	Sexual via direct contact with genital lesions	Interferon-α; liquid nitrogen for warts
Parvovirus B19	Non-enveloped; DNA virus; single-stranded; linear	Erythema infectiosum (fifth disease)—characterized by "slapped cheek" appearance; may cause aplastic crisis in sickle cell disease	Erythema infectiosum—virus causes immune-complex deposition; aplastic anemia: virus infects immature RBCs and kills them	Parvovirus-specific IgG/IgM antibody levels; laboratory analysis for viral DNA	Unknown, may be respiratory or direct contact	Self-limited
Poliovirus	Non-enveloped RNA virus; single-stranded; + polarity	Aseptic meningitis (more common); paralytic poliomyelitis	Replicates in the pharynx and GI tract and spreads to the CNS; death of the anterior horn cells in the spinal cord	Isolation from CSF	Fecal-oral	Salk vaccine: inactivated; Sabin vaccine: attenuated, given in childhood immunizations; no treatment
Rabies virus	Enveloped RNA virus; bullet shape; single-stranded; − polarity RNA; polymerase in virion	Rabies	ACh receptor of neuron binds virus; the virus follows the retrograde direction to invade the CNS and brain, resulting in encephalitis	Negri bodies (eosinophilic inclusion in nerve cell)	Animal (skunks, bats) bites; domestic dogs in third world countries	Before exposure: vaccine; after exposure: anti-rabies immuno globulin plus inactivated vaccine from human cell culture; no treatment

Reovirus (Rotavirus)	Non-enveloped RNA virus; 11 segments; double-stranded; RNA polymerase in virion	Gastroenteritis in children	Resistant to stomach acid, thus infects the small intestine	ELISA detects the virus in stool	Respiratory droplets; fecal-oral route	Rehydration with fluids and electrolytes
Respiratory syncytial virus	Enveloped RNA virus; single-stranded; − polarity; polymerase in virion	Pneumonia or bronchiolitis in children	Immune response to lower respiratory tract infection	Multinucleated giant cells	Respiratory droplets	Ribavirin
Rhinovirus	Non-enveloped RNA virus; single-stranded; + polarity; numerous serotypes	Common cold	Upper respiratory tract mucosa and conjunctiva infected; replicates at temperature <37°C and killed by stomach acid	None	Aerosol droplets with hand-to-nose transmission	None
Rubella virus	Enveloped RNA virus; single-stranded; + polarity	Rubella; congenital: cardiovascular and neurologic malformations, especially if infection occurs during the first trimester	Spreads from the nasopharynx to the skin via the bloodstream; rash caused by replication and immune injury	Growth in cell culture via interference of coxsackievirus; recent infection in the mother is detected by IgM, IgA, or IgG	Respiratory droplets	Attenuated vaccine; no treatment
Varicella-zoster virus	Enveloped DNA virus; linear; double-stranded	Chickenpox (varicella) in children; shingles (zoster) in adults	Infects respiratory tract and spreads to the liver and skin via the blood; an acute episode followed by latency in the sensory ganglia	Intranuclear inclusions; shingles generally follows the distribution of the dermatomes	Chickenpox: respiratory droplets; shingles: reactivation of the latent virus	Attenuated vaccine; famcyclovir valacyclovir

ACh=acetylcholine; *Ag-Ab*=antigen-antibody; *AZT*=azidothymidine; *CNS*=central nervous system; *CSF*=cerebrospinal fluid; *ddC*=dideoxycytosine; *ELISA*=enzyme-linked immunosorbent assay; *GI*=gastrointestinal; *HbcAb*=hepatitis B core antibody; *HbsAg*=hepatitis B surface antigen; *HbsAb*=hepatitis B surface antibody; *HbcAg*=hepatitis B core antigen; *PCR*=polymerase chain reaction; *RBC*=red blood cell; *SSPE*=subacute sclerosing panencephalitis.

Fungi

Name	Morphology	Pathogenesis	Description of Disease	Laboratory Findings, Notes	Transmission	Prevention; Therapy
Aspergillus fumigatus	Filamentous; septate hyphae and dichotomous branching; mold only	Opportunistic; growth of *Aspergillus* in a preexisting cavitary lesion in the lung	Aspergilloma—hemoptysis; invasive aspergillosis in neutropenic individuals	Septate, branching hyphae; "fungus ball" seen on a radiograph	Airborne spores	Amphotericin B, itraconazole; surgery to remove a "fungus ball"
Blastomyces dermatitidis	Dimorphic fungus—mold in the soil, but a yeast in tissue	Invades the respiratory tract and may invade the skin or bone	Blastomycosis—granulomatous and suppurative infection of the respiratory tract	Tissue biopsy showing circular yeast with a broad-based bud	Airborne; endemic to North America	Itraconazole; amphotericin B for serious infections
Candida albicans	Pseudohyphae and hyphae on invasion; yeast in normal flora; germ tubes at 37°C; yeast only	Opportunistic in the immunosuppressed and those with foreign bodies (e.g., catheters); mucocutaneous lesions in children with a T-cell defect	Thrush; chronic mucocutaneous candidiasis; vaginal candidiasis	Colonies on Sabouraud's agar; germ tube formation	Part of the normal flora	Oral form can be prevented by nystatin "swish and swallow"; treatment with nystatin; miconazole; amphotericin B; IV amphotericin B or fluconazole for blood-borne infection
Coccidioides immitis	Dimorphic—mold in the soil, spherule in tissue; barrel-shaped hyphae	Inhalation; spherules, releasing endospores within the respiratory tract	Coccidioidomycosis—an influenza-like illness with fever and cough	Tissue specimen showing spherules	Airborne; endemic to southwestern U.S. and Latin America	Amphotericin B; ketoconazole
Cryptococcus neoformans	Encapsulated; not dimorphic; yeast only	Usually immunocompromised; spread via the bloodstream	Cryptococcosis; cryptococcal meningitis	Organism with a capsule seen on an Indian ink preparation; latex agglutination test	Inhalation of airborne yeast cells	Oral fluconazole as preventative in AIDS patients; amphotericin B with flucytosine
Histoplasma capsulatum	Dimorphic—a mold in the soil, a yeast in tissue; septate hyphae	Inhaled spores are engulfed by macrophages and develop into yeast forms intracellularly	Histoplasmosis—granulomas in the lung tissue	Tissue biopsy showing yeast cells visible in macrophages; radioimmunoassay for histoplasma RNA and DNA	Airborne; endemic to Ohio and Mississippi River valley; found in bird droppings	Amphotericin B; itraconazole
Mucor species	Nonseptate hyphae that branch at near right angles; mold only	Invade the nasal sinuses, lungs, and GI tract	Tissue necrosis	Nonseptate hyphae seen microscopically	Airborne	Amphotericin B; débridement of necrotic tissue
Pneumocystis carinii	Respiratory pathogen	Alveolar inflammation	Pneumonia	Silver stain; confusion about classification: protozoan or fungus	Inhalation by immunocompromised individual	Trimethoprim-sulfamethoxazole; pentamidine
Sporothrix schenckii	Thermally dimorphic fungus	Inflammation and swelling of the lymph nodes and vessels	Sporotrichosis ("rose gardener's disease")	Cigar-shaped budding cells	Thorn prick	Protection during gardening; potassium iodide; ketoconazole

GI=gastrointestinal.

Parasites and Protozoa

Name	Morphology	Pathogenesis	Description of Disease	Laboratory Findings, Notes	Transmission	Prevention; Therapy
Ascaris lumbricoides	Intestinal parasite	Larvae in the lung and a heavy worm burden in gastrointestinal tract	Ascariasis—intestinal obstruction, abdominal pain, coughing, nausea	Eosinophilia; eggs in feces	Contaminated food or soil	Maintain sanitary conditions; mebendazole
Entamoeba histolytica	Intestinal protozoan; cigar-shaped cysts; 4 nuclei	Trophozoite form invades the colon	Amebic dysentery; liver abscess; flask-shaped ulcers	Trophozoites seen in stool	Fecal-oral	Maintain sanitary conditions; metronidazole with diloxanide, steroids exacerbate
Enterobius vermicularis	Intestinal parasite	Worms and eggs (passed in feces) result in perianal pruritus	Pinworm infection—anal pruritus, vaginal irritation, cystitis	Eggs on "Scotch tape" test (tape applied to the anus and then viewed under a microscope)	Reinfection by self; fecal-oral contact; egg ingestion	Mebendazole
Giardia lamblia	Intestinal protozoan; pear-shaped; flagella; tumbling motility; 2 nuclei; 4 flagella	Interfere with fat and protein absorption	Giardiasis—acute diarrhea	Visible in stool	Fecal-oral	Maintain sanitary conditions; metronidazole
Leishmania donovani	Protozoan	Organs of the reticuloendothelial system are destroyed by macrophages infected with the protozoan	Visceral leishmaniasis (kala-azar)—hyperpigmentation of the skin, massive splenomegaly, fever, anemia, and malaise	Biopsy of reticuloendothelial tissue shows the infected macrophages	Female *Phlebotomus* sandfly transmits the disease from the infected host to a human	Protection from sandfly bites; sodium stibogluconate (antimony compound)
Plasmodium species	Blood and tissue protozoan; signet-ring trophozoites in RBCs; Schüffner's dots (red-yellow dots in RBCs); banana-shaped gametocytes	Sporozoites from bite enter the bloodstream and invade hepatocytes (exoerythrocytic phase); merozoites invade the RBCs (erythrocytic phase)	Malaria—fever, chills, hepatomegaly, splenomegaly; symptoms in cyclical pattern (3 days for *malariae*; 2 days for *ovale, falciparum, vivax*); tissue anoxia	Blood smear shows organisms; *P. falciparum* is acute and needs immediate treatment	Female *Anopheles* mosquito	Protection from bites; chloroquine; quinine; mefloquine; chloroquine; insecticides
Schistosoma species	Blood fluke; eggs have spine (*S. mansoni* has large lateral spine, *S. haematobium* has a terminal spine, *S. japonicum* has a small lateral spine); 2 sexes	Eggs lead to inflammation, fibrosis, and granuloma formation	Schistosomiasis—pipestem fibrosis of liver; *S. haematobium* affects the bladder; *S. mansoni* affects the colon	Eggs in the stool or urine	Penetration of the skin by cercariae	Maintain sanitary conditions; praziquantel

Name	Morphology	Pathogenesis	Description of Disease	Laboratory Findings, Notes	Transmission	Prevention; Therapy
Taenia species	Cestode: *T. solium*— pork tapeworm; *T. saginata*—beef; *Diphyllobothrium latum*—fish; 4 suckers and circle of hooks; 5–10 uterine branches	Encyst in tissue (eyes, brain, muscle) resulting in mass lesions	Taeniasis and cysticercosis	Gravid proglottids in stool	Eating raw or undercooked meat	Cook meat and maintain sanitary conditions; niclosamide
Toxoplasma gondii	Tissue protozoan	Infect macrophages; infect the brain, liver, eyes	Toxoplasmosis	Serologic; high morbidity and mortality	Ingestion of cysts; transplacental; cat feces	Cook meat; sulfonamides
Trichinella spiralis	Intestinal parasite	Muscle inflammation	Trichinosis—periorbital edema, myositis, fever, diarrhea	Larvae on muscle biopsy; eosinophilia by 14th day; double-barreled egg	Eating raw or undercooked meat	Cook meat; thiabendazole
Trichomonas vaginalis	Urogenital protozoan; pear-shaped; flagella	Attach to the wall of the vagina	Trichomoniasis—itching and burning with yellow discharge from the vagina (strawberry cervix)	Visible in secretions	Sexual transmission	Treat both partners; metronidazole
Trypanosoma brucei (African)	Blood and tissue protozoan	Infects the brain and leads to encephalitis	Sleeping sickness— Winterbottom's sign, blank look, fever, edema, epilepsy	Visible in the blood	Tsetse fly (in Africa);	Protection from bites; insecticide; suramin
Trypanosoma cruzi (American)	Blood and tissue protozoan	Amastigotes attack cells, especially cardiac muscle cells	Chagas' disease—CHF; Romaña's sign	Visible in the blood	Reduviid bugs (in Latin America)	Protect from bites; insecticide; nifurtimox

CHF=congestive heart failure; *RBC*=red blood cell.

Glossary

ABG • Arterial blood gas

Accuracy • Degree to which a measurement represents the actual value

Acne vulgaris • Simple acne, usually occurs during puberty

AD • Right ear

Addison's disease • Insufficient production of cortisol by the adrenal gland

AFOF • Anterior fontanelle open and flat

AFP • α-Fetoprotein

AKA • Above-knee amputation

Albuminocytologic dissociation • Increased protein in cerebrospinal fluid without an increased cell count, found in Guillain-Barré syndrome

Allotype • Antigenic differences of immunoglobulins that differ among individuals (e.g., variations in H chains are allotypes)

Amenorrhea • Absence or abnormal cessation of menses

Argyll Robertson pupil • Loss of pupillary light reflex, but accommodation retained; found in syphilis

Arthus reaction • A localized allergic inflammatory reaction

AS • Left ear

Asherman's syndrome • Amenorrhea and infertility secondary to scarring of the uterus (usually caused by excessive curettage)

ASO • Antibody to streptolysin O; streptolysin O made by group A β-hemolytic streptococcus

Auer rods • Rod-shaped structures in myeloblasts, found in acute myelogenous leukemia

BE • Barium enema

Bence Jones protein • Immunoglobulin light chains found in the urine of patients with multiple myeloma

BKA • Below-knee amputation

BPD • Biparietal distance; also bronchopulmonary dysplasia

Brushfield spots • Speckled nodules of the iris; found in Down's syndrome

Bullous pemphigoid • Tense skin vesicles with antibodies to the epidermal basement membrane

C & S • Culture and sensitivity

Café au lait spots • Hyperpigmented cutaneous lesions associated with neurofibromatosis type 1 (von Recklinghausen's disease)

Cauda equina syndrome • Sacral pain, pelvic analgesia, and bowel and bladder dysfunction

Chancre • Painless lesion of primary syphilis

Chancroid • Painful genital ulcer caused by *Haemophilus ducreyi*

Chandelier sign • Found in pelvic inflammatory disease; severe pain on pelvic examination (specifically cervical portion of examination) causing a woman to "jump up and hit the chandelier"

Charcot triad • (1) Found in multiple sclerosis: nystagmus, tremor, and scanning speech; (2) found in cholangitis: fever, upper abdominal pain, and jaundice

Charcot-Leyden crystals • Found in asthma; elongated double pyramid-shaped crystals

Chem 7 (Screen 7) • Serum electrolyte tests for sodium, potassium, chloride, bicarbonate, blood urea nitrogen, creatinine, and glucose

Chocolate cysts • Ovarian cyst containing an old hematoma often found in endometriosis

Chvostek sign • Tapping the facial nerve causes a unilateral spasm of the facial muscles; found in hypocalcemic tetany

Clue cells • Cells with a "rough" border and intracellular "dots"; found in bacterial vaginosis

CMT • Cervical motion tenderness

Condyloma lata • Flat-topped papules often in the anal region; found in secondary syphilis

Corrigan's pulse • Also called a "water-hammer pulse"; quickly rising and falling pulse; found in aortic valve regurgitation

Craniotabes • Thinning and softening of the skull; found in syphilis and rickets

CREST • Calcinosis, Raynaud's phenomenon, esophageal disorders, sclerodactyly, telangiectasia

CRI • Chronic renal insufficiency

CTX • Contractions

Cullen sign • Periumbilical ecchymoses; sign of retroperitoneal hemorrhage

CVAT • Costovertebral tenderness

CXR • Chest x-ray

DKA • Diabetic ketoacidosis

Donovan bodies • Clusters of blue or black-staining chromatin condensations seen in mononuclear cells infected with *Calymmatobacterium granulomatis* (granuloma inguinale)

DVT • Deep vein thrombosis

Dysmenorrhea • Painful menses

Dyspnea • Shortness of breath

ECC • Endocervical curettage

Eclampsia • Preeclampsia (hypertension, proteinuria, and edema) and seizures; occurs during pregnancy

Eczema • Acute or chronic inflammation of the skin described as edematous, papular, vesicular, and crusting; often very itchy

Epitope • Simplest antigenic determinant

Erythema chronicum migrans • A spreading circular red rash with a clear center at the bite site; found in Lyme disease

Erythema marginatum • Distinctive rash, often involving the trunk and extremities; rheumatic fever

Erythema multiforme • Macules, papules, or subdermal vesicles often on the hands and arms; can be an allergic or drug-induced reaction; called Stevens-Johnson syndrome if severe

Ewing sarcoma • Malignant neoplasm of bone usually found in young men; associated with 11:22 translocation

Exstrophy • A congenital defect resulting in a hollow organ with inside grossly visible, as in exstrophy of the bladder

Ferruginous bodies • Foreign body in the lungs coated with hemosiderin; found in asbestosis or mesothelioma

FEV • Forced expiratory volume

FEV$_1$ • Volume expired in the first second of forced expiration

FLP • Fasting lipid panel

Foam cell • Histiocytes that have ingested lipid; found characteristically in hypercholesterolemia

Gardner syndrome • Autosomal dominant-inherited disease characterized by multiple tumors of the colon, osteomas of the skull, epidermoid cysts, and fibromas that occur before 10 years of age

Genomic imprinting • Differences in the expression of a gene that depend on whether it has been inherited from the mother or the father

Goiter • Enlarged thyroid gland

Gower maneuver • Using the arms to stand from a prone position because of muscle weakness in the legs; found in muscular dystrophy

Gravid • Pregnancy; cumulative number of times a woman has been pregnant

Grey Turner sign • Flank ecchymosis in a butterfly pattern in the retroperitoneum; found in acute hemorrhage of the pancreas

Hapten • Antigen that must be combined with a carrier protein to induce antibody production

Harrison groove • Rib deformity; found in rickets

Heinz bodies • Intracellular inclusions of denatured hemoglobin in red blood cells; found in thalassemia, enzyme defects, and hemoglobinopathies, especially glucose-6-phosphate dehydrogenase deficiency

HELLP • Hemolysis, elevated liver enzymes, low platelets; associated with eclampsia or preeclampsia

Hematochezia • Bloody stool

Hemoptysis • Coughing up blood

Henoch-Schönlein purpura • Purpuric lesions, joint pain and swelling, colic, and bloody stools; usually found in children

Heterophil antibodies • Antibodies found in mononucleosis, caused by Epstein-Barr virus

Hirsutism • Excessive male pattern body and facial hair found in women

Homer-Wright pseudorosettes • Characteristic arrangement of tumor cells often seen in medulloblastomas

Idiotype • Antigenic determinant in their hypervariable regions, unique to a clonal cell line of antibody-producing cells (e.g., IgG antibodies to measles and mumps viruses are idiotypes)

Impetigo • Superficial infection of the skin caused by *Staphylococcus* or *Streptococcus*; begins as a vesicle that ruptures and becomes yellow and crusty; often occurs on the face

Involucrum • Sheath of new bone that forms around necrotic bone (sequestrum)

Isotype • Antigenic differences of immunoglobulins in their constant regions, but they are found in all members of a given species (e.g., IgM and IgG are isotypes)

IVDU • Intravenous drug use

Jarisch-Herxheimer reaction • Inflammatory reaction induced by antibiotic treatment of syphilis

JVD • Jugular venous distention

Kartagener syndrome • Situs inversus, bronchiectasis, chronic sinusitis, impaired cilia; causes reduced fertility in women and sterility in men; autosomal recessive disease of the dynein arms

Kawasaki disease • Fever, conjunctivitis, pharyngitis, cervical lymphadenopathy, acute necrotizing vasculitis; can lead to coronary artery aneurysms; found in children especially younger than 2 years of age

Kayser-Fleischer rings • Green pigment encircling the cornea; found in Wilson's disease

Keratin pearls • Characteristic microscopic findings in squamous cell carcinoma

Kimmelstiel-Wilson nodules • Characteristic glomerular nodules found in diabetic nephropathy

Koilocytes • Cells with a clear perinuclear halo, characteristic of hepatitis B virus infection

Koplik spots • Red lesions with a blue-white center on the buccal mucosa; characteristic of early measles

Kussmaul breathing • Deep, rapid breathing with an increase in both tidal volume and respiratory rate; often seen in diabetic ketoacidosis or other types of metabolic acidosis

Kussmaul sign • Increase in jugulovenous pressure with inspiration; cardiac tamponade

Lhermitte sign • Flexing of the head causes electriclike shocks to be felt down the spine

Libman-Sacks endocarditis • Aseptic endocarditis with warty lesions of the cardiac valves, found in systemic lupus erythematosus

Lichen planus • Flat, shiny papules on buccal mucosa, male genitalia, and flexor surfaces; unknown cause

Lichen sclerosis • White atrophic patches (leukoplakia) of vulva

LLQ • Left lower quadrant

Lou Gehrig syndrome • Also called amyotrophic lateral sclerosis; disease of the motor tracts of the lateral columns of the spinal cord that causes muscular atrophy

LUQ • Left upper quadrant

Macrosomia • Abnormally large body size

Malar • Cheek or cheek bones

Mallory-Weiss syndrome • Tear of the lower esophagus associated with bloody vomitus, usually found in alcoholics

McBurney point • Located two thirds of the way down on a line connecting the umbilicus with the anterior superior iliac spine; a point of pain in appendicitis

Meigs syndrome • Ovarian fibroma, ascites, and hydrothorax

Menorrhagia • Profuse bleeding during menses

Menorrhalgia • Painful menses

Metrorrhagia • Irregular bleeding from the uterus between menstrual cycles

MMPI • Minnesota Multiphasic Personality Test

Molluscum contagiosum • Disease of the skin caused by a virus characterized by pearl-colored papular lesions

MRSA • Methicillin-resistant *Staphylococcus aureus*

Mycosis fungoides • Progressive lymphoma and inflammatory process of the skin

Myotome • Mesoderm that gives rise to skeletal muscle; innervated by a common nerve

NEC • Necrotizing enterocolitis

Negri bodies • Cytoplasmic inclusion bodies found in nerve cells in rabies; eosinophilic and sharply demarcated

Neurofibrillary tangles • Found in Alzheimer's disease

NIFS • Noninvasive flow study

NPO • Latin for "nothing by mouth"

NSS • Normal saline solution

Obturator sign • Right lower quadrant pain on external rotation of the hip; usually associated with appendicitis

OCP • Oral contraceptive pills

OOBTC • Out of bed to a chair

Opsonization • Process by which bacteria are made easier to phagocytize

Orthopnea • Shortness of breath on lying down

Pancoast tumor • Tumor of the apex of the lung resulting in Horner's syndrome and brachial plexus compression

Pannus • Grayish membrane that covers the upper portion of the cornea; found in trachoma

Parity • Having given birth to a child

Pemphigus vulgaris • Serious illness marked by flaccid vesicles over the entire body

PFOF • Posterior fontanelle open and flat

PFT • Pulmonary function tests

PICC • Peripherally inserted central catheter

Pleurisy • Inflammation of lung pleura

Plummer-Vinson syndrome • Dysphagia with esophageal webs and hypochromic microcytic anemia

PND • Paroxysmal nocturnal dyspnea; often a symptom of heart failure

PO • Latin for "by mouth"

Polymenorrhea • Increased frequency of menstrual cycles

Pott's disease • Tuberculosis of the spine

Precision • Degree to which a measurement is reproducible, but not necessarily correct (e.g., a thermometer that always shows a temperature that is 5 degrees higher than the actual temperature is precise but not accurate)

Psammoma bodies • Microscopic hyalinized concretions surrounded by cells; found in ovarian serous papillary cystadenocarcinoma, thyroid papillary adenocarcinoma, meningioma, and mesothelioma

Pseudocyesis • False pregnancy; psychiatric phenomenon affecting women with a strong unfilled desire for children in which these women exhibit symptoms of pregnancy

Psoas sign • Right lower quadrant pain on hip flexion; often associated with appendicitis

Psoriasis • Reddish maculopapules with silvery scaling; occurs on the flexor surfaces, scalp, and trunk

PVD • Peripheral vascular disease

Rachitic rosary • Junction of the ribs with cartilage looks like beads on a string; found in children with rickets

Raynaud phenomenon • Spasm of arteries of the hand causing blanching, numbness, and pain in the fingers; found in CREST syndrome

Reed-Sternberg cells • Binucleate cells, "owl eyes"; found in Hodgkin's lymphoma

Reinke crystals • Rod-shaped crystals with pointed or rounded ends present in Leydig cell tumors

Reye syndrome • Loss of consciousness, cerebral edema, and fatty change in the liver; often fatal; associated with aspirin ingestion in children with influenza and varicella

RLQ • Right lower quadrant

Romaña sign • Painless edema of the tissue surrounding the orbit; occurs from the bite of the Reduvid bug, which transmits Chagas' disease

Rorschach test • Inkblot test; a psychological test used as a subjective personality assessment

Rouleaux formation • Red blood cells stacked like poker chips; found in multiple myeloma

Rovsing sign • Pain is felt in the lower right quadrant upon palpation of the lower left quadrant; often seen in appendicitis

RUQ • Right upper quadrant

RV • Residual volume

Sensitivity • Number of people who test positive for a disease divided by the total number of people who actually have the disease

Sequestrum • Necrotic tissue, often bone, which has separated from the surrounding tissue

Serum sickness • Immune complex disease appears days after an injection of foreign serum; characterized by urticaria, fever, lymphadenopathy, edema, and joint pain

Sézary syndrome • Variant of mycosis fungoides; characterized by pruritus and exfoliative dermatitis

Sheehan syndrome • Pituitary necrosis and resultant hypopituitarism after parturition

Simmond disease • Anterior pituitary insufficiency, often after parturition, characterized by hypotension, asthenia, loss of weight and hair, and endocrine dysfunction

Sipple syndrome • Multiple endocrine neoplasia (MEN) type 2: pheochromocytoma, medullary thyroid carcinoma, and neural tumors

SLE • Systemic lupus erythematosus

Smith antigen • Highly characteristic antigen found in systemic lupus erythematosus

SOB • Shortness of breath

Somite • Paired embryonic cell masses originating from mesoderm; differentiate into cartilage, bone, muscle, and dermis of the skin

S/P • Status post

Specificity • Number of people who test negative for a disease divided by the total number of people who do not have the disease

Standard deviation • Measure of variation from the central tendency

Standard error • The amount that the mean of a population sample deviates from the true mean of a population

Stein-Leventhal syndrome • Polycystic ovary syndrome

String sign • Narrowed region of small bowel as seen on an abdominal x-ray with contrast

Subcutaneous nodules • Small painless swellings over bony prominences; found in rheumatic fever

Sydenham's chorea • Dancelike movements of the extremities appearing weeks to months after rheumatic fever

Tabes dorsalis • Neurosyphilis; posterior roots of the spinal cord are usually infected, resulting in ataxia, impotence, hypotonic bladder, Romberg's sign, Argyll Robinson pupils, and Charcot joints

Target cells • Erythrocyte with a dark center and a surrounding clearing encircled by a dark border (looks like a target); most commonly found in thalassemias and sickle cell disease

Tinkles • High-pitched bowel sounds; often heard in obstruction of the bowels

Tophi • Uric acid deposition in fibrous tissues such as cartilage; found in gout

TORCHES • Toxoplasmosis, other infections, rubella, cytomegalovirus, herpes, syphilis; causes birth defects if the mother is infected during pregnancy

Trousseau's sign • Carpal pedal spasm, evident when the upper arm is compressed as with a blood pressure cuff; found in hypocalcemic tetany

Turcot's syndrome • Rare disease characterized by multiple intestinal polyps and brain tumors

U/A • Urinalysis

UGI • Upper gastrointestinal

Urticaria • Hives

Vaginismus • Vaginal contraction primarily caused by attempted penile penetration

VC • Vital capacity

Virchow's node • Enlarged, palpable, supraclavicular lymph node, usually on the left; highly suggestive of a thoracic or abdominal malignancy

von Hippel-Lindau disease • Autosomal dominant disease consisting primarily of hemangiomas of the central nervous system and hamartomas of the internal organs

VRE • Vancomycin-resistant enterococcus

Water-hammer pulse • See Corrigan's pulse

Waterhouse-Friderichsen syndrome • Infection, usually meningeal; found mainly in children younger than 10 years of age; characterized by purpura, diarrhea, vomiting, cyanosis, convulsions, circulatory collapse, and hemorrhage into the adrenal glands

WD/WN • Well developed/well nourished

Wegener's granulomatosis • Disease of necrotizing granulomas of the lungs and glomerulonephritis; the underlying cause of disease is a vasculitis

Wermer's syndrome • Multiple endocrine neoplasia (MEN) type 1; characterized by tumors of the parathyroid, pancreatic islets, and pituitary or other endocrine organ

Wernicke's aphasia • Inability to comprehend the spoken word, even though normal hearing is intact

Whipple's disease • A disease characterized by steatorrhea, lymphadenopathy, arthritis, fever, and cough; foamy macrophages are found in the jejunum

Winterbottom's sign • Lymphadenopathy of the posterior cervical chain found in African trypanosomiasis (African sleeping sickness)

Wire-loop glomeruli • Thickened basement membrane of glomeruli; characteristic lesion found in patients with systemic lupus erythematosus

WNL • Within normal limits

y/o • Years old

Zollinger-Ellison syndrome • Gastrin hypersecretion and a tumor of the non–insulin-producing cells of the pancreatic islets

Index

Page numbers in *italic* designate figures; page numbers followed by *t* designate tables; (*see also*) cross-references designate related topics or more detailed topic breakdowns.